Drugs in Sport

Drug use and abuse is perhaps the biggest challenge facing sport today. However, in the eye of the storm of public and press opinion and with medals and morals at stake, it can be difficult to gain a clear perspective on this complex issue. Now available in a fully updated and revised sixth edition *Drugs in Sport* is the most comprehensive and accurate text available on the subject. Taking into account the latest regulations, methods, and landmark cases, the book explores the hard science behind drug use in sport as well as the ethical, social, political, and administrative context. Key topics include:

- Mode of action and side effects of each major class of drugs used in sport
- Discussion of cutting-edge issues such as gene doping and Athlete Biological Passports
- The latest doping control regulations of the World Anti-Doping Agency (WADA)
- Issues surrounding non-prohibited substances and ergogenic aids in supplements
- Medical and pharmaceutical services at major sporting events
- An assessment of the prevalence of drug taking in sport.

Accessibly written, extensively referenced, and supported throughout with illustrative case studies and data, *Drugs in Sport* provides a comprehensive, objective resource for students and researchers, athletes, sports scientists and coaches, journalists, sports administrators, and policymakers.

David R. Mottram is Emeritus Professor of Pharmacy Practice at Liverpool John Moores University, UK. His teaching and research interests have centred on the use of drugs in sport. He is the editor of five previous editions of *Drugs in Sport*. He was a member of the Pharmacy Planning Committee of the London Organising Committee for the 2012 Olympic and Paralympic Games.

Neil Chester is a Senior Research Officer at Liverpool John Moores University, UK. His teaching and research has an anti-doping focus specifically concerning over-the-counter stimulants, sports supplements, and the adverse health effects of long-term use of anabolic agents. He has published widely in the area and is a member of the UK Anti-Doping Research Steering Committee.

6   Peptide hormones, growth factors, and related substances   **86**

DAVID R. MOTTRAM AND NEIL CHESTER

7   Beta-2 agonists   **105**

NEIL CHESTER AND DAVID R. MOTTRAM

8   Hormone and metabolic modulators   **117**

NEIL CHESTER

9   Diuretics and other masking agents   **126**

DAVID R. MOTTRAM

Contents

Drugs in Sport

6th Edition

Edited by David R. Mottram and Neil Chester

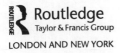
Routledge
Taylor & Francis Group

LONDON AND NEW YORK

First published 2015
by Routledge
2 Park Square, Milton Park, Abingdon, Oxon OX14 4RN

and by Routledge
711 Third Avenue, New York, NY 10017

Routledge is an imprint of the Taylor & Francis Group, an informa business

British Library Cataloguing-in-Publication Data
A catalogue record for this book is available from the British Library

Library of Congress Cataloging-in-Publication Data
Drugs in sport / edited by David R. Mottram and Neil Chester. – 6th.
p. ; cm.
Includes bibliographical references and index.
I. Mottram, D. R. (David R.), 1944- editor. II. Chester, Neil, editor.
[DNLM: I. Doping in Sports. 2. Sports Medicine. 3. Substance-Related
Disorders. QT 262]
RC1230. D783 2015
362.29–dc23
2014017974

ISBN: 978-0-415-71525-6 (hbk)
ISBN: 978-0-415-71528-7 (pbk)
ISBN: 978-1-315-88193-5 (ebk)

Typeset in Times
by Cenveo Publisher Services

SECTION 5
The extent of doping in sport   303

25   Prevalence of drug misuse in sport   305
DAVID R. MOTTRAM

26   Future issues concerning drug use in sport   316
NEIL CHESTER AND DAVID R. MOTTRAM

Appendix: Synopsis of drugs used in sport

DAVID R. MOTTRAM AND NEIL CHESTER

The background to and regulation of drug use in sport

Chapter 1

Drugs and their use in sport

David R. Mottram

1.1. Introduction

In this chapter we will review what is meant by the term *drug*. After establishing how drugs exert their effects and side effects within the body, we will reflect on the various circumstances for which athletes may take drugs. Finally, we will consider why drugs are used by athletes for the purpose of performance enhancement.

1.2. What is a drug?

Definition of a drug

Drugs are chemical substances that, by interaction with biological targets, can alter the biochemical systems of the body. The branch of science investigating drug action is known as pharmacology. For example, drugs such as ephedrine can lead to an increase in the force and rate of beating of the heart. Effects in the central nervous system by drugs such as amphetamines can produce changes in mood and behaviour. Interactions with metabolic processes, with drugs such as insulin, can be used in the treatment of disorders such as diabetes.

Banned drugs in sport

In this chapter, frequent reference is made to drugs that appear on the World Anti-Doping Agency (WADA) Prohibited List of Substances and Methods (http://list.wada-ama.org), the 2014 edition of which is presented in Table 1.1. The Prohibited List is the most visited document on WADA's web site. Mazzoni *et al.* (2011) have provided an excellent description of the structure, review, and update processes for the WADA Prohibited List.

Classification and description of drug names

Drugs are variously classified and described by their

- Generic name (International Non-proprietary Name, INN)
- Proprietary name (manufacturer's name)
- Mechanism of action.

The generic name (INN) is the internationally recognised name of the drug and should normally be used when describing the drug. However, when a pharmaceutical company first

Table 1.1 WADA Prohibited List of Substances and Methods, January 2014

SUBSTANCES AND METHODS PROHIBITED AT ALL TIMES (IN- AND OUT-OF-COMPETITION)

Prohibited Substances
S.0 Nonapproved substances
S.1 Anabolic agents
S.2 Peptide hormones, growth factors, and related substances
S.3 Beta-2 agonists
S.4 Hormone and metabolic modulators
S.5 Diuretics and other masking agents

Prohibited Methods
M.1 Manipulation of blood and blood components
M.2 Chemical and physical manipulation
M.3 Gene doping

SUBSTANCES AND METHODS PROHIBITED IN-COMPETITION

Categories S.0 to S.5 and M.1 to M.3 plus:
S.6 Stimulants
S.7 Narcotics
S.8 Cannabinoids
S.9 Glucocorticosteroids

SUBSTANCES PROHIBITED IN PARTICULAR SPORTS

P.1 Alcohol
P.2 Beta blockers

Source: http://list.wada-ama.org/

develops a new drug, it patents the drug under a proprietary name. When the patent expires, other pharmaceutical companies may produce the same drug, but they give the drug their own proprietary name to distinguish their version of the drug from that of other companies. Some examples of the classification and names of drugs subject to restrictions in sport are presented in Table 1.2.

Drugs may be classified by their mechanism of action (pharmacology) or by the therapeutic use for which the drug is designed. Examples are given in Table 1.3.

Development of new drugs

Over the centuries, herbalists and apothecaries have extracted drugs from plant and animal sources. A few drugs are still derived from natural sources. For example, morphine is extracted from the opium poppy and digoxin from the foxglove plant. However, the majority of drugs are produced by pharmaceutical companies through chemical synthesis. Current

Table 1.2 Examples of the classifications and descriptions of drugs by their names

Class of drug	Generic name	Proprietary name
Androgenic anabolic steroids	Nandrolone	Deca-Durabolin
Diuretics	Furosemide	Lasix
Beta-2 agonists	Salbutamol	Ventolin
Narcotics	Morphine	Sevredol
Beta blockers	Atenolol	Tenormin
Human growth hormone	Somatropin	Humatrope

Table 1.3 Examples of the classification of drugs by their mechanisms of action and uses

Class of drug	Pharmacological action	Therapeutic use
Diuretics	Prevention of re-absorption of water from the kidneys	Heart failure Hypertension
Beta-2 agonists	Bronchodilation through stimulation of beta-2 adrenoreceptors	Asthma Chronic obstructive pulmonary disease
Morphine	Agonist on opioid μ-receptors	Severe pain
Beta blockers	Antagonists on beta adrenoreceptors	Angina Hypertension Cardiac arrhythmias Anxiety

research into gene technology is revolutionising the development of new drugs. The pharmaceutical industry is ideally placed to identify the doping potential of new medicines and to support early development of detection methods (Elliott and Leishman 2012).

The development of new drugs is monitored by government agencies who evaluate the activity and safety of new drugs before awarding a product licence. The product licence states the therapeutic purpose(s) for which the drug may be used. The development of new drugs can take 10–12 years and cost several hundred million dollars.

Dosage forms for drug delivery to the body

There are many different dosage forms through which drugs can be administered to the body. Some examples for drugs that are subject to restrictions in sport are presented in Table 1.4.

The absorption, distribution, metabolism, and elimination of drugs

For a drug to exert its effect, it must reach its site of action. This will involve its passage from the site of administration to the cells of the target tissue or organ. The principal factors that can influence this process are absorption, distribution, metabolism, and elimination – known as the *pharmacokinetics* of drug action.

Table 1.4 Examples of dosage forms for drugs used in sport

Generic drug name	Dosage forms
Testosterone (anabolic androgenic steroid)	Oral capsules Intramuscular injection Transdermal patches
Terbutaline (beta-2 agonist)	Aerosol inhaler Oral tablets Syrup Injection
Hydrocortisone (glucocorticosteroid)	Oral tablets Injection Ear/eye drops Cream/ointment
Pethidine (narcotic analgesic)	Oral tablets Injection

Absorption

The absorption of a drug depends, in part, on its route of administration. Most drugs must enter the bloodstream in order to reach their site of action. The most common route of administration for this purpose is orally, in either liquid or tablet form.

When a drug is required to act more rapidly or is susceptible to breakdown in the gastrointestinal tract, the preferred route of administration is by injection. The main routes of injection are subcutaneous (under the skin), intramuscular (into a muscle), and intravenous (directly into the bloodstream via a vein).

Many drugs can be applied topically for a localized response. This may take the form of applying a cream, ointment, or lotion to an area of skin for treatment of abrasions, lesions, infections, or other such dermatological conditions. Topical applications may also involve applying drops to the eye, the ear, or the nose.

Drugs administered by a topical route are not normally absorbed into the body to the same extent as drugs administered orally. Consequently, the WADA regulations regarding certain drugs take into account the route of administration.

Distribution

Apart from topical administration, a significant proportion of a drug will reach the bloodstream. Most drugs are then dissolved in the water phase of the blood plasma. Within this phase, some of the drug molecules may be bound to proteins and thus may not be freely diffusible out of the plasma. This will affect the amount of drug reaching its target receptors.

An additional obstruction to the passage of drugs occurs at the *blood–brain barrier*, which is a layer of cells that covers the capillary walls of the vessels supplying the brain. This barrier effectively excludes molecules that are poorly lipid soluble. The blood–brain barrier is an important factor to be considered in drug design because a drug's ability to cross this barrier can influence its potential for centrally mediated side effects.

Metabolism

The body has a very efficient system for transforming chemicals into safer molecules, which can then be excreted by the various routes of elimination. This process is known as metabolism, and many drugs that enter the body undergo metabolic change.

Several enzyme systems are responsible for producing metabolic transformations. These enzymes are principally located in the cells of the liver but may also be found in other cells. They produce simple chemical alterations of the drug molecules by processes such as oxidation, reduction, hydrolysis, acetylation, and alkylation.

The consequences of drug metabolism may be seen in a number of ways:

1 An active drug is changed into an inactive compound. This is the most common means for the termination of the activity of a drug.
2 An active drug can be metabolised into another active compound. The metabolite may have the same pharmacological action as the parent drug, or it may have higher or lower potency or a different pharmacological effect.
3 An active drug can be changed into a toxic metabolite.
4 An inactive drug can be converted into pharmacologically active metabolites. This mechanism can occasionally be used for beneficial purposes if a drug is susceptible to

rapid breakdown before it reaches its site of action. In this case, a 'prodrug' can be synthesised, which is resistant to breakdown but will be metabolised to the active drug on arrival at its target tissue.

Generally speaking, the metabolism of drugs results in the conversion of lipid-soluble drugs into more water-soluble metabolites. This change affects distribution because less lipid-soluble compounds are unable to penetrate cell membranes. The kidneys are able to excrete water-soluble compounds more readily than lipid-soluble molecules because the latter can be reabsorbed in the kidney tubules and therefore re-enter the plasma.

Metabolism is a very important factor in determining a drug's activity because it can alter the drug's intrinsic activity, its ability to reach its site of action, and its rate of elimination from the body. Many drugs are completely metabolised before being excreted in the urine. *The WADA testing procedures in doping control detect both the parent drug and its metabolite(s), where appropriate.*

Elimination

There are many routes through which drugs can be eliminated from the body:

- Kidneys (urine)
- Salivary glands (saliva)
- Sweat glands (sweat)
- Pulmonary epithelium (exhaled gases)
- Mammary glands (mammary milk)
- Rectum (faeces).

The most important route for drug excretion is through the kidneys into the urine. *Urine sampling is the principal method used in dope testing.* The methods available for detecting drugs and their metabolites are extremely sensitive and capable of determining both the nature and the concentration of the drug and/or metabolite present.

Pharmacological means have been used in an attempt to mask drug-taking activities. Diuretics have also been used as masking agents by accelerating urine excretion.

Effect of exercise on pharmacokinetics

Under most circumstances, exercise does not affect the pharmacokinetics of drug action. During severe or prolonged exercise, blood flow within the body will be altered, with a decrease in blood supply to the gastrointestinal tract and to the kidneys. However, there is little documented evidence to suggest that such changes significantly affect the pharmacokinetics of the majority of drugs.

Drugs and their targets

Ideally, a drug should interact with a single target to produce the desired effect within the body. However, all drugs possess varying degrees of side effects, largely dependent on the extent to which they interact with sites other than their primary target. During their development, drugs undergo a rigorous evaluation in order to maximise therapeutic effects and minimise side effects. *Designer drugs*, produced by 'backstreet' laboratories to supply the illicit sport market, do not undergo such rigorous testing for safety.

The sites through which most drug molecules interact are known as receptors. These receptors are normally specific areas within the structure of cells, mostly on cell membranes. Receptors are present within cells to enable naturally occurring substances, such as neuro-transmitters, to induce their biochemical and physiological functions within the body. We exploit the fact that receptors exist by designing drugs to stimulate (agonists) or block (antagonists) these receptors, thereby intensifying or reducing biochemical processes within the body, respectively.

The interaction between a drug (ligand) and a receptor is the first step in a series of events that eventually lead to a biological effect. The drug–receptor interaction can therefore be thought of as a trigger mechanism.

There are many different receptor sites within the body, each of which possesses its own specific arrangement of recognition sites. Drugs are designed to interact with the recognition sites of particular receptors. The more closely a drug can fit into its recognition site, the greater the triggering response and therefore the greater the potency of the drug on that tissue.

Agonists and antagonists

A drug that mimics the action of an endogenous biochemical substance (i.e. one that occurs naturally in the body) is said to be an *agonist*. The potency of agonists depends on two parameters:

* *Affinity* – the ability to bind to receptors
* *Efficacy* – the ability, once bound to the receptor, to initiate changes that lead to effects.

Another group of drugs used in therapeutics is known as *antagonists*. They have the ability to interact with receptor sites (affinity) but, unlike agonists, do not trigger the series of events leading to a response. The pharmacological effect of antagonists is produced by preventing the body's own biochemical agents from interacting with the receptors and therefore inhibiting particular physiological processes.

A typical example of this can be seen with beta blockers. They exert their pharmacological effect by occupying beta receptors without stimulating a response; however, by so doing, they prevent the neurotransmitter, noradrenaline (norepinephrine), and the hormone, adrena-line (epinephrine), from interacting with these receptors. Beta blockers therefore reduce heart rate under stress conditions or in exercise.

Many receptor classes can be subclassified. This can be illustrated by looking at how adrenaline (epinephrine) interacts with adrenergic receptors. Five subclasses of adrenergic receptors are known: alpha-1 (α_1), alpha-2 (α_2), beta-1 (β_1), beta-2 (β_2), and beta-3 (β_3). Adrenaline can interact with all of these receptors and produce a variety of physiological effects, some of which are shown in Figure 1.1. Some drugs have selectivity for particular subclasses of receptors. For example, the drug salbutamol was developed to have a selec-tive effect on β-2 receptors. It therefore produces bronchodilation, without the other effects associated with adrenaline. As such, it is a first-line drug in the treatment of asthma. The selective nature of salbutamol is recognised by the WADA; thus, its use is permitted in sport, subject to certain restrictions, whilst other less selective sympathomimetics are banned.

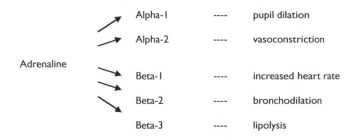

	Alpha-1	----	pupil dilation
	Alpha-2	----	vasoconstriction
Adrenaline	Beta-1	----	increased heart rate
	Beta-2	----	bronchodilation
	Beta-3	----	lipolysis

Figure 1.1 Some physiological effects of adrenaline mediated through the five principal classes of adrenergic receptors.

Side effects of drugs

All drugs produce side effects. Some of these side effects occur at normal, therapeutic dose levels, whilst other side effects are experienced only at higher doses. In many instances, athletes are taking drugs in doses far in excess of those required for therapeutic purposes; in so doing, they are increasing the risk of side effects. Side effects associated with some of the drugs that are commonly misused in sport are shown in Table 1.5.

The side effects of drugs are usually well documented as a result of extensive toxicity studies during the development of the drug and from adverse reaction reporting once the drug is on the market. These predictable toxic effects are more pronounced when the drug is taken in overdose. Accidental toxicity can easily occur with athletes who self-medicate without appreciating the full implications of their actions.

Unpredictable toxicity can also occur following the administration of therapeutic or even subtherapeutic doses of drugs. An example of this is *idiosyncrasy*, in which a drug produces an unusual reaction. This effect is normally genetically determined and is often due to a biochemical deficiency, resulting in a patient's overreaction to a drug. This may be due to an inability to metabolise the drug.

Table 1.5 Side effects associated with some drugs that are commonly misused in sport

Class of drugs	Side effects
Amphetamines	Restlessness, irritability, tremor, insomnia, cardiac arrhythmias, aggression, addiction (Knopp *et al.* 1997)
Beta-2 agonists	Tremor, tachycardia, cardiac arrhythmias, insomnia, headache (Prather *et al.* 1995)
Narcotic analgesics	Constipation, respiratory depression, addiction
Anabolic androgenic steroids	Acne, hypertension, mania, depression, aggression, liver and kidney tumours In females: masculinisation, cliteromegaly In males: testicular atrophy, gynaecomastia (Tucker 1997)
Diuretics	Dehydration, muscular cramps (Caldwell 1987)
Human growth hormone	In children: gigantism In adults: acromegaly (hypertension, diabetes, muscular weakness, thickening of the skin) (Healy & Russell-Jones 1997)
Erythropoietin	Flu-like symptoms, hypertension, thromboses (Drug and Therapeutics Bulletin 1992)

A second type of unpredictable toxicity is *drug allergy*. It differs from normal toxicity to drugs in that the patient only exhibits the reaction after being previously exposed to the drug or a closely related chemical. This initial exposure to the drug, or its metabolite, sensitises the patient by inducing an allergic response. The drug combines with a protein within the body to produce an antigen, which, in turn, leads to the formation of other proteins called antibodies. Subsequent exposure to the drug will initiate an antigen-antibody reaction. This allergic reaction can manifest itself in a variety of ways. An acute reaction is known as anaphylaxis and normally occurs within 1 hour of taking the drug. This response frequently involves the respiratory and cardiovascular systems and is often fatal. Subacute allergic reactions usually occur 1–24 hours after the drug is taken; the most common manifestations involve skin reactions, blood dyscrasia, fever, and dysfunction of the respiratory, kidney, liver, and cardiovascular systems. Examples of drugs known to produce such allergic responses are aspirin and some antibiotics, including penicillins and cephalosporins.

Complex drug reactions

Complex reactions may occur during long-term use of a drug or when more than one drug is being taken simultaneously.

If the frequency of administration exceeds the elimination rate of a drug, then *drug cumulation* occurs, thereby increasing the likelihood of toxicity reactions. The reason for a slow elimination may be related to a slow metabolism, a strong tendency toward plasma protein binding, or an inhibition of excretion (e.g. in patients with kidney disease).

The opposite response to cumulation is seen in patients with *drug resistance*. This drug resistance may be genetically inherited or acquired. Inherited resistance is not common in humans, although it is an increasing problem in antibacterial therapy, in which pathogenic microbes can develop genetic changes in their structure or biochemistry; these changes render them resistant to antibiotic drugs. Acquired resistance to drugs, also known as *tolerance*, can develop with repeated administration of a drug. When tolerance occurs, more of the drug is needed to produce the same pharmacological response. A very rapidly developing tolerance is known as *tachyphylaxis*. This is usually caused by a slow rate of detachment of the drug from its receptor sites, so that subsequent doses of the drug are unable to form the drug–receptor complexes that are required to produce an effect.

A number of drugs acting on the central nervous system, particularly narcotic analgesics, produce tolerance that is accompanied by *physical dependence*. This is a state in which an abrupt termination of the administration of the drug produces a series of unpleasant symptoms, known as the abstinence syndrome. These symptoms are rapidly reversed after the readministration of the drug. A further manifestation of this problem involves psychogenic dependence, in which the drug taker experiences an irreversible craving, or compulsion, to take the drug for pleasure or for relief of discomfort.

If a patient is taking more than one drug, a *drug interaction* may occur. Less commonly, drugs may interact with certain foodstuffs; for example, the calcium in milk products can bind to certain drugs and limit their absorption. The effects of interactions can range from minor toxicity to potential fatality.

Drugs and the law

The manufacture and supply of drugs are subject to legal control. This legislation may vary from country to country, but the principles are the same.

The definition of a medicinal product

A *medicinal product* is any substance that is manufactured, sold, supplied, imported, or exported for use in either or both of the following ways:

- It is administered to human beings or animals for medicinal purposes.
- It is used as an ingredient in the preparation of substances administered to human beings or animals for medicinal purposes.

Medicinal purpose means any one or more of the following:

- Treating or preventing disease
- Diagnosing a disease or physiological condition
- Providing contraception
- Inducing anaesthesia
- Otherwise preventing or interfering with the normal operation of physiological function.

Classes of medicinal products

In many countries, there are three classes of medicinal products:

- General sale list medicines
- Pharmacy medicines
- Prescription-only medicines.

The laws of a country dictate which medicines may be purchased and which can only be obtained through a prescription. In general, these laws are similar from country to country, but exceptions do occur. Regrettably, most drugs can be obtained legally or illegally, without professional advice, through internet sources.

Patients can obtain *prescription-only medicines* from medical practitioners in a hospital, clinic, or community practise. Prescriptions are then dispensed by a pharmacist or, in some cases, by a dispensing doctor. Once the prescription has been dispensed, the medicine becomes the property of the patient.

Over-the-counter (OTC) medicines are available for purchase without a prescription. These medicines are normally only available from a pharmacy (so-called pharmacy medicines), although some medicines, such as aspirin and other analgesics, may be obtained in small pack sizes from other retail outlets (general sale list medicines). OTC drugs pose particular problems for athletes because a number of drugs subject to WADA regulations are available in OTC preparation.

Controlled drugs, normally those drugs with addictive properties, are subject to more extensive legal restrictions. In most countries, controlled drugs include

- Hallucinogenic drugs (e.g. LSD, marijuana)
- Opiates (narcotic analgesics; e.g. morphine, heroin)
- Amphetamines
- Cocaine.

For these drugs, the law states that it is illegal to possess such drugs, except when the user is a registered addict and has obtained the drug legally on prescription. In some countries, anabolic steroids, clenbuterol, and some polypeptide hormones are classified as controlled drugs as a further deterrent to their misuse in sport and bodybuilding.

1.3. Why might athletes take drugs?

There are many reasons why athletes may take drugs. These can be broadly categorised as

- Legitimate therapeutic use for the treatment of medical conditions (prescription drugs or self-medication)
- Social or recreational use (legal and illegal)
- Performance enhancement.

Within each of these categories there are drugs that appear in the WADA list of prohibited substances (see Table 1.1). Both the deliberate and inadvertent use of prohibited drugs carries significant consequences for athletes. It would be easy to suggest that athletes should avoid taking drugs, particularly at the time of competition. However, there are many circumstances when drug use is advisable, if not imperative, for the general health and well-being of the athlete. Athletes should always carefully consider the specific need for taking a drug and the full implications of their action.

Therapeutic use of drugs for the treatment of medical conditions

Like any other person, an athlete is liable to suffer from a major or minor illness that requires treatment with drugs. A typical example might involve a bacterial or fungal infection necessitating the use of an antibiotic or antifungal agent. Apart from side effects, such treatment would be unlikely to affect an athlete's ability to compete, and most drugs are not subject to WADA restrictions. However, some medical conditions for which athletes may require drug treatment involve drugs that appear on the WADA Prohibited List. Examples of these conditions are shown in Table 1.6. For each condition, the commonly used classes of drugs are listed. The classes of drugs subject to WADA regulations are highlighted.

For minor illnesses, such as coughs, colds, gastrointestinal upset, and hay fever, a wide range of preparations can be purchased from a pharmacy without a prescription. Athletes should carefully scrutinise the label on such medication to ensure that banned substances, such as ephedrine, methylephedrine, pseudoephedrine, or cathine, are not included in the medicine.

Athletes frequently experience injuries involving muscles, ligaments, and tendons, for which they may take palliative treatment in the form of analgesic and anti-inflammatory drugs. This treatment enables the athlete to continue to train and even compete during the period of recovery from the injury. The wisdom of such action is perhaps debatable, but the use of analgesics under these circumstances is unlikely to confer an unfair advantage. Doping regulations restrict the types of analgesics that can be used, with narcotic analgesics being prohibited. Regulations also control the methods of administration for drugs, such as glucocorticosteroids.

Table 1.6 Medical conditions for which athletes may require drug treatment involving drugs that appear on the WADA Prohibited List

Type of medical condition	Medical condition	Drug classes commonly used
Long-term chronic conditions	Asthma	Beta-2 agonists* Drugs subject to WADA Prohibited List (2014) regulations. Glucocorticosteroids* Drugs subject to WADA Prohibited List (2014) regulations. Leukotriene antagonists
	Diabetes mellitus (type I)	Insulin* Drugs subject to WADA Prohibited List (2014) regulations.
	Hypertension	Diuretics* Drugs subject to WADA Prohibited List (2014) regulations. Beta blockers* Drugs subject to WADA Prohibited List (2014) regulations. ACE inhibitors Calcium channel blockers Angiotensin II receptor antagonists
Short-term acute conditions	Viral cough and cold	Antitussives Decongestant stimulants* Drugs subject to WADA Prohibited List (2014) regulations. Nonnarcotic analgesics
Sport injuries	Musculoskeletal damage and inflammation	Nonsteroidal anti-inflammatories Nonnarcotic analgesics Narcotic analgesics* Drugs subject to WADA Prohibited List (2014) regulations. Glucocorticosteroids* Drugs subject to WADA Prohibited List (2014) regulations.

*Drugs subject to WADA Prohibited List (2014) regulations.

In the event that an athlete visits a medical practitioner, it is in his or her best interest to discuss the nature of any drug treatment to avoid the prescribing of prohibited substances whenever possible.

The WADA regulations related to the drugs listed in Table 1.6 are described in subsequent chapters.

Therapeutic use exemption

If an athlete needs to be prescribed a drug that appears on the WADA Prohibited List, the athlete and his or her medical practitioner must obtain a Therapeutic Use Exemption (TUE; https://elb. wada-ama.org/en/what-we-do/science-medical/therapeutic-use-exemptions) to avoid an adverse analytical finding during anti-doping testing.

The following broad criteria are considered when granting a TUE:

- The athlete would experience a significant impairment to health if the prohibited substance or prohibited method were to be withheld in the course of treating an acute or chronic medical condition.
- The therapeutic use of the prohibited substance or prohibited method would produce no additional enhancement of performance other than that which might be anticipated by a return to a state of normal health following the treatment of a legitimate medical condition.
- There is no reasonable therapeutic alternative to the use of the otherwise prohibited substance or prohibited method.
- The necessity for the use of the otherwise prohibited substance or prohibited method cannot be a consequence, wholly or in part, of the prior use, without a TUE, of a substance or method that was prohibited at the time of use.

TUEs are normally granted to athletes by international federations or national anti-doping organisations. Requests are dealt with by a panel of independent physicians (Therapeutic Use Exemption Committee). Professor Ken Fitch, as Chair of the International Olympic Committee's Therapeutic Use Exemption Committee, provided an interesting insight into the medical indications and pitfalls in the TUE process (Fitch 2012).

How to identify if a medicine contains a prohibited substance

It is in the athlete's interest to ensure that accurate identification of medicines containing prohibited substances is undertaken on each occasion that a medicine is taken. The Global Drug Reference Online (DRO; http://www.globaldro.com) provides an up-to-date reference source for athletes and health care professionals to identify whether or not a medicine contains a prohibited substance. Global DRO was developed through a partnership between UK Anti-Doping, the Canadian Centre for Ethics in Sport, and the United States Anti-Doping Agency. Visitors to the site can search for specific information on products sold in the United Kingdom, Canada, and the United States.

Global DRO asks the user to provide information on

- User type (e.g. athlete, coach, health care professional)
- The user's sport
- The country in which the medicine was obtained
- The name of the medicine.

From this information, the web site provides details on the active ingredients of the medicine and their permitted or prohibited status (in competition or out of competition), relative to the country of purchase and sport within which the medicine is to be used.

Social or recreational use of drugs

Many cultures, throughout the ages, have used drugs for social and recreational purposes. These drugs include those that are generally socially tolerated, such as nicotine, alcohol, cannabinoids, and caffeine (a constituent of beverages frequently consumed in many societies), and drugs that are addictive, such as narcotic analgesics that are related to heroin and morphine, and psychomotor stimulants like cocaine. Although these drugs may be taken in a social or recreational setting, they can all affect sporting performance; hence, many are subject to WADA regulations. The social/recreational drugs that are subject to WADA regulations are shown in Table 1.7.

Amphetamines

Amphetamines are used socially to produce alertness and energy. However, they also impair judgement and mental concentration with excessive use, leading to depression and anxiety. There is a risk of addiction with regular use of amphetamines (Knopp *et al.* 1997).

Cocaine

Cocaine is a powerful stimulant. It is usually inhaled as a powder, but a crystalline ('crack') form of cocaine can be smoked as a vapour, which increases the absorption and effect of the drug. The complex pharmacology of cocaine leads to a wide spectrum of adverse effects, including a negative effect on glycogenolysis, paranoid psychosis, seizures, hypertension, and myocardial toxicity, which could lead to ischaemia, arrhythmias, and sudden death, especially following intense exercise (Conlee 1991; Eichner 1993). After regular use, addictive cravings for cocaine can persist for a period of months.

Caffeine

Perhaps the most widely used social drug is caffeine, which is present in many beverages that we consume daily. Caffeine was on the International Olympic Committee banned list but was removed by WADA in January 2004. However, it is still part of the WADA Monitoring Program (https://wada-main-prod.s3.amazonaws.com/resources/files/WADA-Monitoring-Program-2014-EN.pdf).

Narcotics

Narcotics are potent drugs that primarily affect the central nervous system. The discovery of opiate receptors within the brain has helped in the understanding of the mode of action of morphine, heroin, and other related narcotic analgesics. These drugs appear to be mimicking the effect of certain endogenous opiates, known as endorphins and enkephalin. Narcotics are renowned for their ability to cause tolerance and dependence in the regular user.

Alcohol

Even when alcohol is taken for recreational purposes, its effects may well be manifested in the field of sport. Some sporting events even take place in an environment where alcohol is

Table 1.7 Drugs used socially or recreationally that are subject to WADA regulations

Drug	WADA regulation
Amphetamines	Prohibited: class S6 (stimulants)
Cocaine	Prohibited: class S6 (stimulants)
Narcotics	Prohibited: class S7
Alcohol	Prohibited in particular sports: class P1
Cannabinoids	Prohibited: class S8

freely available to both the spectator and the performer. Alcohol suppresses inhibitions but also impairs judgement and reflexes. Alcohol is prohibited in particular sports.

Cannabinoids

The precise mode of action of cannabinoids is not fully understood, but the effects produced are principally euphoria and elation accompanied by a loss of perception of time and space. Although marijuana is unlikely to be used as a performance-enhancing substance in sport, it may be used as part of the lifestyle of many athletes. Cannabinoids are prohibited by WADA in all sports.

The use of social and recreational drugs, particularly in Western cultures, is widespread. This is reflected in the numbers of positive test results, particularly for cannabinoids, from WADA-accredited laboratories (see Chapter 15).

1.4. The use of drugs for performance enhancement

What are the factors that influence athletic performance?

Many factors may influence an athlete's attempt to reach the peak of his or her chosen sport. In addition to an athlete's innate ability and commitment to training, many external influences come into play. These include:

- Coaches
- Sponsorship deals
- Resources and equipment
- Sports nutritionists
- Sports psychologists
- Physiotherapists
- Sports physicians.

Inevitably, many athletes achieve excellence in their sport but never reach their ultimate goal. These athletes, as well as those who seek a shortcut to glory, may be tempted to experiment with performance enhancement through pharmacological means. The culture of using substances to enhance performance in sport dates back more than 2,000 years to the ancient Olympic Games.

What is performance enhancement?

The performance-enhancing effects of substances are for the most part directly related to the following (Barroso *et al.* 2008):

- Ergogenic effects (enhanced strength, higher energy production, improved recovery)
- Anabolic potential (increased protein synthesis)
- Stimulating properties (improved attention, decreased anxiety).

How are performance-enhancing substances classified?

Prohibited performance-enhancing substances have two origins. Exogenous substances are produced synthetically and are not normally produced by the body, whereas endogenous substances are produced naturally in the body. Anti-doping detection methods for exogenous substances are clear cut. However, for endogenous substances, the proof of substance use is more problematic.

Substances that are used in an attempt to enhance performance can be broadly divided into two types:

• Legal supplements
• Illegal performance-enhancing drugs.

Legal supplements

Anecdotal evidence suggests that the majority of today's athletes, regardless of their level of sporting achievement, use supplements. A study by Backhouse *et al.* (2013) concluded that doping use is three-and-a-half times more prevalent in nutritional supplement users than in nonusers. The authors suggested that their results offered support for the gateway hypothesis, whereby athletes who engage in legal performance-enhancement practices embody an at-risk group for transition toward doping.

Are supplements safe to use?

A landmark study by Geyer *et al.* (2004) of 634 nonhormonal nutritional supplements purchased in thirteen countries showed that 14.8 per cent contained anabolic androgenic steroids, which were not declared on the label. Athletes are therefore vulnerable to the inadvertent use of prohibited substances. Many cases of athletes recording adverse analytical findings after supplement use have been reported. One of the most recent cases involved a Syrian hurdler, Ghfran Almouhamad, who tested positive at the London 2012 Olympic Games for methylhexaneamine, a substance found in certain supplements.

Advice regarding supplement use

WADA advises the use of extreme caution with supplement use (https://www.wada-ama.org/en/questions-answers/supplements):

> The use of dietary supplements by athletes is a concern because in many countries the manufacturing and labelling of supplements may not follow strict rules. This may lead to a supplement containing an undeclared substance that is prohibited under anti-doping regulations. A significant number of positive tests have been attributed to the misuse of supplements and taking a poorly labelled dietary supplement is not an adequate defence in a doping hearing.

Checking supplements

Informed-Sport (http://www.informed-sport.com) is an organisation that provides a risk-minimisation programme for sports nutrition products. The programme certifies that specified batches of nutritional supplements and/or ingredients that bear the Informed-Sport logo have been tested for banned substances in their laboratory. However, this still does not guarantee a supplement is completely free from prohibited substances because there can even be differences in ingredients within a single batch.

Illegal performance-enhancing drugs

The detailed criteria for substances and methods on the WADA prohibited list are specified in the World Anti-Doping Code (https://wada-main-prod.s3.amazonaws.com/resources/files/wada_anti-doping_code_2009_en_0.pdf) and can be summarised as follows.

A substance or method is considered for inclusion on the prohibited list if WADA determines that the substance or method meets any two of the following three criteria:

1 The substance or method, alone or in combination with other substances or methods, has the potential to enhance or enhances sport performance.
2 The use of the substance or method represents an actual or potential health risk to the athlete.
3 WADA determines that the use of the substance or method violates the spirit of sport.

The WADA Prohibited List is subject to annual review, with revised lists coming into force each January.

Why do athletes use prohibited performance-enhancing substances?

The reasons that athletes use drugs that appear on the WADA Prohibited List are manifold, complex, and vary from athlete to athlete and from sport to sport.

In a review of thirty-three studies published between 2000 and 2011, Morente-Sánchez and Zabala (2013) reported that the initial reasons given by elite athletes for using banned substances included the following:

• Achievement of athletic success by improved performance
• Financial gain
• Improving recovery
• Prevention of nutritional deficiencies
• The idea that others use them.

In addition, this study found that there is a belief by athletes about the inefficiency of antidoping programmes, and athletes criticised the way tests are carried out.

The differences in athletes' motivation for illicit drug use between sports were demonstrated by Bilard *et al.* (2011). In this study, the main motivations were preserving health for cyclists, increasing muscular strength for bodybuilders, and personal recreation for footballers.

Some of the compounding factors that encourage the use of prohibited substances are the following:

• *Media coverage*: In their attempt to sell newspapers and other promotional material, the media tend to give extensive coverage to doping scandals within sport. This may give the athlete a misleading impression of the extent to which performance-enhancing drugs are used in sport.
• *Peer pressure*: Athletes may directly observe or may hear of the practices of fellow athletes who use performance-enhancing drugs. Alternatively, athletes may be offered performance-enhancing drugs by their fellow competitors or team members.

- *Support team pressure*: The people who support athletes, such as family members, coaches, and health care professionals, may instil additional pressure on athletes to improve performance by whatever means are available.
- *Availability of substances*: In addition to the more traditional sources of drug supply, athletes can now obtain virtually any product they wish through the internet.
- *Misleading information*: Some apparently safe supplements may contain traces of prohibited substances. In addition, the labelling of some supplements may not be complete or accurate.
- *Lack of understanding*: Athletes are not pharmacologists, and the plethora of information that appears on medicinal products can be confusing to the untrained eye.

Specified substances

There are occasions when an athlete may take a prohibited substance inadvertently. For this reason, WADA has introduced a Specified Substances clause, which applies to certain classes of substances and methods on the Prohibited List. For Specified Substances, sanctions should be made more flexible when an athlete or other person associated with an adverse analytical finding can clearly demonstrate that he or she did not intend to enhance sport performance.

1.5. Summary

- Drugs are potent substances that are used widely in modern society.
- The mechanisms by which drugs are taken and interact within the body are complex. All drugs produce side effects, the severity of which largely depends on dose and frequency of use.
- There are many reasons why athletes may take drugs, including accepted social use, therapeutic use for the treatment of medical conditions, and the use of supplements and illegal use of drugs for performance enhancement.
- The prescribing of drugs that appear on the WADA Prohibited List, when used by athletes for legitimate medical conditions, may invoke Therapeutic Use Exemption procedures.
- The factors that may influence athletes to take illegal performance-enhancing drugs are complex, varying from athlete to athlete and from sport to sport.
- Athletes are subject to severe penalties for inappropriate use of prohibited drugs.

The remaining chapters of this book provide a detailed analysis of the substances and methods that are used for performance enhancement in sport, as well as the past and present attempts at doping control.

1.6. References

Backhouse, S. H., Whitaker, L., and Petróczi, A. (2013). Gateway to doping? Supplement use in the context of preferred competitive situations, doping, attitude, beliefs, and norms. *Scandinavian Journal of Medical Science in Sports* 23(2):244–252.

Barroso, O., Mazzoni, I., and Rabin, O. (2008). Hormone abuse in sports: The antidoping perspective. *Asian Journal of Andrology* 10(3):391–402.

Bilard, J., Ninot, G., and Hauw, D. (2011). Motives for illicit use of doping substances among athletes calling a national anti-doping phone-help service: An exploratory study. *Substance Use and Misuse* 46(4):359–367.

Conlee, R. K. (1991). Amphetamine, caffeine, and cocaine. In *Perspectives in Exercise Science and Sports Medicine* Ed. Lamb, D.R., and Williams, M.H., New York, Brown & Benchmark.

Eichner, E. R. (1993). Ergolytic drugs in medicine and sports. *American Journal of Medicine* 94(2):205–211.

Elliott, S., and Leishman, B. (2012). Abuse of medicines for performance enhancement in sport: Why is this a problem for the pharmaceutical industry? *Bioanalysis* 4(13):1681–1690.

Fitch, K. (2012). Proscribed drugs at the Olympic Games: Permitted use and misuse (doping) by athletes. *Clinical Medicine* 12(3):257–260.

Geyer, H., Parr, M. K., Mareck, U., Reinhart, U., Schrader, Y., and Schanzer, M. (2004). Analysis of non-hormonal nutritional supplements for anabolic-androgenic steroids: Results of an international study. *International Journal of Sports Medicine* 25(2):124–129.

Knopp, W. D., Wang, T. W., and Bacch, B. R. (1997). Ergogenic drugs in sports. *Clinics in Sports Medicine* 16(3):375–392.

Mazzoni, I., Barroso, O., and Rabin, O. (2011). The list of prohibited substances and methods in sport: Structure and review process by the World Anti-Doping Agency. *Journal of Analytical Toxicology* 35(9):608–612.

Morente-Sánchez, J., and Zabala, M. (2013). Doping in sport: A review of elite athletes' attitudes, beliefs, and knowledge. *Sports Medicine* 43(6):395–411.

Tucker, R. (1997). Abuse of anabolic-androgenic steroids by athletes and body builders: A review. *Pharmaceutical Journal* 259(6954):171–179.

Chapter 2

The evolution of doping and anti-doping in sport

David R. Mottram

2.1. Introduction

Organised sport has a history dating back to ancient Greece. By the seventh century BC, religion, culture, and sport were all an integral part of Greek society; this tradition continued through to the Roman era. There is little documented evidence for organised sport between the fall of the Roman Empire and the mid-nineteenth century. At this time, sport comprised recreational activities associated with religious, cultural, and seasonal events (Australian Sports Drug Agency 2001). By the end of the nineteenth century, urbanisation and industrialisation had transformed sport into a more organised activity with associated rules and the formation of sporting clubs and institutions. As the twentieth century progressed, participation in sport increased. More people became spectators and commercial interests developed.

After the Second World War, international pharmaceutical companies expanded the armoury of medicines available to tackle ill health. Drugs that had hitherto been derived principally from plant and animal sources were now manufactured in the laboratory. Athletes turned to these new, potent drugs to enhance performance.

Attempts to control substance misuse in sport began around the 1950s. However, ignorance of the extent of the problem, a lack of sophisticated testing procedures, and uncoordinated systems for legislating against doping meant that those intent on introducing anti-doping measures were initially playing catch-up. It was not until the beginning of the twenty-first century, with the formation of the World Anti-Doping Agency (WADA), that the anti-doping movement gained the upper hand.

Figure 2.1 shows a timeline of the significant events related to sport, doping, and anti-doping from the ancient Olympics to the current time. These events are described in more detail in the rest of this chapter. A number of landmark doping cases, from which key lessons have been learned, are highlighted in this chapter.

2.2. The ancient Olympic and Roman Games

The Ancient Olympic Games began in 776 BC and were the most important of the Panhellenic Games. Initially, the Games comprised just running events. Over the centuries, other sports were introduced, such as wrestling, boxing, chariot racing, long jump, javelin, and discus throwing. Participants represented their city-states and the victors were rewarded with rich prizes and high esteem. Even in those days, athletes resorted to cheating in order to reap the rewards of victory.

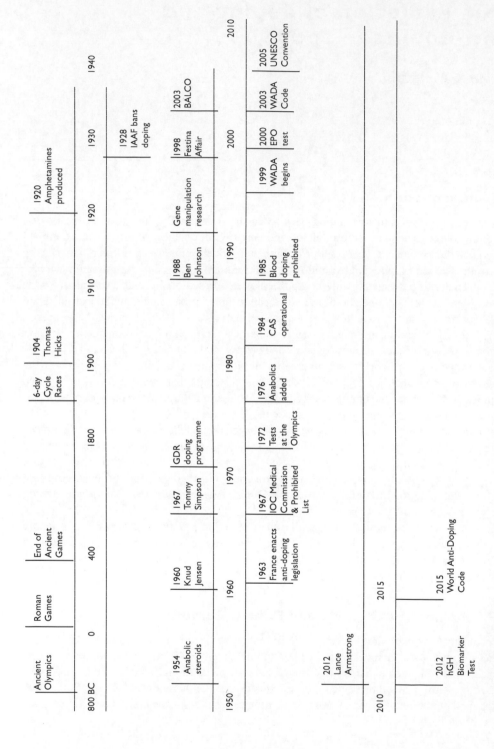

Figure 2.1 Time-line for significant events related to sport, doping, and anti-doping.

2.3. Nineteenth century

At the beginning of the nineteenth century, sport reflected a rural way of life, including boxing, races, football, and sports involving animals, such as cockfighting (Australian Sports Drug Agency 2001). The increasing industrialisation of society altered peoples' lifestyles. Transport systems improved and leisure time increased along with peoples' disposable income. All of these factors had an impact on the development of sport, which became more organised with the formation of clubs and societies. Some sports became more professional, and stadia were built so spectators could pay to watch their heroes.

Most drugs were still extracted from plant and animal sources. Those used by athletes included stimulants such as caffeine (from tea and coffee), strychnine (from the seeds of *Strychnos nux-vomica*), and cocaine (from the leaves of the coca plant). The analgesic morphine (from the opium poppy) and the depressant, alcohol (brewed and/or distilled from a variety of sources) were also used. It is widely accepted that the word *doping* is derived from 'dop,' an alcoholic beverage made from grape skins that was used in South Africa and exported by the Dutch in the nineteenth century.

Few reports of drug use in sport were recorded, although cycle racing, a sport long associated with substance misuse, had its roots in the late nineteenth century. Gruelling 6-day cycle races took place in Europe and involved cyclists taking cocktails of the types of drugs mentioned previously.

2.4. Early twentieth century

One of the earliest reports of drug use in the Modern Olympics occurred in the 1904 Games in St. Louis, when a marathon runner, Thomas Hicks, received doses of strychnine and brandy during the race (Holt *et al.* 2009). Drugs were still crude products because the international pharmaceutical companies did not yet exist.

In 1920, amphetamine became one of the first drugs to be produced synthetically in the laboratory. By 1935, it was used to treat narcolepsy, depression, anxiety, and hyperactivity in children (George 2005). Athletes were free to access whatever substances were available because there was little regulation in sport. The first international sport federation to ban the use of doping (stimulants) was the International Amateur Athletic Federation in 1928; however, restrictions remained ineffective because no tests were available (Fraser 2004).

2.5. The 1940s and 1950s

Amphetamine was used widely in society to enhance mental awareness – a property that was exploited during the Second World War to delay fatigue in combat troops and air crew. This nontherapeutic use of drugs was then mirrored in sport, where athletes experimented with amphetamines to enhance performance (Verroken 1996).

The use of anabolic steroids in sport dates back to the 1950s. Dr. John Ziegler, a physician for the American weightlifting team, suspected the Soviet team of using testosterone at the 1954 World Weightlifting Championships in Vienna (Hoberman 1992). Dianabol was synthesized in 1958 and was used by the American weightlifters at the 1962 World Championships.

In the 1950s, multinational drug companies evolved and invested huge sums of money on research into new classes of drugs for the treatment of diseases. It was not long before athletes tapped into this rich source of potential performance-enhancing drugs.

2.6. The 1960s

Several major new classes of drugs were developed by the pharmaceutical industry in the 1950s and marketed in the 1960s. These drugs included oral contraceptives, corticosteroids, beta blockers, tranquilizers, and antidepressants. The 1960s heralded the era of experimentation into the nontherapeutic use of drugs, both socially and in sport.

Although it is difficult to attribute mortality and morbidity directly to drug use because there may be other contributory factors, there were a number of deaths of athletes directly associated with drug-taking during the 1960s. The cyclist Knud Jensen died in the 100-km team time trial at the 1960 Rome Olympic Games, and Tommy Simpson died during the 1967 Tour de France. Both deaths were associated with amphetamine use, but both occurred under exceptional conditions of heat and exhaustion (George 2005).

The fear of bringing sport into disrepute meant that many sporting authorities denied the possibility that doping took place. Therefore, anti-doping testing was haphazard, at best. The Fédération Internationale de Football Association and Union Cycliste Internationale (UCI) introduced doping tests into their respective world championships in 1966. In 1967, the International Olympic Committee (IOC) instituted a medical commission and set up a list of prohibited substances (Table 2.1). The first mandatory tests at Olympic events were in 1968 at the Winter Olympics in Grenoble and at the Summer Games in Mexico (Fraser 2004).

Table 2.1 Major changes to the IOC Prohibited List, 1967–2003

Year	Classes of substances and methods prohibited	Major changes
1967	I. Central nervous system stimulants II. Psychomotor stimulants III. Sympathomimetic amines IV. Narcotic analgesics	
1976		Anabolic steroids added
1985		Beta blockers and diuretics added
		Prohibited methods added, including blood doping and pharmacological, chemical, and physical manipulation
1987		Probenecid and other masking agents added
1988	I. Doping classes Stimulants Narcotic analgesics Anabolic steroids Beta blockers Diuretics II. Doping methods Blood doping Pharmacological, chemical, and physical manipulation III. Classes of drugs subject to certain restrictions Alcohol Local anaesthetics Corticosteroids	Central nervous system and psychomotor stimulants and sympathomimetics grouped under Stimulants Classes of drugs subject to certain restrictions added
1989		Peptide hormones and analogues added

Table 2.1 Major changes to the IOC Prohibited List, 1967–2003 (Continued)

Year	Classes of substances and methods prohibited	Major changes
1993		Beta blockers moved to Drugs Subject to Certain Restrictions
		Anabolic steroid class renamed as Anabolic Agents to incorporate clenbuterol
		Codeine removed from the list
1998		Insulin added
2000		Oxygen carriers and plasma expanders added
		Erythropoietin added to Peptide Hormones
2003	I. Prohibited classes of substances	The IOC and WADA produce a joint Prohibited List
	Stimulants	
	Narcotics	Agents with antioestrogenic activity added
	Anabolic agents	A separate class of masking agents added
	Diuretics	Gene doping added as a prohibited method
	Peptide hormones, mimetics, and analogues	Enhancement of oxygen transfer added to include blood doping and the administration of products that enhance the uptake, transport, or delivery of oxygen
	Agents with antioestrogenic activity	
	Masking agents	
	II. Prohibited methods	
	Enhancement of oxygen transfer	
	Pharmacological, chemical, and physical manipulation	The title of Section III changed
	Gene doping	Marijuana changed to cannabinoids
	III. Classes of prohibited substances in certain sports	
	Alcohol	
	Cannabinoids	
	Local anaesthetics	
	Glucocorticosteroids	
	Beta blockers	

2.7. The 1970s

The paper by Franke and Berendonk (1997), written after the reunification of Germany, provides a startling account of state-controlled doping by the German Democratic Republic during the late 1960s and 1970s.

German Democratic Republic Doping Programme (1970s and 1980s)

Key Factors	Lessons Learned
• Over 2,000 athletes, preparing for international competition, were systematically dosed with performance-enhancing drugs, including androgenic hormones. • Special emphasis was placed on administering androgens to women and adolescent girls.	• State-controlled doping can occur. • Athletes are exposed to significant health risks arising from doping. • Physicians and scientists may collaborate in doping.

Scientists and physicians undertook research into the systematic doping of thousands of athletes, with particular emphasis on the use of anabolic steroid administration to adult women and adolescent girls, despite documentation of serious side effects.

Most international sports federations had introduced systems for drug testing by the 1970s. However, the IOC's prohibited list only comprised narcotic analgesics and three classes of stimulants (sympathomimetic amines, psychomotor stimulants, and central nervous system stimulants). The first comprehensive testing at an Olympic Games took place in Munich in 1972. Nine positive results for stimulants were detected from more than 2,000 tests.

The use of anabolic steroids was known to be widespread, but a reliable method for testing was not available in the early 1970s. The IOC added anabolic steroids to its prohibited list in 1976 as testing improved. Ground-breaking research by Brooks *et al.* (1975) used radio-immunoassays to identify androgenic anabolic steroids. Steroid testing was conducted for the first time at the 1976 Montreal Olympic Games.

Whilst anti-doping measures to control stimulants and anabolic steroids were beginning to have an impact, the 1970s witnessed the use of blood doping as a method to increase the oxygen-carrying capacity of the blood.

2.8. The 1980s

The 1980s was a turbulent time for sport, with political differences being manifested through boycotts at the Olympic Games of 1980 in Moscow and 1984 in Los Angeles. In addition, there were accusations of a cover-up at the 1983 World Track and Field Championships and the withdrawal of athletes from the Pan American Games when word got through that drug testing was to be included (Hunt 2008).

In 1985, blood doping was the first doping method to be added to the IOC's prohibited list, following reports of its use by the US cycling team at the 1984 Los Angeles Olympics. In 1985, the IOC amended the prohibited list to include beta blockers and diuretics as doping agents and pharmacological, chemical, and physical manipulation as prohibited methods. Despite this, in the 1988 Tour de France, the cyclist Pedro Delgado tested positive for probenecid, a masking agent that was banned according to the IOC's prohibited list but was not on the banned list for the UCI. This inconsistency between sporting authorities meant that Delgado was not disqualified and eventually won the race.

During the 1980s, the decisions by the IOC's medical commission to prohibit diuretics, beta blockers, and glucocorticosteroids were the catalyst for the introduction of what has become known as Therapeutic Use Exemptions (TUEs) to allow athletes to take prohibited drugs for genuine medical conditions and still compete in sport (Fitch 2012).

During the late 1980s, a number of countries, particularly in Scandinavia, developed national anti-doping organisations in an attempt to strengthen anti-doping activity across the boundaries of individual sports (Vance 2007). However, although there was an increase in cooperation between international sports authorities and various governmental agencies, debate still took place regarding definitions, policies, and sanctions. A result of this dishar-mony was that doping sanctions were often disputed and sometimes overruled in civil courts (World Anti-Doping Agency 2009). The Court for Arbitration for Sports became operational in June 1984.

The most significant event of the 1980s occurred at the Seoul Olympic Games in 1988, when Ben Johnson tested positive for the anabolic steroid, stanozolol. The Ben Johnson affair drew the attention of the world to the issue of doping in sport. This event showed that athletes in disciplines other than pure strength events were using steroids and that athletes who thought that they could avoid detection were vulnerable to testing regimes.

Ben Johnson Case (1988)

Key Factors	Lessons Learned
• Johnson won the 100m Olympic gold medal, then tested positive for stanozolol. • The general public was alerted to doping in sport.	• Doping occurs at the highest levels of sport. • Anabolic steroids may be used in any sport. • Physicians and scientists may collaborate in doping. • The Dubin inquiry was set up (Dubin 1990).

Subsequent events implicated six of the eight sprinters who competed in the Seoul 100m final in activities involving performance-enhancing substances (Cooper 2012). In the late 1980s, a cluster of sudden deaths of European cyclists was associated with the appearance of recombinant erythropoietin (EPO) on the market (Eichner 2007).

2.9. The 1990s

The incidence of high-profile doping cases continued into the 1990s. Many of these illustrated the inconsistencies that existed between the IOC and individual sports federations regarding their respective prohibited lists and the application of regulations.

Evidence that the hormone EPO enhances oxygen transport by increasing red blood cell production, led to the addition of EPO to the IOC's prohibited list, despite the absence of a validated test.

In 1992, the sprinter Diane Modahl received a 4-year ban when she tested positive for testosterone during an event in Portugal. However, after a protracted appeal, her suspension was lifted because the laboratory failed to follow the accredited procedures for testing.

The IOC first operated a Therapeutic Use Exemption Committee to approve or reject TUE applications by athletes at the 1992 Olympic Games (Catlin *et al.* 2008).

The testing of two British weightlifters prior to the 1992 Olympic Games in Barcelona lead to their ban for using clenbuterol. This drug is a beta-2 agonist, classified as a stimulant. However, clenbuterol was being used, in this case, for its anabolic effects – a secondary pharmacological property that a number of beta-2 agonists possess. The chemical nature of beta-2 agonists does not permit their classification as anabolic steroids. Consequently, in 1993, the IOC added to its prohibited list the class of anabolic agents, including anabolic steroids and other agents with anabolic properties, principally the beta-2 agonists.

Blood testing of athletes was first implemented at the 1994 Winter Olympic Games in Lillehammer, Norway. Initially, blood testing was used to define acceptable upper limits for blood parameters in an attempt to control the use of drugs such as EPO, for which a validated urine test was not available. An example where upper limits were used was the "no-start" rule in cycling, in which a level of red blood cells (the haematocrit) greater than 50% precluded a cyclist from competing (Saugy *et al.* 2011). Blood testing led to the development of the athlete's "biological passport" (see Chapter 12 for further explanation of biological passport).

Although unpublished evidence existed, particularly in East Germany, that anabolic steroids were effective as doping agents, it was not until 1996 that scientifically robust evidence showed that increased muscle bulk and strength resulted from supraphysiological doses of testosterone (Bashin *et al.* 1996).

The culture of athletes taking substances to enhance performance has meant that the majority of athletes use legal supplements. These may be nutritional, such as vitamins, or ergogenic, such as protein supplements. However, the production and marketing of supplements are not always robust. In the late 1990s, a spate of positive dope tests for the anabolic steroid nandrolone occurred, which, it was claimed, had been taken inadvertently in supplements. This was substantiated by a study showing that many supplements do contain hormonal-based constituents that may lead to athletes testing positive (Schänzer 2002).

In 1963, the French government enacted national anti-doping legislation, which allowed the French police to undertake a raid during the 1998 Tour de France. This became known as the Festina Affair.

The Festina Affair (1998)	
Key Factors	**Lessons Learned**
• A French police raid revealed significant quantities of prohibited substances in a Festina team car. • Several drugs were identified, particularly erythropoietin (EPO).	• Willy Voet (2001) published a revealing account of the affair. • Teams undertook systematic doping. • This affair highlighted the need for a worldwide anti-doping agency.

By the end of the 1990s, questions were being asked as to whether the IOC's prohibited list needed updating (Mottram 1999). More significantly, the whole question of the harmonization of doping control was called into question. In February 1999 in Lausanne, Switzerland, the IOC convened the World Conference on Doping in Sport, resulting in the Lausanne Declaration on Doping in Sport. The World Anti-Doping Agency (WADA) was then established on 10 November 1999 as a direct result of the Lausanne Declaration (WADA, 2014).

WADA was created for several reasons. Different international sport federations and national anti-doping organisations were operating under different rules, leading to doping cases being contested in courts. In addition, there was a lack of a coordinated research policy, particularly with respect to new analytical methods. Finally, little had been done to promote anti-doping activities internationally (Catlin *et al.* 2008). WADA provided harmonisation among anti-doping agencies. Its creation triggered the foundation of national and regional anti-doping organisations, which are key agencies in the worldwide fight against doping in sport (Kamber 2011).

2.10. The early twenty-first century

The first decade of the new millennium heralded a number of significant events associated with doping and anti-doping. A validated test for EPO was introduced at the 2000 Olympic Games in Sydney (Lasne and Ceaurriz 2000). This may have prompted the withdrawal of six Chinese female track-and-field athletes from these games. Despite the introduction of the test, many athletes continued to use EPO, particularly in the sport of cycling.

Athletes began to test positive for darbepoetin, a second-generation EPO, in 2002. At the 2008 Beijing Olympics, five athletes were disqualified for using a third-generation EPO, a continuous erythropoietin receptor activator (Fitch 2012).

Improvements continued to be made in testing procedures, including the development of isotope ratio mass spectrometry for the detection of testosterone misuse (Aguilera *et al.* 2001).

The use by athletes of over-the-counter (OTC) medicines to treat minor conditions has created serious problems. Many of these products contain minor stimulants, such as ephedrine. A number of high-profile athletes tested positive, including Andrea Răducan, a gymnast who lost her gold medal from the Sydney Olympics in 2000 for using pseudoephedrine, and Alain

Baxter, a skier who tested positive for levomethamphetamine at the 2002 Winter Olympics in Salt Lake City (Armstrong and Chester 2005).

Alain Baxter Case (2002)

Key Factors	Lessons Learned
• Baxter tested positive for levomethamphetamine from a medicine purchased over-the-counter (OTC). • He was stripped of his Olympic medal, but an appeal hearing acknowledged that he had not attempted to cheat.	• OTC medicines pose a significant problem to athletes. • All medications taken by athletes should be checked by a healthcare professional. • WADA introduced the 'Specified Substances' clause for those prohibited substances that may be taken inadvertently.

These and other cases led to the removal of most of these OTC drugs from the first prohibited list produced by WADA in 2004. The drugs were placed on a monitoring list, and their use is still recorded by some WADA laboratories. However, evidence has suggested that some of these drugs are now perceived as a fair target for performance enhancement (Mottram *et al.* 2008), leading WADA to reconsider their prohibited status. In January 2010, WADA reintroduced pseudoephedrine to the prohibited list, where an adverse analytical finding is recorded if a urinary threshold of 150 µg/ml is exceeded.

With the increasing robustness and sensitivity of testing procedures, illicit drug suppliers attempted to produce 'designer' drugs that were ostensibly undetectable. The most notorious of these was tetrahydrogestrinone, produced by the Bay Area Laboratory Co-operative (BALCO; Catlin *et al.* 2004). An extensive investigation was undertaken by US government agencies, resulting in the revelation that numerous top-level athletes were listed in BALCO files, several of whom were prosecuted for doping offences in the absence of any adverse analytical chemical evidence – an unprecedented event in the history of doping at that time (Marclay *et al.* 2013).

The Bay Area Laboratory Co-operative (BALCO) Affair (2003)

Key Factors	Lessons Learned
• The BALCO laboratory supplied drugs, including the 'undetectable' steroid tetrahydrogestrinone (TGH; 'The Clear'). • A test was developed for TGH and several high-profile athletes were sanctioned. • Governmental law enforcement agencies were used to investigate doping.	• Back-street laboratories produce 'designer' drugs. • Athletes are prepared to take drugs that have not undergone strict safety checks. • Athletes can be prosecuted for doping offences in the absence of any adverse analytical chemical evidence.

Research into gene technology had been undertaken to develop non-drug-based prevention and treatment of disease. Such technology was also being used to improve drug design by more precisely targeting drugs to their therapeutic site of action. In anticipation of this technology being applied to enhance sporting performance, the IOC and WADA added gene doping to the prohibited list in 2003. However, by the end of the decade, it was suggested that, although gene transfer in humans could theoretically lead to gene doping, the prospect remained theoretical (Wells 2008). Monitoring technological advances in this field remains imperative.

WADA produced the World Anti-Doping Code in 2003, which was endorsed in the same year by over 1,000 delegates at the Second World Conference on Doping in Sport in Copenhagen, Denmark. WADA became responsible for the prohibited list in January 2004 (Table 2.2). WADA invited all stakeholders to comply with the code, including athletes and their supporters, sports federations, the Olympic movement, and governments.

The World Anti-Doping Code was implemented for the first time at the Olympic Games in Athens in 2004. By the end of the decade, most sports (apart from some professional sports in the United States) had declared their support for WADA, and many governments had signed up in support of the International Convention Against Doping in Sport (United Nations Organization for Education, Science and Culture 2005).

Since 2006, WADA has been working closely with international enforcement agencies to uncover doping activities, such as trafficking, which would not come to light through the athlete testing procedures. This was exemplified by the US Drug Enforcement Administration's operation, called Raw Deal, which involved ten countries; the operation resulted in 124 arrests and the seizure of large quantities of steroids from fifty-six laboratories across the United States, mainly supplied from companies in China (Vance 2007). Another law enforcement agency swoop, *Operación Puerto*, involved an investigation of a laboratory in Spain (Soule and Lestrelin 2011).

Operación Puerto (2006)

Key Factors	Lessons Learned
• The Spanish Police discovered a laboratory with frozen blood packs and prohibited substances, such as anabolic steroids and growth hormones. • Several cyclists were implicated and many were withdrawn from the Tour de France.	• This case showed the effectiveness of collaboration between anti-doping organisations and criminal investigation authorities. • Further evidence emerged of medical practitioners involved in doping.

In 2007, the sprinter Marion Jones admitted to steroid use leading up to the 2000 Sydney Olympic Games. She also admitted to using the BALCO steroid 'The Clear.' The IOC stripped Marion Jones of the three gold and two bronze medals she won in 2000.

A further strengthening of the testing procedures was implemented by having athletes declare their whereabouts for a 1-hour period each day to facilitate no-notice, out-of-competition testing with penalties for missed tests. Testing authorities increased their use of 'intelligence' testing which, instead of testing athletes at random, focusses on athletes who are either in higher risk sports and/or who trigger an element of suspicion by their own behaviour or biological profile (i.e. Athlete Biological Passports; Vance 2007; Schumacher *et al.* 2012).

The Global Drug Reference Online (http://www.globaldro.com) was established through the partnership of United Kingdom Anti-Doping, Canadian Centre for Ethics in Sport, and the United States Anti-Doping Agency (USADA). It provides athletes and support personnel with the prohibited status of medicines commonly used in the three partner countries.

Since 2004, WADA has undertaken an annual review of its prohibited list, the major changes to which are presented in Table 2.2. A review of WADA's prohibited list, outlining the substances and methods included on the list and the processes involved in its annual revision, was presented by Mazzoni *et al.* (2011).

A significant advance in anti-doping was achieved at the London 2012 Olympic and Paralympic Games when the biomarker test for human growth hormone (Erotokritou-Mulligan

Table 2.2 Major changes to the WADA Prohibited List, 2004–2014

Year	Classes of substances and methods prohibited	Major changes
2004	I. Substances and methods prohibited in-competition S1 Stimulants S2 Narcotics S3 Cannabinoids S4 Anabolic agents S5 Peptide hormones S6 Beta-2 agonists S7 Agents with antioestrogenic activity S8 Masking agents S9 Glucocorticosteroids M1 Enhancement of oxygen transfer M2 Pharmacological, chemical, and physical manipulation M3 Gene doping II. Substances and methods prohibited in- and out-of-competition Sections S4 to S8 and M1 to M3 above III. Substances prohibited in particular sports P1 Alcohol P2 Beta blockers P3 Diuretics IV. Specified substances	Beta-2 agonists now a separate class Diuretics included in S8 as masking agents but also prohibited in sports (P3) when used to reduce weight Most over-the-counter stimulants (e.g. caffeine, pseudoephedrine) removed but placed on a monitoring list Therapeutic Use Exemption (TUE) introduced for some classes, such as beta-2 agonists and glucocorticosteroids Specified substances added where some classes or specific substances within classes are subject to reduced sanctions if taken inadvertently Glucocorticosteroids now prohibited in all sports
2005		Rearrangement of how substances and methods prohibited in-competition and out-of-competition were presented Beta-2 agonists now prohibited in- and out-of-competition Diuretics removed from Section III and specifically mentioned with masking agents
2008		Class S4 changed to Hormone Antagonists and Modulators to include other groups of drugs that affect endogenous hormones Selective androgen receptor modulators added to S1 Anabolic Agents
2009		The Section IV Specified Substances removed as the definition was changed Abbreviated TUEs removed
2010		Class S2 changed to Peptide Hormones, Growth Factors and Related Substances Salbutamol and salmeterol no longer require a TUE Pseudoephedrine returned to the list
2011		Class S0 added to cover drugs with no official approval Methods that consist of sequentially withdrawing, manipulating, and reinfusing whole blood added to M2 Chemical and Physical Manipulation
2012		Formoterol excepted from prohibition, subject to restrictions on administration S4 Hormone Antagonists and Modulators changed to S4 Hormone and Metabolic Modulators

(Continued)

Table 2.2 Major changes to the WADA Prohibited List, 2004–2014 (Continued)

Year	Classes of substances and methods prohibited	Major changes
2013	I. Substances and methods prohibited at all times (in- and out-of-competition) S0 Nonapproved substances S1 Anabolic agents S2 Peptide hormones, growth factors, and related substances S3 Beta-2 agonists S4 Hormone and metabolic modulators S5 Diuretics and other masking agents M1 Manipulation of blood and blood components M2 Chemical and physical manipulation M3 Gene doping II. Substances and methods prohibited in-competition All categories in Section I plus S6 Stimulants S7 Narcotics S8 Cannabinoids S9 Glucocorticosteroids III. Substances prohibited in particular sports P1 Alcohol P2 Beta blockers	Insulins moved from S2 to S4 Hormone and Metabolic Modulators M1 Enhancement of Oxygen Transfer changed to M1 Manipulation of Blood and Blood Components
2014		Reclassification of some stimulants to reflect their use in society and in sport

et al. 2007; Powrie *et al.* 2007) was introduced, resulting in the eviction from the games of two Paralympic athletes.

Perhaps the most significant doping case revealed to date came on 24 August 2012, when the USADA announced that it had imposed on Lance Armstrong a sanction of lifetime ineligibility and disqualification of competitive results achieved since 1 August 1998 (Mottram 2013). Then, on 10 October 2012, the USADA (2012) published their 'reasoned decision' on the Lance Armstrong case, stating that the evidence shows beyond any doubt that the US Postal Service Pro Cycling Team 'ran the most sophisticated, professionalized and successful doping program that sport has ever seen.' On 22 October 2012, UCI accepted the USADA findings and formally stripped Lance Armstrong of his seven Tour de France titles.

Lance Armstrong Case (2012)

Key Factors	Lessons Learned
• USADA announced a lifetime ban and disqualification of Armstrong's results since 1998. • Armstrong was stripped of his seven Tour de France titles. • Evidence was based primarily on sworn testimonies.	• This case provided further confirmation of extensive team doping in sport. • Sanctions can be applied for anti-doping rule violations other than urine/blood analytical tests. • Commercial sponsorship can be rapidly withdrawn when doping is proven.

Lance Armstrong claimed to have been one of the most frequently tested athletes in the world and that the results of his tests had never shown the presence of a prohibited drug. The presence of a prohibited substance is just one of the eight anti-doping rule violations, as specified in the World Anti-Doping Code, for which athletes can be sanctioned. USADA's charge against Lance Armstrong was based on a wide variety of evidence, including the following:

- Sworn statements from professional cyclists
- Banking and accounting records
- E-mail communications
- Laboratory test results and expert analysis.

Considering the weight of the evidence, one could ask why Lance Armstrong and his team were not sanctioned earlier. There are two principal reasons:

- The nature of the substances and methods used
- The inadequacies of the testing procedures.

The substances and methods used included testosterone, erythropoietin, blood transfusions, human growth hormone, and corticosteroids. These are substances and methods for which there is a naturally occurring component in the body and for which analytical testing provides significant challenges to the testers. Regarding inadequacies of the testing procedures, it was reported in USADA's reasoned decision document that the team riders overcame what little out-of-competition testing there was at the time by simply using their wits to avoid the testers.

2.11. The future

Anti-doping policies continue to be centred on a strategy of testing and punishment (Mazanov and Connor 2010; Hunt *et al*. 2012). This fact has been acknowledged by WADA who, in 2012, established a working group to investigate and report on the 'lack of effectiveness of testing programs' (WADA 2013).

With respect to WADA's policy of global harmonization of anti-doping work, a survey of the members of associations of national anti-doping organisations revealed that, in many countries, the WADA Code was not implemented in accordance with prescribed policy with regard to registered testing pools, the requirements of availability for testing athletes, and the requirements on sanctions (Hanstad *et al*. 2010).

WADA and its partner anti-doping agencies continue to strive for even more robust and accurate analytical testing procedures. These include the development of whereabouts filing (WADA 2010) to more efficiently target athletes for out-of-competition testing and a wider adoption by sports federations of the Athlete Biological Passport (WADA 2012) to improve detection of blood doping and erythropoietin use.

Anti-doping organisations are increasingly developing collaborative partnerships with governments and other institutions (WADA 2011) to coordinate investigations and share anti-doping information and evidence to control the trafficking, supply, and use of performance-enhancing substances. WADA has consolidated several agreements with representatives from the pharmaceutical and biotechnological industries to facilitate the identification and transfer of information on drugs and biotechnological methods under development (Rabin 2011).

In the coming years, it will be interesting to see who gains the upper hand in the battle between the dopers and the anti-dopers.

2.12. Summary

- The use of substances and methods to attempt to improve sport performance dates back to the Ancient Olympics.
- The first recorded instance of drug use in the modern Olympics occurred in 1904, when strychnine with brandy was used.
- Some athletes began to experiment with amphetamines and anabolic steroids in the mid-twentieth century.
- The first IOC list of prohibited substances was introduced in 1967, with mandatory testing at the Olympic Games in 1968.
- Landmark doping cases at the individual athlete, team, and even national level were prevalent through the late twentieth and early twenty-first centuries.
- By the end of the 1990s, it was clear that a more harmonised approach to combatting doping was required. The First World Conference on Doping in 1999 led to the establishment of the World Anti-Doping Agency.
- Significant changes to the WADA Prohibited List and improvements in testing regimes were introduced during the early twenty-first century. However, remarkable revelations of doping cases persisted.
- The current strategy for anti-doping agencies is to continue with robust analytical testing regimes, supported by collaboration with governments and other organisations, to implement a more targeted, intelligence-based anti-doping approach.

2.13. References

Aguilera, R., Chapman, T. E., Starcevic, B., *et al.* (2001). Performance characteristics of a carbon isotope ratio method for detecting doping with testosterone based on urine diols: Controls and athletes with elevated testosterone/epitestosterone ratios. *Clinical Chemistry* 47(2): 292–300.

Armstrong, D. J., and Chester, N. (2005). Drugs used in respiratory tract disorders. In D. R. Mottram (Ed.), *Drugs in Sport* (4th ed.). London, UK: Routledge.

Australian Sports Drug Agency. (2001). The history of drug use in sport. Available online at http://www.ausport.gov.au/fulltext/2001/asda/drugsinsporthistory.asp (accessed 15 July 2014).

Bashin, S., Storer, T. W., Berman, N., *et al.* (1996). The effects of supraphysiological doses of testosterone on muscle size and strength in normal men. *New England Journal of Medicine* 335(1): 1–7.

Brooks, R. V., Firth, R. G., and Sumner, N. A. (1975). Detection of anabolic steroids by radioimmunoassay. *British Journal of Sports Medicine* 9(2):89–92.

Catlin, D. H., Fitch, K. D., and Ljungqvist, A. (2008). Medicine and science in the fight against doping in sport. *Journal of Internal Medicine* 264(2):99–114.

Catlin, D. H., Sekera, M. H., Ahrens, B. D., *et al.* (2004). Tetrahydrogestrinone: Discovery, synthesis and detection in urine. *Rapid Communications in Mass Spectrometry* 18(12):1245–1249.

Cooper, C. (2012). Prologue: A tale of two races. In *Run, Swim, Throw, Cheat*. Oxford, UK: Oxford University Press.

Dubin, C. L. (1990). *Commission of Inquiry into the Use of Drugs and Banned Practices Intended to Increase Athletic Performance*. Ottawa, Ontario, Canada: Canadian Publishing Centre.

Eichner, E. R. (2007). Blood doping: Infusions, erythropoietin and artificial blood. *Sports Medicine* 37 (4–5):389–391.

Erotokritou-Mulligan, I., Bassett, E. E., Kniess, A., *et al.* (2007). Validation of the growth hormone (GH)-dependent marker method of detecting GH abuse in sport through the use of independent data sets. *Growth Hormone and IGF Research* 17(5):416–423.

Fitch, K. (2012). Proscribed drugs at the Olympic Games: Permitted use and misuse (doping) by athletes. *Clinical Medicine* 12(3):257–260.

Franke, W. W., and Berendonk, B. (1997). Hormonal doping and androgenization of athletes: A secret program of the German Democratic Republic government. *Clinical Chemistry* 43(7): 1262–1279.

Fraser, A. D. (2004). Doping control from a global and national perspective. *Therapeutic Drug Monitor* 26(2):171–174.

George, A. J. (2005). CNS stimulants. In D. R. Mottram (Ed.), *Drugs in Sport* (4th ed.). London, UK: Routledge.

Hanstad, D. V., Skille, E. A., and Loland, S. (2010). Harmonization of anti-doping work: Myth or reality. *Sport in Society* 13(3):418–431.

Hoberman, J. M. (1992). Faster, higher, stronger. A history of doping in sport. In J. M. Hoberman (Ed.), *Mortal Engines: The Science of Performance and Dehumanization of Sport.* Toronto, Ontario, Canada: Maxwell Macmillan Canada.

Holt, R.I.G., Erotokritou-Mulligan, I., and Sonksen, P.H. (2009) The history of doping and growth hormone abuse in sport. *Growth Hormone & IGF Research* 19(4):320–326.

Hunt, T. M. (2008). The lessons of crisis: Olympic doping regulations during the 1980s. *Iron Game History* 10(2):12–25.

Hunt, T. M., Dimeo, P., and Jedlicka, S. R. (2012). The historical roots of today's problems: A critical appraisal of the international anti-doping movement. *Performance Enhancement and Health* 1(2): 55–60.

Kamber, M. (2011). Development of the role of national anti-doping organisations in the fight against doping: From past to future. *Forensic Science International* 213(1–3):3–9.

Lasne, F., and Ceaurriz, J. D. (2000). Recombinant erythropoietin in urine. *Nature* 405 (6787):635.

Marclay, F., Mangin, P., Margot, P., *et al.* (2013). Perspectives for forensic intelligence in anti-doping: Thinking outside the box. *Forensic Science International* 229(1–3):133–144.

Mazanov, J., and Connor, J. (2010). Rethinking the management of drugs in sport. *International Journal of Sport Policy and Politics* 2(1):49 63.

Mazzoni, I., Barroso, O., and Rabin, O. (2011). The list of prohibited substances and methods in sport: Structure and review process by the World Anti-Doping Agency. *Journal of Analytical Toxicology* 35(9):608–612.

Mottram, D. R. (1999). Banned drugs in sport. Does the International Olympic Committee (IOC) list need updating? *Sports Medicine* 27(1):1–10.

Mottram, D. (2013). The Lance Armstrong case: The evidence behind the headlines. *Aspetar Sports Medicine Journal* 2(1):60–65.

Mottram, D., Chester, N., Atkinson, G., *et al.* (2008). Athletes' knowledge and views on OTC medication. *International Journal of Sports Medicine* 29(10):851–855.

Powrie, J. K., Bassett, E. E., Rosen, T., *et al.* (2007). Detection of growth hormone abuse in sport. *Growth Hormone and IGF Research* 17(3):220–226.

Rabin, O. (2011). Involvement of the health industry in the fight against doping in sport. *Forensic Science International* 213(1–3):10–14.

Saugy, M., Robinson, N., Grimm, K., *et al.* (2011). Future of the fight against doping: Risk assessment, biological profiling and intelligence. *Forensic Science International* 213(1–3):1–2.

Schänzer, W. (2002). Analysis of non-hormonal nutritional supplements for anabolic-androgenic steroids: An international study. Available online at http://www.olympic.org/Documents/Reports/EN/en_report_324.pdf (accessed 15 July 2014).

Schumacher, Y. O., Saugy, M., Pottgiesser, T. *et al.* (2012). Detection of EPO, doping and blood doping: The haematological module of the Athlete Biological Passport. *Drug Testing and Analysis* 4(11):846–853.

Soule, B., and Lestrelin, L. (2011). The Puerto Affair: Revealing the difficulties of the fight against doping. *Journal of Sport and Social Issues* 35(2):186–208.

United Nations Organization for Education, Science and Culture. (2005). International Convention against Doping in Sport. Available online at http://www.unesco.org/new/en/social-and-human-sciences/themes/anti-doping/international-convention-against-doping-in-sport (accessed 15 July 2014).

United States Anti-Doping Agency. (2012). US Postal Service Pro Cycling Team Investigation. Available online at http://cyclinginvestigation.usada.org (accessed 15 July 2014).

Vance, N. (2007). Developments in anti-doping in elite sports. *Journal of Exercise Science and Fitness* 5(2):75–78.

Verroken, M. (1996). Drug use and abuse in sport. In D. R. Mottram (Ed.), *Drugs in Sport* (2nd ed.). London, UK: Spon.

Voet, W. (2001). *Breaking the Chain*. London, UK: Yellow Jersey Press.

Wells, D. J. (2008). Gene doping: the hype and the reality. *British Journal of Pharmacology* 154(3): 623–631.

World Anti-Doping Agency. (2009). A short history of anti-doping. Available online at https://www.wada-ama.org/en/resources/play-true/play-true-magazine-special-tenth-anniversary#.VA7i8csg_X4 (accessed 7 September 2014).

World Anti-Doping Agency. (2010). Athlete whereabouts. Available online at https://www.wada-ama.org/en/resources/anti-doping-community/at-a-glance-athlete-whereabouts#.VA7kB8sg_X4 (accessed 9 September 2014).

World Anti-Doping Agency. (2011). Coordinating investigations and sharing anti-doping information and evidence. Available online at https://www.wada-ama.org/en/resources/world-anti-doping-program/coordinating-investigations-and-sharing-anti-doping-information#.VA7ky8sg_X4 (accessed 9 September 2014).

World Anti-Doping Agency. (2012). Athlete biological passport operating guidelines and compilation of required elements. Available online at https://wada-main-prod.s3.amazonaws.com/resources/files/WADA-ABP-Operating-Guidelines_v3.1-EN.pdf (accessed 9 September 2014).

World Anti-Doping Agency. (2013). Lack of effectiveness of testing programs. Available online at https://wada-main-prod.s3.amazonaws.com/resources/files/2013-05-12-Lack-of-effectiveness-of-testing-WG-Report-Final.pdf (accessed 9 September 2014).

World Anti-Doping Agency. (2014) Who we are. Available online at https://www.wada-ama.org/en/who-we-are (accessed 4 September 2014).

Chapter 3

Regulation of anti-doping in sport

International and national operational frameworks

Neil Chester and Nick Wojek

3.1. Introduction

Ever since drug use has been recognised as a significant issue in sport, the need to regulate it has been seen as an important step in safeguarding both the welfare of athletes and the integrity of sport. As the prevalence of doping grew, it was evident that sports-governing bodies needed to impose rules and regulations to provide clear direction regarding the use of drugs by athletes. Following on from this was a clear need to impose a framework by which governance and sanctions may be applied. Whilst the need for regulation was apparent, the difficulty in establishing such an operational framework was evident in light of the numerous sports-governing bodies and cultural differences that existed. In recent years the creation of the World Anti-Doping Agency (WADA) has helped to provide much uniformity to the anti-doping movement. Nevertheless, challenges remain in ensuring parity from an anti-doping governance perspective, both nationally and internationally across different sports.

3.2. Why regulate drug use in sport?

As discussed in Chapter 1, there are a number of reasons that athletes might use drugs. It is also evident that there exists a distinction between those used to enhance performance and those used for what they have been designed to do (i.e. treat illness or injury). It is for this distinction that anti-doping regulation exists, to deter athletes from using drugs to enhance performance. Whether regulation should exist at all is typically viewed as an ethical issue and has been the topic of much philosophical debate.

Maintenance of the proverbial 'level playing field' is often quoted as a major reason to prohibit the use of drugs in sport, as athletes who use performance-enhancing drugs are deemed to proffer an advantage over those who do not. However, it is argued that even without drugs, the level playing field does not exist due to both biological and environmental inequalities (Kayser *et al.* 2007). Debate often surrounds the fact that the use of many performance-enhancing drugs is not illegal under state law yet is prohibited under the rules laid down by WADA. This generally means that anyone not competing in organised sport may freely use such drugs to enhance performance and not fear any sanctions. There is clearly an ethical issue surrounding the use of drugs for nontherapeutic purposes. However, the use of performance-enhancing drugs is often left to an individual decision that is not legislated outside of organised sport, unless the drug is deemed to have a significant impact on public health (e.g. some recreational psychoactive drugs, such as amphetamine or cocaine).

A major argument in support of the regulation of drug use in sport is related to the welfare of athletes in terms of protecting their health. Despite the lack of empirical evidence, it is widely accepted that athletes who use drugs (and methods) to enhance sports performance are putting their health at significant risk. However, the opposing argument might be that participation in sport, particularly at an elite level, increases the chances of developing serious health problems such as injury (Kayser *et al.* 2007). One might argue that the risks of participating in sport might be more apparent, allowing an individual to make a more informed decision as to whether he or she partakes or not.

Whether one agrees with the ethical arguments put forward to justify the legislation of drug use in organised sport is often irrelevant. According to the rules of particular sports, the use of performance-enhancing drugs (and in most cases, recreational drugs) is against the rules. Therefore, much like handball in soccer, the use of such drugs is prohibited. The whole basis of competitive sport relies on rules; without such rules, sport would cease to function. The ethical arguments around drug use in sport therefore become secondary but nonetheless no less important.

3.3. The history of the anti-doping movement

Anti-doping has been a reactive movement in response to key incidents in sport, which highlighted not only the use of drugs as performance enhancers but also the dangers surrounding their use from a health perspective.

The International Association of Athletics Federations, formerly known as the International Amateur Athletics Federation, was the first sports federation to implement anti-doping regulations when it banned stimulants in 1928. However, it was not until the 1960s, after the untimely death of the Danish cyclist Knud Jenson in the Rome Olympics (allegedly as a consequence of amphetamine use), that other sports federations took significant steps to legislate against the use of drugs in sport. In 1966, the Fédération Internationale de Football Association (FIFA) introduced a list of prohibited substances; the following year, the Union Cycliste Internationale (UCI) and the International Union of Modern Pentathlon followed suit (Mazzoni *et al.* 2011). In the same year, the International Olympic Committee (IOC) formalised its battle against drug misuse in sport by establishing a medical commission to oversee doping maters and introduce anti-doping regulations.

In 1967, the British cyclist Tom Simpson died shortly after his collapse close to the summit of Mont Ventoux during the thirteenth stage of the Tour de France, which was attributed to the use of amphetamine and alcohol. At this time, the UCI and FIFA were the first to introduce drug tests as a deterrent to its athletes in their respective world championships in 1966 (WADA 2010). The IOC followed suit in 1968 by introducing a list of prohibited substances and drug testing in time for the Winter Olympic Games in Grenoble and the Summer Games in Mexico City. Initial urine tests could only detect the use of stimulants, such as amphetamine; it was not until the mid-1970s that a test was established for the detection of anabolic androgenic steroids. Further advances in analytical chemistry enabled a growing list of prohibited substances to be detected in urine; however, problems remained in terms of the effectiveness of doping control methods.

In 1988, one of the most famous episodes of drug misuse in sport led the anti-doping movement to consider its efficacy once more. The Canadian track-and-field athlete Ben Johnson tested positive for the anabolic androgenic steroid stanozolol immediately after the 100m Olympic final, which led to a large review of the use of performance-enhancing drugs by athletes. This review was led by the Canadian lawyer Charles Dubin and became known as the Dubin Inquiry. The inquiry lasted a year and unearthed widespread doping amongst athletes, as well as marked inadequacies from a doping control perspective. It also put forward numerous recommendations in an attempt to control performance-enhancing drug use in sport (Moriarty *et al.* 1992).

In addition to improved testing and stricter penalties to act as a deterrent to those partaking in doping or considering it in the future, the Dubin Inquiry also put forward several ambitious recommendations that would attempt to stem the tide of widespread doping. Such recommendations focused on maintaining ethical standards, including shifting emphasis away from extrinsic rewards, such as gold medals, toward intrinsic rewards and incorporating ethics and morality into coach education (Moriarty *et al.* 1992). Many of the recommendations made in the report form the basis of the anti-doping education that exists today. However, as elite sport attracts a wider audience, the rewards that come with success continue to grow; therefore, a huge cultural change may be needed for motivation to shift toward rewards that are more intrinsically based.

Although the failed drug test of Ben Johnson put doping in sport in the media spotlight, this was not an isolated case. Indeed, less than 2 years later, reports of systematic doping in the former German Democratic Republic (GDR) were uncovered as the reunification of Germany was reached. Shocking evidence was uncovered of a state-run doping programme that was central to GDR's success from the mid-1960s until the reunification of Germany in 1990.

Despite the horrific reports of systematic doping in the GDR, it is interesting to note that the sporting community did relatively little in the aftermath to address such atrocities. The international federations and the IOC did not address the humanistic issues that the investigation into the GDR system unearthed, nor did they look to rescind any of the medals or records that were achieved by known doped athletes. Franke and Berondonk (1997) provided a comprehensive review of the doping practices in the former GDR; in doing so, they offered a sobering reflection that doping was unlikely to be isolated to such a small state or that individuals with similar support would not have done the same.

It was not until after the events of the Tour de France in 1998, when large-scale team doping was uncovered, that the anti-doping movement would be pushed to make a monumental shift and establish WADA. This allowed anti-doping as a movement to function both independently of sports federations and, most importantly, globally to harmonise the fight against doping in sport. On 10 November 1999, the IOC convened the first World Conference on Doping in Sport in Lausanne, Switzerland, which led to the formation of WADA.

In the subsequent years, after extensive consultation, WADA produced the first draft of the World Anti-Doping Code (WADC), which would provide the framework for the anti-doping movement throughout the twenty-first century. The second World Conference on Doping in Sport was held in November 2003 in Copenhagen, Denmark. In addition to major international sports federations, stakeholders from eighty governments were represented, who formally agreed on the Copenhagen Declaration on Anti-Doping in Sport. This declaration was a formal acceptance of the WADC (and of WADA) by governments, which was to come into effect on 1 January 2004. As part of the WADC, international standards were introduced, including the new List of Prohibited Substances and Methods (formerly produced by the IOC Medical Commission).

Because the WADC is a nongovernment document and therefore not legally binding for governments, the Copenhagen Declaration was further developed by the United Nations Educational, Scientific and Cultural Organisation (UNESCO) to address this shortcoming. The UNESCO International Convention Against Doping in Sport was developed to provide an internationally recognised legal framework for governments to attend to doping in sport and to recognise the WADC. On 19 October 2005, the UNESCO Convention was adopted and took effect from 1 February 2007.

Future World Conferences on Doping in Sport in 2007 and 2013 have seen two revisions of the WADC and International Standards to adapt to the ever-changing doping landscape and further harmonise anti-doping regulations.

3.4. Anti-doping structure

Anti-doping from an organisational perspective is led by WADA, which links both international sporting organisations and state governments. There are few institutions that successfully combine such varied organisations with a unified goal. WADA's goal is to protect athletes against doping and provide a level playing field globally, across all sports. By combining both sports organisations and governments, the fight against doping in sport benefits from not only a unified and consistent approach, but also from the resources that each organisation brings to the table.

Whilst WADA brings together both sports organisations, such as the IOC, and state governments in a unique partnership, its role is largely to manage the World Anti-Doping Program, which has been developed to ensure that the World Anti-Doping Code is adhered to by all those who sign up to it (Figure 3.1). As an independent body, WADA facilitates and monitors the efforts of all signatories (i.e. governments and sports federations) in terms of their compliance with the WADC; where necessary, sanctions may be imposed if noncompliance is evident. A set of international standards have also been developed to help to operationalise the code together with models of best practice, which provide guidelines and solutions for many anti-doping issues.

Regional anti-doping organisations (RADOs) and national anti-doping organisations (NADOs) are in place to ensure that countries comply with the WADC. States that do not have the funds to commit to a fully operational NADO may be served by a RADO, which ensures code compliance across several states within a particular region. In the United Kingdom, UK Anti-Doping is the NADO responsible for managing all anti-doping matters and ensuring effective governance of a national anti-doping programme set up to enable compliance with the code.

The power afforded to WADA lies in the fact that the participation of specific sports and nations at major international competitions including the Olympics, Paralympics, and world championships of various sports is dependent on both the acceptance and implementation of the WADC. From a legislative perspective, some countries have specific laws to help govern drug use in sport (e.g. France and Spain), whilst others have laws to help govern societal drug use as a whole that may be applied to doping (e.g. the United Kingdom and Germany). Nevertheless, the UNESCO convention is in place to provide a legal framework for governments that have ratified it.

3.5. The World Anti-Doping Agency

In 1999 at the first World Conference on Doping in Sport, the World Anti-Doping Agency was founded. According to its constitution (WADA 2009b), the organization's purpose, at an international level, is to

1   Promote and coordinate anti-doping in sport both in and out of competition
2   Enforce ethical principles to underpin doping-free sport and protect the health of athletes
3   Establish and update annually a list of prohibited substances and methods in sport

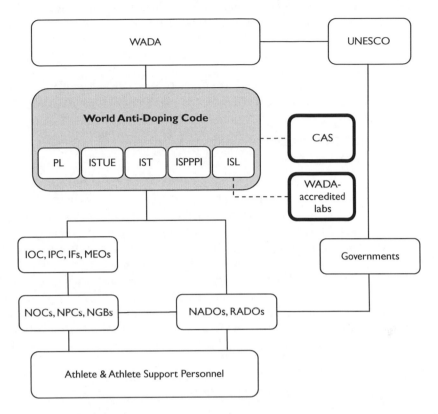

Figure 3.1 A schematic representation of the structure of anti-doping within the context of the World Anti-Doping Code.

CAS, Court of Arbitration in Sport; IOC, International Olympic Committee; IPC, International Paralympic Committee; ISL, International Standard for Laboratories; ISPPPI, International Standard for Protection of Privacy and Personal Information; ISTUEs, International Standard for Therapeutic Use Exemptions; IST, International Standard for Testing; MEOs, Major Event Organisers; NADO, National Anti-Doping Organisation; NGBs, National Governing Bodies; RADO, Regional Anti-Doping Organisation; NOCs, National Olympic Committees; NPCs, National Paralympic Committees; PL, Prohibited List; UNESCO, United Nations Educational, Scientific and Cultural Organisation.

4 Support and coordinate an out-of-competition drug testing programme
5 Develop and harmonise a scientific approach to drug testing through technical standards and procedures in sampling and analysis
6 Promote harmonised rules, disciplinary procedures, and sanctions to combat doping in sport
7 Develop an education programme to promote doping-free sport based on ethical principles
8 Promote and coordinate research into anti-doping.

Members of the WADA Foundation Board are generally representatives from the IOC and public authorities (i.e. government) who form an equal partnership. The president of WADA is an honorary position that lasts for a maximum of two 3-year terms. The position, appointed by the Foundation Board, alternates between representation from the IOC and public authorities. In addition to the Foundation Board, an executive committee takes charge of the actual management and running of the organisation. There are also several additional committees with specialist roles, including the athlete committee; the education committee; the finance and administration committee; and the health, medical, and research committee. Further groups have been formed to provide expert opinion in specialist areas and serve important roles with respect to the WADC, including for the prohibited list, therapeutic use exemptions, laboratories, gene doping, and ethical issues.

As a partnership between governments and the IOC, WADA's budget is funded equally by both parties. In 2012, the WADA budget amounted to more than US $26 million (WADA 2013a).

3.6. The UNESCO international convention against doping in sport

UNESCO introduced the International Convention Against Doping in Sport on 1 February 2007. The convention provides the legal framework to enable governments to address anti-doping in sport. Whilst sports organisations may be able to progress so far with regards to anti-doping and sanctioning athletes, there is a necessity for government to be able to support this work. Indeed, the nature of many doping programmes are so extensive that only governments have the authority to deal with them.

To tackle a doping culture, there is a need to focus on issues surrounding drug availability and distribution and to address the part that athlete support personnel play in a doping case. Essentially, the convention highlights the importance of anti-doping and ensures that governments make a concerted effort to tackle the problem. According to the 2012 WADA Annual Report, 172 countries, including all European Union member states, have ratified the UNESCO convention (WADA 2013a).

3.7. The World Anti-Doping Code

Since its inception in 2004, more than 630 organisations have signed up to the World Anti-Doping Code (WADA 2011a), including, amongst others, the IOC, the International Paralympic Committee (IPC), international sports federations (IFs), national Olympic and Paralympic committees, RADOs and NADOs, and event organisations (e.g. Commonwealth Games Federation, World Transplant Games Federation).

The WADC provides a universal standard for anti-doping practice, which includes a wide range of activities ranging from drug testing to education and research. In addition to the WADC, there are a number of mandatory documents that outline the international standards of operation for the key activities of anti-doping organisations and personnel, including the following:

- The List of Prohibited Substances and Methods
- Therapeutic Use Exemptions
- Testing
- Laboratories
- Protection of privacy and personal information.

Models of best practices and guidelines relating to the WADC and its implementation are also available to use by signatories, but they are not mandatory (WADA 2009a).

As the anti-doping landscape changes, WADA must adapt accordingly. It does this most notably through regular revisions to the code. The first WADC was introduced in 2004, and then a revised code was developed through a widespread consultation process amongst stakeholders and approved in 2007 at the Third World Conference on Doping in Sport in Madrid, Spain. The revised code came into effect as of 1 January 2009.

Following a similar consultation process, a third revision of the code was adopted at the Fourth World Conference on Doping in Sport in Johannesburg, South Africa, in 2013. The new code comes into effect on 1 January 2015 and will include several changes to the current version. The most significant changes include increased sanctions for those who commit a first doping offence, a recognition of the role of nonanalytical evidence in investigations into potential anti-doping rule violations (ADRVs), and the role of athlete support personnel in doping offences. Further details on the new code are outlined in Chapter 26.

Compliance to the code is essential and thus a major element of the WADC. For the anti-doping movement to function, all signatories of the code must adhere to the rules and regulations set out in the document. In doing so, signatories must put in place policies that ensure that the rules, regulations, and procedures set out in the WADC are followed by all stakeholders. Governance relating to code compliance is therefore an important aspect of WADA's role.

The following sections provide a brief description of the key elements of the WADC, including doping control, education and research, roles and responsibilities, and compliance.

Doping control

A major portion of the WADC is focused on anti-doping rules and regulations and the procedures required to enforce such rules. The code outlines a wide range of rules and regulations that athletes must follow and sports organisations must implement. Further details on doping control procedure are provided in Chapter 4.

What is doping?

According to the code (WADA 2009a), the definition of *doping* is specified as the occurrence of one or more of the following anti-doping rule violations (ADRVs):

1   The presence of a prohibited substance or its metabolites or markers in an athlete's sample
2   The use of or attempted use by an athlete of a prohibited substance or method
3   Refusing or failing to provide a sample after notification without compelling justification
4   Violation of applicable requirements regarding athlete availability for out-of-competition testing, including failure to file sufficient whereabouts information and missed tests
5   Tampering or attempted tampering with any part of the doping control procedures
6   Possession of prohibited substances or methods
7   Trafficking or attempted trafficking in any prohibited substance or method
8   Administration, attempted administration, or assisting in the administration of any prohibited substance or method.

With the introduction of the new code in 2015, the definition of doping will be extended to better reach athlete support personnel who are involved in doping through the introduction of two new ADRVs (WADA 2014a):

9   Intentional complicity (e.g. aiding, abetting, conspiring, covering up) to commit an ADRV
10   Association in a professional or sport-related capacity of an athlete with support personnel who are serving a period of ineligibility or who have been convicted in a criminal proceeding for conduct that would constitute doping.

In light of the wide range of ADRVs, proof can be rather difficult to establish. Because many ADRVs do not involve the determination of a prohibited substance or use of a prohibited method via a positive drug test, evidence may be gathered from a variety of sources, including an admission by an athlete, the testimony of a third person, or documentary evidence. When an ADRV is alleged to have occurred, an anti-doping organisation (typically the NADO) must establish that the proof is greater than the balance of probability for a case to proceed. The individual accused of an ADRV may then refute the claims at a hearing.

The prohibited list

Whilst not all ADRVs involve the use of a prohibited substance or method, the Prohibited List is fundamental to doping control because it clearly outlines what is deemed to be unacceptable, both in and out of competition (see Chapter 1; Table 1.1). As with the Code, the Prohibited List is an evolving document. New pharmacological agents and potential performance-enhancing methods are continually being developed and becoming available. Therefore, the list must be updated regularly to keep pace with the rapidly changing landscape.

A specific expert committee has been established by WADA to oversee the development of the Prohibited List and consider the inclusion or exclusion of specific substances or methods on an annual basis. Each year, the Prohibited List committee initiates a consultation process with all WADA stakeholders, asking them to consider potential modifications to the list. Modifications may take the form of changes to the terminology of the document (including the use of particular drug names) to help in the understanding and thus compliance of the list or changes to the actual content in terms of introducing or removing substances or methods to the list. In addition, the committee also considers the inclusion of particular thresholds for specific substances or the reclassification of particular substances.

The criteria by which the Prohibited List committee makes decisions as to whether a substance or method is to be considered for inclusion on the list are as follows:

1   The use of a substance or method has the potential to enhance performance in sport.
2   The use of a substance or method has the potential to adversely affect health.
3   The use of a substance or method contravenes the spirit of sport.

In addition, substances or methods that have the potential to mask the presence or use of a prohibited substance or method would also be considered for inclusion on the Prohibited List.

The Prohibited List committee considers the comments made during the consultation process and the data made available to them from WADA-accredited laboratories, the WADA monitoring programme, and research publications, particularly those funded by WADA research grants.

The monitoring programme

In addition to the List of Prohibited Substances and Methods, WADA also conducts a monitoring programme, which allows for the monitoring of substances beyond that of the Prohibited List to determine patterns of use that may reflect possible misuse (WADA 2014b). The programme typically includes substances that are not prohibited but have the potential to be misused in sport for possible performance-enhancing purposes. A number of substances that are part of the monitoring programme are also present on the Prohibited List, although they are subject to only partial prohibition (i.e. only in-competition and/or above a particular threshold).

Therapeutic use exemption

Doping by athletes is not to be confused with the use of drugs for therapeutic purposes. Whilst drug use in sport is synonymous with doping, there are numerous instances when drug use by athletes is entirely legitimate. Indeed, WADA has outlined a process whereby athletes may apply for and be granted an exemption for the use of a particular prohibited substance or method specifically for therapeutic purposes. This process is known as Therapeutic Use Exemption (TUE) and is outlined in detail in the International Standard for Therapeutic Use Exemptions (WADA 2011b).

The procedure for obtaining a TUE requires an athlete to make a request with supporting medical evidence. Each application is then considered, according to the guidelines set out by the international standards document, by an independent TUE committee that is formed by the respective NADO, IF, or major event organiser. TUE committees are made up of physicians with experience in the field of sports medicine and specialists with expertise in treating specific medical conditions. TUE committees make decisions as to whether to grant a TUE based on the following three criteria (WADA 2011b):

1   The athlete would experience significant health problems without taking the prohibited substance or method.
2   The therapeutic use of the substance would not produce significant enhancement of performance.
3   There is no reasonable therapeutic alternative to the use of the otherwise prohibited substance or method.

Decisions made by each committee are reported to WADA, who may decide to confirm or rescind the initial decision according to whether or not the TUE committee complied with procedures set out in the international standards document. There is also an appeals process that can be used by athletes to contest the committee's decision.

Testing

To enforce the rules set out in the WADC and the international standards, a robust testing procedure is necessary. So that the Prohibited List may serve as an effective deterrent, testing is required to be a covert operation that follows strict guidelines in terms of sampling and analysis as outlined in the International Standard for Testing (WADA 2012a) and the International Standard for Laboratories (WADA 2012b).

Sample analysis is carried out in specific laboratories that follow approved procedures and are formally accredited by WADA. Strict accreditation and regular assessment procedures ensure both validity and harmonisation of test results across all laboratories and that the highest standards are maintained. There are currently thirty-two WADA-accredited laboratories that are distributed in cities across the globe (WADA 2014c). More than half (nineteen) of the accredited laboratories are based in Europe, whereas the African and South American regions are considered to be underserved. As a result, WADA is discouraging the setup of further laboratories in Europe and is exploring opportunities to establish additional laboratories in South America and Africa (WADA 2013b).

Results management

Associated with the high standards maintained by a laboratory is a results management system that ensures a clear chain of events, whereby an athlete is notified as soon as his or her sample returns an adverse analytical finding that is not supported by a valid TUE. Likewise, there should not be any reported deviation from the procedures outlined in the international standards for testing or laboratories. The athlete may then request an analysis of the B-sample; if it confirms the analytical results of the A-sample, an adverse analytical finding is established (at the time of collection, urine is split into A- and B-samples and stored separately; see Chapter 4).

In the event of an adverse analytical finding, there is a requirement for an anti-doping organisation to provide a fair hearing process to establish if an ADRV has occurred and what sanctions are to be imposed. If the hearing confirms the evidence put forward by the anti-doping organisation and a sanction is applied, an appeals process must be made available. A disciplinary case for doping might be dealt with initially between the NADO, IF, and the athlete. A subsequent appeal might be lodged with the Court of Arbitration for Sport (CAS).

Sanctions

The WADC clearly outlines the sanctions to be imposed on individuals, teams, and sporting organisations implicated in an ADRV. The provision of clear sanctions is imperative to ensure harmonisation and act as a real deterrent to all those tempted by doping. Current sanctions include disqualification and forfeiture of points, medals, and prizes when an ADRV has occurred in competition. In addition, a period of ineligibility is typically imposed, which varies according to the nature of the ADRV and whether the athlete has committed a previous ADRV. The criteria for increasing or reducing the standard 2-year period of ineligibility can be rather complex; they are outlined in Chapter 4.

A public disclosure of those individuals committing an ADRV is arguably the most impactful from both a professional and personal perspective. An athlete who is deemed to have committed an ADRV should be publically identified after a hearing and any subsequent appeals have concluded.

In addition to sanctions imposed on individuals, there are circumstances whereby a team may be sanctioned, particularly in circumstances where more than one member of a team commits an ADRV. In such instances, likely sanctions would include loss of points or disqualification from a competition.

Whereabouts

As a means of conducting an effective and efficient out-of-competition testing programme, a system has been established whereby athletes must report their prospective location for one hour a day, each day throughout their competitive career. This system, in which athletes notify either their IF or NADO of their location, is known as *whereabouts*. Only elite athletes competing at the highest levels who have been identified by their respective IF or NADO are required to undertake such reporting; as such, they are part of a registered testing pool.

The accuracy of the information provided is critical. Athletes who fail to file information or file inaccurate information (i.e. they are found not to be at the location at the time they stated in the whereabouts information) on three separate occasions in an 18-month period are deemed to have committed an ADRV. Under the new code, three filling failures and/or missed tests over a 12-month period are deemed to be an ADRV (WADA 2014a).

Doping control for animals competing in sport

Sports that involve animals, such as horse racing, implement anti-doping rules and procedures specific to the animals via their international federation. However, the testing of humans is under the jurisdiction of WADA when the specific federation has signed up to the WADC.

Statute of limitations

There is a period of 8 years during which an alleged anti-doping violation may have taken place and throughout which action against an athlete may proceed. In addition, when multiple ADRVs are to be considered in determining the sanction (i.e. length of period of ineligibility), these must occur within the same 8-year period. Under the new code, the statute of limitations has been extended to 10 years to acknowledge that sophisticated doping can sometimes take a long time to uncover (WADA 2014a).

Education and research

A key element of the WADC is the promotion of proactive or preventative measures in an attempt to limit both intentional and unintentional ADRVs. In the code, both research and education are highlighted as key preventative measures in which all signatories are expected to engage. Further detail regarding both education programmes and research supported by WADA is provided in Chapter 4.

Roles, responsibilities, and compliance

One of WADA's key roles is to monitor and ensure that its signatories adhere to the rules and procedures set out in the WADC. Nevertheless, ultimately each organisation that is governed by the code must not only ensure its own compliance with the code but also that of the organisations it governs. The consequences of noncompliance should also be visible with a clear penalty for perpetrators, such as ineligibility to participate in major competitions or to bid to host such an event (WADA 2009a).

There is a clear chain of command in terms of roles and responsibilities from a code compliance perspective, which filters down from WADA, the IOC, and the IPC to IFs, NADOs, National Olympic Associations, National Paralympic Associations, and ultimately to National Governing Bodies and athletes. The chain of command, which also includes governments and major event organisers, is a complex one (see Figure 3.1), yet it is essential if anti-doping is to be effective. Devolution of governance ensures that there is engagement with anti-doping at all levels.

Whilst acceptance of the code by signatories has been particularly encouraging, Houlihan (2014) argued that the degree of compliance is less so. Clearly, such an issue places the core WADA principle of harmonisation in doubt. Further efforts are required to address issues concerning the capacity and commitment of stakeholders in terms of code compliance. Such a challenge highlights the importance of individual state legislation that addresses the use of prohibited substances and methods. Legislation that tackles issues, such as trafficking, provides the necessary weight to assist NADOs in their efforts to ensure the necessary code compliance (WADA 2013a).

3.8. Court of Arbitration for Sport

The CAS has an important role within the structure of anti-doping because it provides an independent means, where necessary, for the resolution of disputes associated with ADRVs and related sanctions. It is available to both athletes and federations for all sports-related disputes, including those linked to disciplinary charges, such as doping, and those that are commercial in nature, such as sponsorship and relationship disputes between athletes, coaches, clubs, and agents.

The concept of CAS was introduced by the IOC and established in 1984. Based in Lausanne, it was comprised of sixty members who were appointed by the IOC, IFs, and national Olympic associations. However, the independence of CAS was later questioned. In 1994, following major reform, it became both structurally and financially autonomous.

3.9. Summary

The anti-doping movement has made huge strides over recent decades in an attempt to address the increasingly complex nature of doping practice. The establishment of policies and practices to address doping in sport is now led by the World Anti-Doping Agency through the World Anti-Doping Code. International federations, international and national Olympic and Paralympic committees, major event organisations, and national anti-doping organisations are all signatories to the code. Governments accept the WADC by signing up to the UNESCO Convention, which provides the legal framework to enable governments to address anti-doping in sport. Whilst sports organisations may be able to progress so far with regards to anti-doping and sanctioning athletes, there is a necessity for governments to be able to support this work by aligning their domestic policies with the code. However, challenges exist to guarantee that such a model can be implemented across all states, thus ensuring harmonisation – a fundamental objective of the WADC.

3.10. References

Franke, W. W., and Berendonk, B. (1997). Hormonal doping and androgenization of athletes: A secret program of the German Democratic Republic government. *Clinical Chemistry* 43(7):1262–1279.

Houlihan, B. (2014). Achieving compliance in international anti-doping policy: An analysis of the 2009 World Anti-Doping Code. *Sport Management Review* 17(3):265–276.

Kayser, B., Mauren, A., and Miah, A. (2007) Current anti-doping policy: A critical appraisal. *BMC Medical Ethics* 8(2):1–10.

Mazzoni, I., Barroso, O., and Rabin, O. (2011). The List of Prohibited Substances and Methods in Sport: Structure and Review Processby the World Anti-Doping Agency. *Journal of Analytical Toxicology* 35(9):608–612.

Moriarty, D., Fairall, D., and Galasso, P. J. (1992) The Canadian Commission of Inquiry into the use of drugs and banned practices intended to increase athletic performance. *Journal of Legal Aspects of Sport* 2(1):23–31.

World Anti-Doping Agency. (2009a). World Anti-Doping Code. Available online at https://www.wada-ama.org/en/resources/the-code/2009-world-anti-doping-code#.VAyy6ssg_X4 (accessed 6 September 2014).

World Anti-Doping Agency. (2009b). Constitutive instrument of foundation of the World Anti-Doping Code. Available online at http://www.wada-ama.org/Documents/About_WADA/Statutes/WADA_Statutes_2009_EN.pdf (accessed 9 February 2014).

World Anti-Doping Agency. (2010). A brief history of anti-doping. Available online at https://elb.wada-ama.org/en/who-we-are/a-brief-history-of-anti-doping (accessed 6 September 2014).

World Anti-Doping Agency. (2011a). Code compliance and reporting. Available online at http://www.wada-ama.org/en/World-Anti-Doping-Program/Sports-and-Anti-Doping-Organizations/The-Code/Code-Compliance-Reporting (accessed 9 February 2014).

World Anti-Doping Agency. (2011b). International standard for Therapeutic Use Exemptions. Available online at https://www.wada-ama.org/en/resources/science-medicine/international-standard-for-therapeutic-use-exemptions-istue#.VAzIecsg_X4 (accessed 5 September 2014).

World Anti-Doping Agency. (2012a). International standard for testing. Available online at https://wada-main-prod.s3.amazonaws.com/resources/files/WADA_IST_2012_EN.pdf (accessed 6 September 2014).

World Anti-Doping Agency. (2012b). International standard for laboratories. Available online at https://wada-main-prod.s3.amazonaws.com/resources/files/WADA_Int_Standard_Laboratories_2012_EN.pdf (accessed 5 September 2014).

World Anti-Doping Agency. (2013a). 2012 annual report. Available online at https://elb.wada-ama.org/en/media/2013-06/wada-publishes-2012-annual-report#.VAzI-8sg_X4 (accessed 5 September 2014).

World Anti-Doping Agency. (2013b). Laboratory network strategy. Available at https://wada-main-prod.s3.amazonaws.com/resources/files/WADA-ExCo-Decisions-Lab-Strategy-Oct2013-EN.pdf (accessed 9 September 2014).

World Anti-Doping Agency. (2014a). World Anti-Doping Code 2015. Available online at https://elb.wada-ama.org/en/resources/the-code/2015-world-anti-doping-code#.VAzKZcsg_X4 (accessed 7 September 2014).

World Anti-Doping Agency. (2014b). The 2014 monitoring program. Available online at https://elb.wada-ama.org/en/resources/science-medicine/monitoring-program#.VAzLBcsg_X4 (accessed 7 September 2014).

World Anti-Doping Agency. (2014c). List of WADA Accredited Laboratories. Available online at https://www.wada-ama.org/en/node/4619#.VAzMo8sg_X5 (accessed 7 September 2014).

Chapter 4

Doping control in sport

Neil Chester and Nick Wojek

4.1. Introduction

There is a need to implement a set of rigorous procedures to ensure that doping control in sport is both fair and consistent across different nations and sports and acts as an effective deterrent. From Chapter 3, it is clear that doping is defined by the violation of any of the anti-doping rules set out in the World Anti-Doping Code (WADC). Doping control procedures are therefore centred on the detection of those who contravene these rules but also on effective preventative mechanisms. Whilst detection of anti-doping rule violations (ADRVs) and subsequent sanctioning may act as a deterrent to those who are tempted by doping, it is envisaged that anti-doping education is able to act as an effective preventative measure.

As laid out in the WADC, anti-doping organisations must ensure that an effective doping control programme is implemented. All signatories and stakeholders of the code, including international sports federations, major event organisations, national sports governing bodies, sports clubs, and athletes and their support staff, have a responsibility to comply with this programme. In addition, all signatories must ensure that education forms part of any anti-doping programme as a preventative measure against both intentional and unintentional ADRVs.

In recent years, the anti-doping movement has focused attention on intelligence-based investigations in an attempt to address a wider range of ADRVs in addition to those that rely on more traditional drug-testing methods (i.e. urine and blood analysis). Whilst such investigations have helped to provide a more targeted approach to drug testing, they have also enabled anti-doping organisations to direct attention toward the manufacture, distribution, and supply of substances and methods on the World Anti-Doping Agency (WADA) Prohibited List.

This chapter seeks to provide an overview of how anti-doping organisations implement doping control procedures from the point of test planning to the collection and analysis of athlete samples. An overview of the results management process following the analysis of a sample and how nonanalytical information is used to enhance the uncovering of ADRVs will also be explained.

4.2. Education and research

A key element of the WADC is the promotion of preventative measures in an attempt to limit both intentional and unintentional ADRVs. In the Code, both research and education are highlighted as key preventative measures in which all signatories are expected to engage.

Education programmes should be viewed as an important aspect of an anti-doping strategy. As such, the code outlines the following key topics (WADA 2009) that should be included:

- The List of Prohibited Substances and Methods
- Anti-doping rule violations and sanctions
- Doping control procedures
- The potential health consequences of doping
- The Therapeutic Use Exemption process
- The risks associated with supplement use and how to minimise them
- The rights and responsibilities of athletes and athlete support personnel
- Doping and its impact on the spirit of sport.

In addition to athletes, education should be directed toward all athlete-support personnel, including parents, coaches, officials, and medical support staff, in an attempt to foster an environment that is conducive to drug-free sport.

WADA has established two funding streams in an attempt to promote research in the physiological and analytical sciences and the social sciences. Funding is assigned to the two programmes on an annual basis, and researchers are encouraged to apply for funds through an application process involving the submission of a detailed project proposal. Following review by the appropriate WADA committee, approval is given to researchers who seek to answer important questions or add key information to new and emerging areas within the field of anti-doping. Funds committed to research since 2001 have totalled more than US $51 million, with $3.2 million allocated in 2012 (WADA 2013a).

The criticism levelled at many research studies that attempt to examine the reputed effects of prohibited substances and methods is that findings are from recreational or nonelite athletic subjects and thus are not representative of elite athletes. Whilst there might be a drive to address this issue, there is a need to be cognisant of the issues that could result. Recruiting athletes to studies that include the supplementation of a prohibited substance or use of a prohibited method should be avoided due to the potential performance-enhancing effects and adverse side effects, as well as the potential of a failed drug test as a consequence of participation in a research study (Howman 2013).

4.3. Drug detection

As outlined in Chapter 3, doping is defined as the infringement of at least one of several anti-doping rules. Whilst the most notable rules relate to the prohibition of substances and methods as specified by the Prohibited List (WADA 2014a), other rules relate to the requirement of all athletes to engage appropriately in doping control procedures, including routine urine and blood collection.

In cases where there is evidence of an ADRV as a consequence of a positive drug test, the principle of strict liability is upheld. Only in exceptional circumstances is the potential sanction eliminated, when athletes can provide evidence to demonstrate that they bear no fault or negligence and can prove how the prohibited substance has entered their body (WADA 2009).

Test distribution plan

An important aspect of an effective doping control programme is the development of a test distribution plan, which not only has the best chance of success (i.e. detection of those athletes who practice doping) but is also the most cost effective. Traditional methods of doping control are inherently ineffective, particularly when it is considered that the percentage of positive drug tests is approximately 2 per cent, yet the prevalence of doping is considered to be much higher (Hermann and Henneberg 2013).

Previously, it was assumed that increased testing would lead to greater success in terms of exposing those involved in doping; however, the cost of increasing the number of tests is not economically viable. Moreover, the distribution of tests as opposed to the volume of tests is thought to have a much greater impact on the effectiveness of a testing programme.

This change in philosophy has led to the focus of current testing programmes being centred on increasing the proportion of target tests. Target tests are essentially tests that target specific individuals and sports at particular times according to the reputed risk of likely doping practice. Whilst random testing still has a place in drug testing, the development of a target testing scheme enables a much more proactive approach toward doping control.

According to the International Standard for Testing (WADA 2011a), the following factors are considered when determining whom tests should be targeted toward:

- Athletes showing abnormal biological parameters arising from the Athlete Biological Passport
- Injured athletes
- Athletes who withdraw or are absent from competition
- Retiring athletes or those deciding to come out of retirement
- Athletes behaving in a manner that might suggest involvement in doping
- Athletes who show sudden improvements in performance
- Athletes repeatedly failing to file whereabouts information
- Athletes whose whereabouts information might suggest involvement in doping (e.g. a move to an isolated location)
- Athletes who are moving into a different age category (e.g. junior athletes moving into the senior ranks and those athletes approaching retirement)
- Athletes whose test history might suggest potential doping practice
- Reinstated athletes following a period of ineligibility
- Athletes who are subject to significant financial incentives for improvements in performance
- Athletes who are associated with support personnel who have a history of involvement in doping
- Athletes who are highlighted by information obtained from a third party.

As part of an effective doping control strategy, a risk assessment is performed to assess which sports or specific athletes might be liable to doping practice and whether this is likely at particular times of the year. A risk assessment to evaluate the potential doping practice of a particular sport should be based upon the following factors, as outlined in the International Standard for Testing (WADA 2011a):

- The demands of the sport and the potential performance-enhancing effects of doping
- Drug testing statistics attributed to the specific sport
- Research on doping trends and the history of doping in the specified sport
- The training and competition calendar of the sport
- Any available information on doping practice attributed to the sport.

This information is imperative in informing a robust target testing strategy. In addition to prioritising target testing and a test distribution plan, the national anti-doping organisation (NADO) must also establish criteria for the sports that require a registered testing pool and implement an effective number of in- and out-of-competition tests for athletes included in this pool. Registered testing pools are developed by both international federations (IFs) and NADOs and consist of those athletes competing at the highest level. Athletes selected for respective registered testing pools are required to provide whereabouts information (see Chapter 3).

Sample provision

The key stages and procedures for sample provision are outlined in the International Standards for Testing (WADA 2011a). However, some variations will occur depending on the testing authority (i.e. NADO, IF, or major event organiser). Key stages in sample provision include selection, notification, chaperoning, reporting to the doping control station, and sample collection. These stages are carried out by authorised individuals known as doping control officers (DCOs) and chaperones.

Selection

When the test is random, a specific selection process must be performed. The selection draw will often involve a lead DCO in addition to an IF or national sports governing body representative or additional doping control staff member. The draw may take several forms, including assigning numbers to named athletes prior to a random number selection. Alternatively, selection may be based on finishing position, such as the winner, runner-up, and fifth position.

Notification

Strict procedures are followed when an athlete is notified and vary slightly according to whether an athlete is an adult or a minor (i.e. under 18 years of age) or has a disability, such as a visual impairment. As soon as possible after a competition, a doping control staff member approaches selected athletes to notify them of their selection for a drug test. At this stage, the athletes are informed of their rights and responsibilities, which include the right to have a representative with them and an interpreter where available, as well as the responsibility to report to the doping control station immediately, to be chaperoned at all times until the sample provision has been completed, and to comply with doping control procedures, including the provision of the first urine sample passed subsequent to notification (WADA 2011a).

If an athlete selects to have a representative, this representative can be any individual he or she chooses, such as a friend, training partner, family member, coach, or team doctor. In the event that an athlete is a minor, there is a requirement that notification, chaperoning, and actual sample provision is performed under the supervision of an additional individual. Whilst at notification and up until the athlete reports to the doping control station (DCS), this individual might be a selected representative. Once inside the DCS, additional doping control staff may fulfil this role.

Chaperoning

From the instant that an athlete is notified, he or she must be chaperoned by a doping control staff member at all times until sample collection procedures are completed. The chaperoning process involves observation of the athlete in full view of a doping control staff member.

Reporting to the doping control station

Athletes are required to report to the DCS immediately after notification. The DCS is a designated facility that might ordinarily be a medical or physiotherapist treatment room or a hotel
room. The DCS is a controlled environment with a strict policy for both entry and exit of
specified individuals. It is essential that the facility allows the privacy of an athlete to be
maintained during sample collection; where possible, the DCS should be used solely for the
purpose of sample provision. A lead DCO must ensure that a designated DCS is able to
maintain sample integrity and that no part of the collection process is compromised.

A delay in reporting to the DCS is acceptable in specific circumstances, such as when an
athlete is required to attend an awards ceremony, undertake media commitments, collect
identification documents (e.g. passport), locate a representative or interpreter (where necessary), compete in further competitions, complete a cool-down or training session (in the case of
out-of-competition tests), or receive medical treatment. When medical treatment is required,
the lead DCO will assess (through consultation with medical staff) whether the athlete is fit
enough to continue with the test and determine whether it is appropriate to abort the test.
Delayed reporting for other reasons must be approved by the lead DCO. Reasons typically
deemed to be unacceptable include showering and meeting family and friends.

Sample collection

On arrival at the DCS, athletes will typically wait in a designated area until they are ready to
provide a sample. Whilst formal notification has occurred, further details may be obtained from
the athlete to complete the notification process. When blood collection is required, athletes are
required to sit for a designated period (a minimum of 10 minutes) before a sample can be taken.
For urine collection, athletes are required to wait only as long as is necessary until they are able
to provide a sample. If athletes are considered to be dehydrated, they might be encouraged to
drink fluids (in moderation) to promote diuresis.

When athletes are ready, they will be asked to select a collection vessel and provide a
sample under the supervision of a DCO of the same sex of the athlete. Athletes are required to
remove sufficient clothing to enable direct observation of sample provision by the supervising
DCO. A minimum volume of 90 ml of urine is required for analysis. Once collected, this is
divided into A- and B-sample bottles. If less than 90 ml is collected, additional samples are
required. An additional sample is added to the previous sample(s) until the minimum volume
is reached.

The concentration of the sample is determined through the assessment of specific gravity
using a digital refractometer. In the event that specific gravity is less than 1.005, further samples
will be collected until the specified range (i.e. ≥ 1.005) is met. This ensures that any potential
substances (on the Prohibited List or part of the monitoring program) can be determined using
current analytical technologies. In the event that further samples are required, athletes will be
encouraged not to consume further fluids in an attempt to increase urine concentration.

In the cases where blood collection is required, a qualified phlebotomist (blood collection
officer; BCO) will perform the procedure. Athletes are required to be seated for a minimum
period of 10 minutes prior to blood collection via venipuncture of an antecubital vein. Blood
collection uses evacuated tubes that enable a specific amount of blood to be collected. If the
BCO is unable to collect a sample or collects insufficient volume, a maximum of three
attempts are performed before sampling is terminated. All samples collected are then sealed
into a tamperproof transport vessel by the athlete, ready for shipment.

Following sample collection, athletes will be asked to declare on a doping control form (DCF) any medication and supplements that they have taken over the previous 7 days, any Therapeutic Use Exemptions that they may currently hold, and any blood transfusions that they may have received within the previous 6 weeks. This information is essential in providing the necessary detail to supplement any potential adverse analytical finding. Following a declaration of the athlete's approval (or not) for the sample to be used in anonymised anti-doping research, the DCF is checked and signed by the athlete and DCO to confirm that satisfactory procedure has been followed and all necessary detail is present and correct. Athletes receive a duplicate copy of the form for their records; the NADO or organisation that authorised the test receives a copy, and an anonymised version is stored with the sample for shipment to the WADA-accredited laboratory.

Athletes are directed throughout the whole process by the DCO including (in the case of urine samples) the apportioning of sample into A and B storage bottles and the packaging of those bottles ready for shipment. This is to ensure that the procedure and sample are not compromised, and at no stage is there any possibility of anyone other than the athlete tampering with the sample.

Shipment of sample

Urine samples are stored in identical glass bottles (labelled A and B) with tamperproof lids. Similarly, blood samples are also sealed in tamperproof A and B bottles, but these must be stored temporarily in a cool storage container until despatched to the laboratory via a refrigerated courier. All sealed samples remain in the custody of the DCO until they are signed over to the courier responsible for delivering the samples to a WADA-accredited laboratory. A chain-of-custody form is transported along with the samples to ensure the integrity of the samples is not compromised. Guidelines are in place to ensure that samples arrive at the laboratory within set timeframes related to the type of analysis. For example, blood passport samples must arrive at the laboratory within 36 hours of collection (WADA 2013b).

Sample analysis

WADA-accredited laboratories endeavour to analyse samples and report the results in a timely manner, which is normally within 15 working days of receipt of a sample. Laboratories use gas or liquid chromatography separation coupled with mass spectrometry detection to identify the majority of substances on the WADA Prohibited List (WADA 2010). Exceptions include use of the following:

- Isoelectric focusing and sarcosyl polyacrylamide gel electrophoresis or sodium dodecyl sulphate polyacrylamide gel electrophoresis to detect recombinant erythropoietin and its analogues (WADA 2013c)
- Immunoassays used to detect recombinant human growth hormone (WADA 2014b)
- Isotope ratio mass spectrometry to detect exogenous testosterone (WADA 2014c).

If a prohibited substance or marker of a prohibited substance or method is detected during the initial testing procedure, the laboratory is required to perform a confirmation step to confirm the identity of the substance and quantify the concentration present in the sample (Figure 4.1). The type of substance identified (i.e. a threshold or nonthreshold substance)

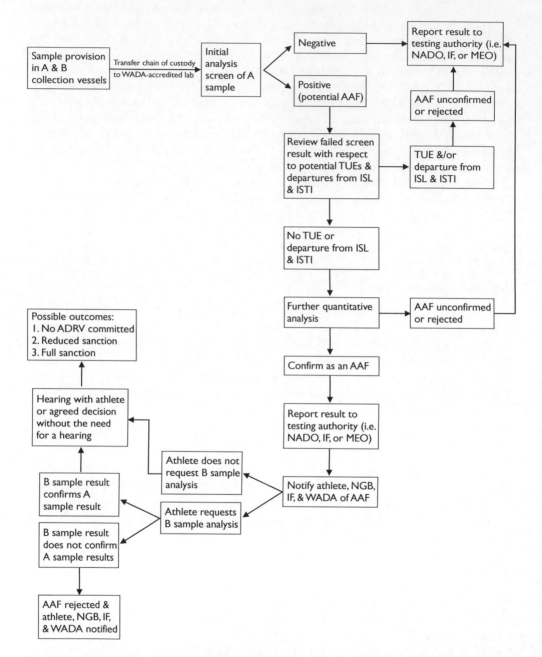

Figure 4.1 A flow diagram illustrating the chain of events with respect to sample provision, analysis, and potential sanctioning in the confirmation of an anti-doping rule violation.

AAF, Adverse Analytical Finding; IF, International Federation; ISL, International Standard of Laboratories; ISTI; International Standard of Testing and Investigations; MEO, Major Event Organiser; NADO, National Anti-Doping Organisation; NGB, National Governing Body; WADA, World Anti-Doping Agency.

will then determine whether the quantity present in the sample can be reported to the testing authority as an adverse analytical finding (AAF).

It is a requirement of WADA that all laboratories have the ability to routinely detect and identify nonthreshold substances at a defined concentration, which is known as the minimum reported performance level (MRPL; WADA 2013d). A laboratory that is not able to detect nonthreshold substances at the MRPL may have their accreditation suspended or even revoked by WADA. As the MRPL is not a threshold or a limit of detection, laboratories with more sensitive techniques can also report an AAF at a concentration below the established MRPL for that particular substance (WADA 2013d).

MRPL values do not apply to threshold substances. The detection and identification of a threshold substance can only be reported as an AAF when the specific threshold limit for the substance is exceeded and the concentration quantified is greater than WADA's agreed decision limit. In reality, a laboratory can only report an AAF for the presence of a threshold substance when the threshold value for that substance has been exceeded with a statistical confidence of at least 95% (WADA 2013e). Decision limits for the reporting of AAFs for threshold substances are set to protect both the athlete and laboratory because a measure of uncertainty exists with the confirmation of any scientific measurement.

The WADA laboratory system

The ability of anti-doping laboratories to reliably identify and quantify the substances prohibited in sport is vital in the fight against doping. The WADA laboratory programme is designed to continuously monitor the capabilities of the laboratories, evaluate laboratory proficiency, and improve test result consistency among laboratories. Laboratories must demonstrate their compliance with the following two international standards: the International Organisation for Standardisation/International Electrotechnical Commission 17025:2005 (ISO/IEC 17025:2005) and the International Standard for Laboratories (ISL) and its related technical documents.

The ISO/IEC 17025:2005 standard contains all of the requirements that a laboratory has to meet in order to demonstrate that they operate a management system, are technically competent, and are able to generate technically valid results. In the United Kingdom, the United Kingdom Accreditation Service is the national accreditation body recognised by government to assess UK-based laboratories against this standard.

The ISL and its related technical documents include requirements for obtaining and maintaining WADA laboratory accreditation and set out the required operating standards that laboratories must achieve. WADA also sets mandatory performance requirements through a series of technical documents. These technical documents provide direction to the laboratories on specific technical issues, such as advances in methodology, and prevent the need for the ISL to be updated every time this occurs.

The accreditation process

A laboratory must go through the following steps to become accredited (WADA 2012):

1 Express interest to WADA.
2 Submit an initial application form so that WADA can complete background checks.
3 Submit anti-doping organisation support letter(s).
4 Obtain laboratory ISO/IEC 17025 accreditation.
5 Obtain final sign-off from the WADA Executive Committee.

External quality assessment scheme

WADA monitors the performance of accredited anti-doping laboratories through an external quality assessment scheme (EQAS). Participation in the EQAS is mandatory; it allows WADA to evaluate laboratory competency through continual assessment of the laboratory's performance and provides laboratories with opportunities to compare their results to improve test result consistency among laboratories. Each laboratory must also analyse at least 3,000 urine samples per year to maintain its accreditation.

Urine or blood samples are periodically distributed by WADA to accredited laboratories to be tested for the presence of prohibited substances and markers. These samples may be sent blind or double-blind, which means that the content is unknown to the laboratories. Laboratories receive points if they fail to correctly identify or accurately measure the presence of the prohibited substance or marker within an EQAS sample. A false-positive EQAS result earns a laboratory 25 points and automatic suspension, whereas a false-negative EQAS result earns a laboratory 10 points. As of 1 January 2015, if a laboratory receives 20 or more points in a single EQAS round, its WADA accreditation will be suspended. When a laboratory receives 30 or more points over the previous 12-month period, its accreditation will be either suspended or revoked (WADA 2014d). WADA's EQAS also incorporates educational opportunities by sending open samples where the content of the sample is known.

Athlete Biological Passport

Blood samples collected as part of the Athlete Biological Passport (ABP) scheme require the athlete to be in a rested state. Whilst samples are collected following 10 minutes of rest in a seated position, athletes must also not have trained or competed in the 2 hours prior to collection. If this is not the case, athletes must remain in the DCS until the 2-hour period has elapsed. Blood samples collected as part of the ABP scheme are used to assess haematological parameters. Since 1 January 2014, urine samples have been included in the ABP scheme to assess androgen profiles as part of a new steroidal module. Further details on the ABP scheme can be found in Chapter 10.

Alcohol testing

Breath analysis is performed in those sports where alcohol is prohibited in competition (e.g. motor sports). Breath analysis may be performed immediately prior to a competition or after the competition has been completed.

Whilst the protocol is similar to both blood and urine sample provision in terms of selection and notification, the actual analysis is performed using an alcometer that records breath alcohol content in milligrams per litre. A reading that is equal to or greater than the level stated by the national governing body/international federation rules is considered to be a positive result. A second reading is then carried out to confirm the positive result. Significant presence is generally considered to be greater than 0.05 mg/l. Further details on alcohol can be found in Chapter 17.

4.4. Nonanalytical approach

Whilst drug detection will always remain an integral part of the anti-doping effort, many ADRVs identified in the code (e.g. possession, administration, trafficking) can only be identified and pursued through the gathering and investigation of nonanalytical anti-doping intelligence. Anti-doping intelligence is mainly used by anti-doping organisations for the following purposes (WADA 2014d):

- To assist test distribution planning
- To identify which athletes to target test
- To decide when to set up an investigation to determine whether an ADRV has been committed
- To investigate after the establishment of an ADRV for an athlete and determine whether athlete support personnel or other persons may have been involved in that violation.

Many high-profile ADRVs were only uncovered by anti-doping organisations after the receipt of information from public authorities, such as law enforcement agencies, customs and borders officials, and other sport regulatory agencies. Examples of seminal cases taken from WADA's guidelines on coordinating investigations (WADA 2011b) include the following:

- The 2003 federal investigation into the trafficking of doping substances by the Bay Area Laboratory Co-Operative, which led to the uncovering of information that was used by the United States Anti-Doping Agency to sanction track-and-field athletes Michelle Collins, Tim Montgomery, and Chrystie Gaines, as well as coaches Trevor Graham and Remi Korchemny
- The Italian police raid that caught Austrian cross-country ski athletes and team officials in possession of blood doping paraphernalia at the Turin Olympic Games, providing the International Olympic Committee and International Ski Federation with evidence to bring proceedings against those involved
- The sanction imposed by the International Tennis Federation on American tennis player Wayne Odesnik in 2010 for the possession of human growth hormone, which was the result of Australian customs officials alerting the Australian Anti-Doping Agency to their search findings.

These cases demonstrate the need for NADOs to establish effective partnerships and information-sharing protocols with law enforcement agencies so that intelligence uncovered during public authority investigations can be shared to enable doping sanctions to be pursued under the WADC. Such relationships also allow for anti-doping organisations to share intelligence in the other direction to tackle the manufacture, distribution, and supply of certain prohibited substances that are also considered to be public health issues. Tackling upstream perpetrators normally falls outside of the jurisdiction of sport, which means that anti-doping regulators are often reliant on the prosecution of these individuals under national laws.

Obtaining information about new medicines from the pharmaceutical industry is another key strategy used to minimise the misuse of these compounds in sport. WADA has established an active cooperation agreement with the International Federation of Pharmaceutical Manufacturers and Associations (2012) and its member pharmaceutical companies that alerts WADA when medicinal compounds have been identified through clinical trials to have doping potential. Receiving this information from the pharmaceutical industry enables WADA to develop detection methods far sooner than would occur if WADA only found out about them on launch to market.

4.5. Sanctions

Sanctions are determined by the severity of the ADRV and any previous convictions within an 8-year period. In most cases, the sanction is determined by a hearing whereby an athlete will put forward a reasoned defence toward the accusations placed in front of his or her. The hearing will determine whether an ADRV has occurred and establish the degree of liability and the intention to dope. Sanctions usually include a period of ineligibility from sport or, at the very least, a warning and reprimand (see Figure 4.1). Sanctions can also include disqualification from an event and forfeiture of points, medals, and prizes.

An ADRV involving the possession or use or attempted use of a prohibited substance or method will typically involve a standard sanction of 2 years of ineligibility. A deviation from the standard sanction might occur in response to a varied set of circumstances considered during a hearing. A reduction in the period of ineligibility may occur as a result of the following situations:

1. It may be established that the athlete bears no fault or no significant negligence in terms of the presence of a prohibited substance in the sample. This may be as a consequence of the contamination of a dietary supplement where due care has been taken to avoid such risk or through sabotage by a fellow competitor. If the prohibited substance detected is classified as a specified substance, then an athlete may be able to establish that there was no intent to enhance performance by administering the substance. In such cases, the period of ineligibility may even be eliminated completely, and the athlete may just receive a warning and reprimand, which is still an ADRV.

2. If an athlete admits to an ADRV voluntarily without a case being called to answer, or the athlete committed an ADRV but offers substantial assistance in determining a further ADRV by another athlete, a reduction in his or her suspension from sport may be considered. In such cases, any reduced sanction may only occur following consultation with WADA and the respective IF.

In addition to a reduced sanction, athletes may receive an increased sanction according to the type of ADRV committed or other circumstances, including their previous history of doping convictions. For example, trafficking (or attempted trafficking) and administration (or attempted administration) are both ADRVs that currently carry a 4-year suspension from sport. The period of ineligibility may also be increased if aggravated circumstances are believed to have occurred, in which an athlete has doped using multiple substances or has committed multiple ADRVs (e.g. use or attempted use and possession).

4.6. Summary

In view of the varied ADRVs that constitute doping, the strategies and procedures involved in its control are diverse. The major goal of such strategies is the prevention of doping through both education and drug testing. Drug testing serves two purposes. First, it enables the implementation of an effective sanctioning system, which provides culpability to those who dope. Most importantly, drug testing acts as a deterrent to those who might be tempted to dope in the future.

The challenge to the anti-doping movement is the implementation of drug testing that is both cost-effective and a real deterrent to athletes. New strategies in doping control involve a nonanalytical approach that uses intelligence amassed from a wide range of sources through the development of key partnerships, including law enforcement agencies, the pharmaceutical industry, and other sport regulatory agencies. Such evidence is proving fruitful in the conviction of individuals and organisations that fall a [afoul] foul of the wide range of ADRVs not involving sample analysis.

4.7. References

Hermann, A., and Henneberg, M. (2013). Anti-doping systems in sports are doomed to fail: A probability and cost analysis. Available online at http://www.adelaide.edu.au/news/news63461.html (accessed 30 March 2014).

Howman, D. (2013). Scientific research using elite athletes: WADA point of view. *Journal of Applied Physiology* 114(10):1365.

International Federation of Pharmaceutical Manufacturers and Associations. (2012). 2 Fields 1 Goal: Protecting the integrity of science and sport. Available online at http://www.ifpma.org/fileadmin/content/Publication/2012/FINAL_2_FIELDS_1_GOAL_Points_to_Consider_Booklet_20120717_.pdf (accessed 26 March 2014).

World Anti-Doping Agency. (2009) 2009 World Anti-Doping Code. Available online at https://www.wada-ama.org/en/resources/the-code/2009-world-anti-doping-code#.VAj34csg_X4 (accessed 4 September 2014).

World Anti-Doping Agency. (2010). Technical document: Identification criteria for qualitative assays – Incorporating column chromatography and mass spectrometry. Available online at https://wada-main-prod.s3.amazonaws.com/resources/files/WADA_TD2010IDCRv1.0_Identification%20Criteria%20for%20Qualitative%20Assays_May%2008%202010_EN.doc.pdf (accessed 7 September 2014).

World Anti-Doping Agency. (2011a). International standard for testing. Available online at https://wada-main-prod.s3.amazonaws.com/resources/files/WADA_IST_2012_EN.pdf (accessed 14 February 2014).

World Anti-Doping Agency. (2011b). Guidelines: Coordinating investigations and sharing anti-doping information and evidence. Available online at https://www.wada-ama.org/en/resources/world-anti-doping-program/coordinating-investigations-and-sharing-anti-doping-information#.VA7ky8sg_X4 (accessed 9 September 2014).

World Anti-Doping Agency. (2012). International standard for laboratories. Available online at https://www.wada-ama.org/en/resources/international-standards/international-standard-for-laboratories-isl#.VAzTs8sg_X4 (accessed 7 September 2014).

World Anti-Doping Agency. (2013a). 2012 annual report. Available online at https://elb.wada-ama.org/en/media/2013-06/wada-publishes-2012-annual-report#.VAzI-8sg_X4 (accessed 5 September 2014).

World Anti-Doping Agency. (2013b). Athlete biological passport operating guidelines (version 4.0). Available online at https://wada-main-prod.s3.amazonaws.com/resources/files/WADA-ABP-Operating-Guidelines_v4.0-EN.pdf (accessed 9 September 2014).

World Anti-Doping Agency. (2013c). Harmonization of the method for the identification of recombinant erythropoietins and analogues. Available online at https://wada-main-prod.s3.amazonaws.com/resources/files/WADA-TD2013EPO-Harmonization-Analysis-of-Recombinant-Erythropoietins-EN.pdf (accessed 9 September 2014).

World Anti-Doping Agency. (2013d). Minimum required performance levels. Available online at https://wada-main-prod.s3.amazonaws.com/resources/files/WADA-TD2013MRPL-Minimum-Required-Performance-Levels-v1-2012-EN.pdf (accessed 9 September 2014).

World Anti-Doping Agency. (2013e). Technical document: Decision limits for the confirmatory quantification of threshold substances. Available online at https://wada-main-prod.s3.amazonaws.com/resources/files/WADA-TD2013DL-Decision-Limits-for-the-Confirmatory-Quantification-Threshold-Substances-2.0-EN.pdf (accessed 9 September 2014).

World Anti-Doping Agency. (2014a). The 2014 WADA Prohibited List. Available online at https://wada-main-prod.s3.amazonaws.com/resources/files/WADA-Revised-2014-Prohibited-List-EN.PDF (accessed 9 September 2014).

World Anti-Doping Agency. (2014b). Guidelines: hGH isoforms differential immunoassays. Available online at https://wada-main-prod.s3.amazonaws.com/resources/files/WADA-Guidelines-for-hGH-Differential-Immunoassays-v2.1-2014-EN.pdf (accessed 9 September 2014).

World Anti-Doping Agency. (2014c). Technical document: Endogenous anabolic androgenic steroids. Available online at https://wada-main-prod.s3.amazonaws.com/resources/files/WADA-TD2014-EAAS-Endogenous-Anabolic-Androgenic-Steroids-Measurement-and-Reporting-EN.pdf (accessed 9 September 2014).

World Anti-Doping Agency. (2014d). International standard for laboratories: Final (2015). Available online at https://wada-main-prod.s3.amazonaws.com/resources/files/WADA-ISL-2015-Final-v8.0-EN.pdf (accessed 9 September 2014).

Substances and methods prohibited in sport

Chapter 5

Anabolic agents

Neil Chester

5.1. Introduction

Anabolic agents are a classification of substances on the World Anti-Doping Agency (WADA) Prohibited List comprised largely of anabolic androgenic steroids (AAS). These substances have become synonymous with the term *performance-enhancing drugs* and remain one of the most prevalent groups of doping agents in sport. In addition, they are widely used by those involved in sport and exercise at a recreational level due to their image-enhancing properties.

Despite the fact that these substances have been available for over 50 years, their efficacy is such that they remain a popular choice of doping agent. Whilst research over recent decades has confirmed the anecdotal evidence and belief that many users held in terms of their efficacy, there remains some conjecture regarding their purported side effects. Research conducted to mirror their use by athletes and recreational users alike is difficult as a consequence of the extremely high, supraphysiological doses administered in practice. However, the availability of substandard preparations via the internet has led to much wider public health concerns.

Whilst methods of detection for such substances have developed throughout the years, athletes have attempted to circumvent such methods by turning to designer steroids. Such substances are designed to combat current detection methods simply as a consequence of the fact that their existence from a doping control perspective is unknown. In addition, the use of endogenous AAS, such as testosterone, androstenedione, and dehydroepiandrosterone (DHEA) pose their own specific problems with regards to detection as a consequence of their natural occurrence in the body.

As therapeutic agents, AAS use is limited but tends to centre on their anabolic properties. Potential clinical uses include combating cachexia associated with postoperational recovery and conditions such as human immunodeficiency virus (HIV)/acquired immunodeficiency syndrome (AIDS), renal failure, chronic obstructive pulmonary disease, and burns. In addition, AAS have been used to treat osteoporosis in postmenopausal women and aplastic anaemia.

In addition to AAS, the WADA Prohibited List includes the following under the classification of anabolic agents: β_2-agonists, including clenbuterol and zilpaterol, selective androgen receptor modulators (SARMs), and tibolone and zeranol (Table 5.1). The SARMs are a class of pharmacological agents that are currently under development and offer an advantage over AAS in being selective to specific tissue types.

Table 5.1 Class S1 of the 2014 WADA List of prohibited substances and methods

S1. Anabolic Agents
   1. Anabolic androgenic steroids (AAS)
      a. Exogenous AAS
      b. Endogenous AAS when administered exogenously
   2. Other anabolic agents, including but not limited to:
      Clenbuterol, selective androgen receptor modulators (SARMs), tibolone, zeranol, zilpaterol

Source: World Anti-Doping Agency (2013b).

5.2. Anabolic androgenic steroids

Anabolic androgenic steroids are typically defined as compounds that are structurally and functionally related to the hormone testosterone. They may be categorised according to whether they exist endogenously or whether they are synthetically derived.

Whilst testosterone was first isolated in 1935 it was soon realised that, when administered orally or parenterally, testosterone was broken down rapidly by the liver by first-pass metabolism. This would clearly have a severe effect on its use as a therapeutic agent and thus paved the way toward the development of an exogenous AAS that would resist first-pass metabolism.

Because the effects of testosterone were perceived to be extensive, both from an androgenic and an anabolic perspective, there was great interest in its potential as a therapeutic agent. However, as a nontherapeutic agent, its use as an anabolic agent was to be exploited in sport.

Testosterone

Testosterone is the primary male androgenic hormone that is responsible for the control of a wide range of processes, most notably the development and maintenance of male characteristics. Such characteristics include those that develop during puberty, such as growth of the penis and testes; the development of secondary sex characteristics, such as body hair growth (particularly that of facial, pubic, and axillary hair); and the deepening of the voice, as a consequence of vocal cord thickening and enlargement of the larynx. Testosterone is produced largely in the testes by the Leydig cells (95%) but also by the adrenal glands and via conversion from weaker androgens, such as androstenedione (also produced by the adrenal glands) in the periphery. It is also present in females and is produced in much smaller amounts by the ovaries, the adrenal glands, and via the conversion of androstenedione produced by the adrenal glands. After puberty, plasma testosterone levels are approximately 250–1,045 ng/dl in men and 1–44 ng/dl in women, with levels declining steadily in males over the age of 60 years (Salameh *et al*. 2010). As with males, testosterone has an important role in the development and maintenance of lean body mass (i.e. muscle and bone) in females. Testosterone also affects the central nervous system (CNS) and has a significant role to play in human behaviour, particularly sexual behaviour, namely libido.

Whilst testosterone is considered the primary androgen, it is by no means the only one; a number of androgens serve important roles in both the development and maintenance of sex-determining characteristics. Several weak androgens are synthesised by the adrenal cortex, most notably DHEA and androstenedione. In females, these act as an important circulating pool of more potent androgen precursors, and their conversion is via several intracellular enzymes (Figure 5.1). After testosterone, 5α-dihydrotestosterone (DHT) is probably the

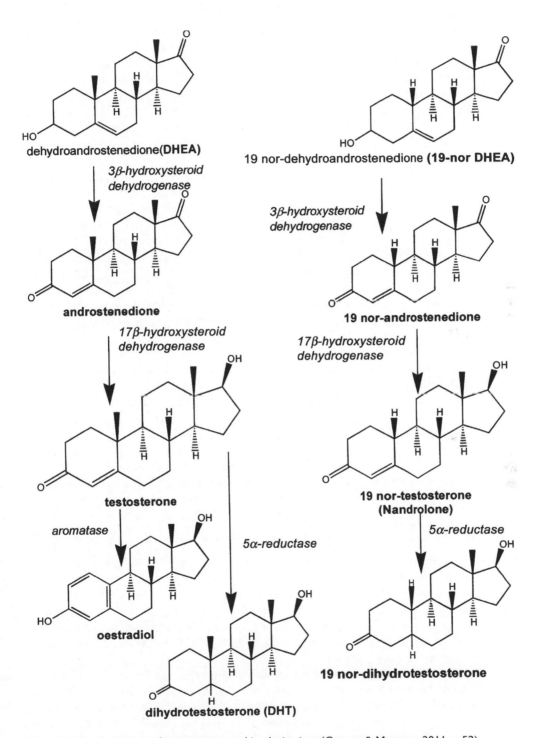

Figure 5.1 The formation of testosterone and its derivatives (George & Mottram 2011; p 52).

most notable androgen; with a greater affinity to the androgen receptor, it has a direct role in the development of secondary sex characteristics. Indeed, testosterone typically acts as a precursor to DHT in reproductive tissue and the skin, where the presence of 5α-reductase mediates its conversion, promoting prostate gland and hair growth, respectively.

The presence of androgens at a cellular level is determined by enzyme action. In addition to the intracellular enzyme 5α-reductase in the skin and reproductive tissue, the presence of aromatase converts testosterone into oestradiol in adipose tissue (Figure 5.1). In skeletal muscle, however, 5α-reductase is undetectable (Thigpen *et al.* 1993); therefore, testosterone exerts its effect directly via androgen receptors. Thus, not only is the presence of androgen receptors important in determining the effects of androgens, but so too is the expression of specific enzymes.

The immediate precursor of testosterone in the biosynthetic sequence is androstenedione, which is converted to testosterone via the action of 17β-hydroxysteroid dehydrogenase (Figure 5.1). This enzyme also acts on other steroids with similar structures, including 19-norandrostenedione, to form 19-nor testosterone, which is otherwise known as nandrolone (Figure 5.1).

Testosterone production is controlled by the hypothalamic-pituitary-gonadal axis. Specifically, testosterone is produced in response to luteinising hormone (LH) and follicle-stimulating hormone (FSH) secreted by the pituitary gland. Gonadotropin-releasing hormone (GnRH) produced by the hypothalamus stimulates the release of LH and FSH from the pituitary gland. This integrated system enables regulatory feedback control, whereby increased levels of circulating testosterone inhibit the release of GnRH, LH, and FSH. Androgen production from the adrenal gland is less clear. Control involves adrenocorticotropin and other factors, including gonadal sex steroids, insulin, growth hormone, and other signalling molecules (Alesci *et al.* 2001).

Testosterone circulates in the bloodstream either freely (approximately 2–3 per cent) or bound to proteins, such as sex hormone-binding globulin (SHBG) or albumin. Testosterone bound to SHBG (approximately 44 per cent; Dunn *et al.* 1981) is essentially inactive due to the high binding affinity of these molecules and the fact that testosterone in this state is unable to penetrate the cell walls of target cells. However, free testosterone and testosterone that is weakly bound to albumin is deemed to be bioavailable because, in its free form, testosterone may penetrate the cell wall and bind with the androgen receptor (AR).

5.3. Pharmacology of anabolic androgenic steroids

The structural modifications of testosterone to create synthetic AAS have been introduced in order to achieve one or more of the following: maximise anabolic effects, minimise androgenic effects, increase metabolic half-life, limit first-pass metabolism, and/or reduce the absorption rate from an intramuscular depot. These modifications aim to improve both the efficacy of testosterone as an anabolic agent and its mode of administration. Whilst the anabolic potency, compared to testosterone, may have been increased in some AAS, the disassociation from androgenic effects has not been achieved; therefore, as performance- and image-enhancing drugs (PIEDs), they all carry potential androgenic side effects.

Testosterone has a 19-carbon skeleton consisting of four fused rings, which may be commonly modified at three positions to create synthetic AAS (Figure 5.2; positions A, B, and C). Such modifications include esterification of the 17β-hydroxyl group (A) to form a group of AAS collectively known as testosterone esters. Testosterone esters have enhanced lipid

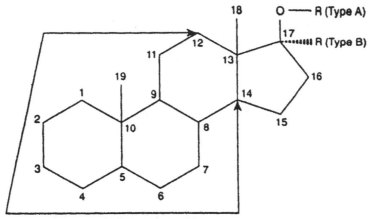

Figure 5.2 The molecular structure of testosterone illustrating the major sites of modification in the formation of synthetic anabolic androgenic steroids (adapted from Wilson 1988).

solubility; when administered intramuscularly, they are released slowly into the circulation, thus enabling prolonged activity and reduced hepatotoxicity. Alkylation at the 17 [17a]α position (B) produces 17α-alkylated AAS, which are orally active due to their ability to limit first-pass metabolism. Structural modifications to other positions on the testosterone skeleton (C) will tend to increase anabolic potency. Examples of AAS categorised according to their modifications and routes of administration are provided in Table 5.2.

Besides oral or parenteral administration via injection, AAS may also be administered topically as gels or creams. Unmodified testosterone is available as a dermal gel or patch, which must be administered daily due to its short half-life (Table 5.2).

Table 5.2 Categorisation of anabolic androgenic steroids (AAS) according to their route of administration and their structural modification from testosterone

AAS	Trade name	Route of administration
Unmodified testosterone		
Testosterone	Androgel, Testim	Topical gel
Testosterone	Androderm, Testoderm	Dermal patch
Testosterone esters		
Testosterone enanthate	Delatetryl	Intramuscular injection
Testosterone cypionate	Depo-Testosterone	Intramuscular injection
Testosterone propionate	–	Intramuscular injection
17α-alkylated AAS		
Methyltestosterone	Android, Virilon	Oral
Fluoxymesterone	Halostestin	Oral
Stanozolol	Winstrol	Oral
Methandrostenelone	Dianabol	Oral
19-nor testosterone esters		
Nandrolone deconate	Deca-durabolin	Intramuscular injection
Nandrolone phenylproprionate	Durabolin	Intramuscular injection

Adapted from Clark (2009).

In addition to testosterone, the naturally occurring 18-carbon AAS, 19-nortestosterone (otherwise known as nandrolone), is considered to be a doping agent; so too are its modifications, particularly its decanoate ester known as deca-durabolin (Table 5.2). As a PIED, nandrolone is attractive because it has fewer androgenic effects than other AAS, so it is not converted to DHT. Also, its 5α-reductase metabolite, 19 nor-dihydrotestosterone, has a low binding affinity to the androgen receptors (ARs; Toth and Zakar 1982).

5.4. Clinical uses of anabolic androgenic steroids

Despite the wide-ranging effects of AAS in terms of stimulating not only muscle growth but also bone and red blood cell production, their current use in clinical settings is limited. Whilst the traditional use of AAS was to promote muscle growth in those with degenerative conditions, their effectiveness has been questioned. Indeed, since the late 1980s, the licences of many AAS have been revoked. The remaining AAS are typically used for hormone replacement therapy in males with hypogonadism. However, the use of AAS to combat muscle atrophy has been reconsidered. Both testosterone esters and 17α-alkylated steroids may now be considered as useful therapeutic agents for the treatment of muscle wastage associated with HIV/AIDS, severe burns, and renal failure (Basaria *et al.* 2001). Nevertheless, although evidence exists to support AAS use in postoperative recovery and in those with chronic conditions such as HIV/AIDS, further research is needed to establish the effects of sustained use on health and well-being before clear recommendations can be made (Woerdeman and de Ronde 2011).

5.5. Anabolic androgenic steroids as performance- and image-enhancing agents

Despite the wealth of anecdotal evidence supporting the efficacy of AAS as performance enhancers, it has only been in recent decades that the scientific community has provided confirmation. Indeed, until the landmark study by Bhasin *et al.* (1996), research involving AAS had significant shortcomings, which limited its potential for making a significant impact on the field. The work by Bhasin *et al.* was able to clearly demonstrate that individuals who were not deficient in testosterone could increase both muscle mass and function following the administration of supraphysiological doses of testosterone enanthate. Their work was also able to shed light on the likely mechanisms involved in such enhancements. Whilst exercise training was shown to have an additive effect on muscle growth and function, significant increases were still demonstrated in those who did not perform exercise training. These findings suggested that AAS were able to exert their effects by traditional genomic action via the ARs without the need for anticatabolic effects.

Regarding genomic action, AAS bind with the ARs; through interaction with the DNA, they mediate transcription, thus leading to protein synthesis. AAS passively diffuse into the cells of target tissues, bind to ARs, translocate into the nucleus, and link with additional AAS–AR complexes to form homodimers. DNA-binding domains on the ARs and then bind with steroid response elements on the DNA; with the addition of co-regulators, gene activation is initiated. Gene activation then leads to gene transcription, translation, and ultimately the production of contractile protein and muscle hypertrophy.

The potential anticatabolic effect relates to the fact that the release of cortisol in response to heavy exercise has a catabolic effect on skeletal muscle. Cortisol is released from the adrenal cortex in response to stress to aid energy provision. This is achieved by promoting gluconeogenesis in the liver and the provision of gluconeogenic substrate in the form of protein through the breakdown of skeletal muscle protein. Clearly, the ability of AAS to limit the effects of cortisol might have a profound effect on skeletal muscle growth and function. It has been suggested that AAS act as antagonists to glucocorticoid receptors, thus reducing the effects of cortisol. However, AAS are generally considered to have a low binding affinity to glucocorticoid receptors (Hickson *et al*. 1990). It is now thought that AAS might affect the gene expression of glucocorticoid receptors (Kicman 2008).

Hypertrophy through genomic pathways is reliant on the apparatus within myonuclei. Muscle fibres contain hundreds of myonuclei; however, there is thought to be a ceiling in terms of the level of skeletal muscle hypertrophy, supported by a finite number of myonuclei. It is therefore suggested that by increasing myonuclei number, AAS are able to enhance hypertrophy (Kadi 2008).

Research recently has provided evidence in support of the view held by many that the performance-enhancing effects of AAS last for much longer than the period of administration. Egner *et al*. (2013) demonstrated, in an animal model, that increased myonuclei numbers following the administration of AAS are not lost during atrophy in response to AAS abstinence; after subsequent training, there was significant hypertrophy compared to a control group. This research suggests that the increased myonuclei are an important reserve that directly relate to hypertrophic potential, which is much greater in those who have used AAS. Further research is clearly needed to determine whether these findings might be transferable to humans. If this is found to be the case, then it would be particularly significant from an anti-doping perspective in terms of the consideration of appropriate sanctions imposed on those caught misusing AAS (i.e. challenging the length of ban from competition).

Whilst the work by Bhasin *et al*. (1996) was able to show unequivocally that AAS were effective as PIEDs, the mechanisms by which this result is achieved are complex. It is likely that positive results in terms of muscle hypertrophy and improvements in function are a consequence of a combination of both physiological and behavioural responses. In addition to the mechanisms directly within skeletal muscle, activation of the CNS via ARs and non-genomic actions to promote psychological effects may be particularly useful as indirect mechanisms by increasing exercise training intensity and volume (Kicman 2008).

AAS, which are known to play an important role in sexual behaviour in both men and women, are also believed to be important in elevating mood and reducing depression. Conversely, reports of increased aggression in those misusing AAS (Yates *et al*. 1992) might be useful to promote increased exercise tolerance and competitiveness in the sporting arena.

5.6. Adverse effects following anabolic androgenic steroid use

As the mismatch between anecdotal and scientific evidence in support of AAS as effective ergogenic aids fuelled the mistrust between users and the scientific and medical community, so has the limited scientific evidence with regards to potential serious adverse health effects. The general acceptance by the medical community that AAS are indeed hazardous is a clear attempt to discourage nontherapeutic use of AAS.

Nevertheless, whilst the paucity of conclusive evidence to link AAS use directly with serious health effects remains, scientific evidence appears to be growing in support of many of the initial claims. However, difficulties remain in obtaining good scientific evidence due to the constraints relating to ethics and problems controlling many of the confounding variables that exist, including concomitant supplement use, the practice of polypharmacy amongst users, and the difficulty in establishing the authenticity of products used.

The adverse effects associated with AAS use in humans have been reported in a number of ways, including surveys, case studies, and placebo-controlled trials involving subjects with hypogonadism. Despite the obvious shortcomings of such research, evidence surrounding the effects of AAS is building as their use becomes more widespread. Nevertheless, prospective, longitudinal studies are required to address the possible development of pathology following long-term AAS use.

The main reported side effects of AAS use are widespread and may be categorised accordingly, as discussed in the following sections.

Liver effects

The 17α-alkylated AAS seems to offer the largest threat of liver damage as a consequence of first-pass metabolism. Hepatotoxicity attributed to AAS use may take several forms, including transient elevations in liver enzyme concentrations, cholestasis, vascular injury, and hepatic tumours. Numerous studies have reported increased concentrations of liver enzymes amongst AAS users (Sanchez-Osorio *et al.* 2008; Nasr and Ahmad 2009). Whilst raised hepatic enzymes may signal toxicity, they may fall over time and hide the real extent of injury during prolonged AAS exposure. Alternatively, raised hepatic enzymes may simply reflect muscle damage as a consequence of heavy training (Hoffman and Ratamess 2006). However, in individuals with liver damage, other symptoms may predominate, such as jaundice and pruritus (itchiness) (Sanchez-Osorio *et al.* 2008; Elsharkawy *et al.* 2012). Such symptoms are typical of cholestasis, a condition where there is retention of bile in the biliary capillaries of the hepatic lobules.

Whilst there are reports of vascular injury in individuals using AAS, these tend to be rare. The condition of peliosis hepatis is a vascular condition that is characterised by the development of blood-filled cysts throughout the liver; it has been reported in numerous cases involving AAS use (Cabasso, 1994). Reports of carcinomas attributed to AAS use are uncommon and only following prolonged use (Shahidi 2001).

Cardiovascular effects

Numerous reports have shown that the use of AAS has diverse effects on the cardiovascular system. The most severe effects include death as a consequence of cardiovascular disease (CD), with a developing body of evidence to link such events with chronic AAS use (Angell *et al.* 2012a; Montisci *et al.* 2012). Evidence of CD is based upon incidence of acute myocardial infarction, heart failure, coronary disease, or cerebrovascular accidents (i.e. stroke), which were all reported via case studies.

There is a growing body of research that links AAS use with CD and the prevalence of numerous CD risk factors; however, the mechanisms behind such effects are unclear (Angell *et al.* 2012c). Reports of the incidence of hypertension (Freed *et al.* 1975; Kuipers *et al.* 1991; Riebe *et al.* 1992), adverse blood lipid profiles (Lenders *et al.* 1988; Lane *et al.* 2006), cardiac hypertrophy (Sachtleben *et al.* 1993; Angell *et al.* 2012b), and electrocardiogram abnormalities (Maior *et al.* 2013) amongst AAS users are numerous. However, there is a distinct lack of more controlled prospective cohort studies, which are necessary to establish possible causal mechanisms.

Reproductive system effects

Hypogonadotropic hypogonadism is a side effect of AAS use as a consequence of the hypo-thalamic negative feedback loop responding to increased circulating androgens. Testicular atrophy and impaired spermatogenesis are symptomatic of a reduced release of gonadotro-phins. In females, suppressed secretion of gonadotrophins leads to menstrual irregularities and increased circulating androgens lead to clitoral hypertrophy following long-term AAS use. The inhibition of spermatogenesis may persist for many months after anabolic steroid withdrawal; however, such side effects are deemed to be reversible. Similarly, in females, the menstrual cycle will recommence soon after AAS use is discontinued. However, side effects such as clitoral hypertrophy appear to be less reversible (Clark 2009).

Cosmetic effects

Cosmetic effects are most pronounced in females because AAS result in an overall masculinis-ing effect, which may be irreversible following the discontinuation of the drugs (Clark 2009). These effects include hirsuitism and deepening of the voice. Chronic use of AAS may produce male pattern baldness, which has been reported in both males and females. Acne is a common condition reported by many AAS users due to androgenic stimulation of the sebaceous glands.

High-dose AAS regimes practised by men may result in high levels of circulating oestro-gens as a consequence of aromatisation of androgens. These high levels of oestrogen may result in gynecomastia, which is the development of breast tissue. Consequently, users will often co-administer tamoxifen, a SERM, to combat such side effects (see Chapter 8).

Psychological effects

One of the most reported side effects attributed to AAS misuse is that relating to the CNS. Increased aggression may be regarded as a positive effect in terms of facilitating increased training load. However, numerous reports have cited episodes of aggression, violence, and mania being common amongst AAS users (Pope and Katz 1988). During abstinence from AAS, users have been reported to exhibit anxiety and depression (Kanayama *et al.* 2009), which is deemed to be attributed to the low circulating levels of endogenous AAS as a consequence of reduced production occurring because of prior sustained circulating exogenous AAS. However, some researchers believe that individuals exhibiting marked changes in mood and behaviour are predisposed to such psychological effects, which are only heightened by AAS use (van Amsterdam *et al.* 2010).

Other side effects

Among adolescents, the administration of AAS can result in the premature closure of epiph-yseal growth plates, leading to stunted growth (Johnson 1990). Other musculoskeletal issues are related to the potential for AAS to inflict problems associated with ligament and tendon damage (Giannotti *et al.* 2014). This is thought to be associated with the development of dysplasia of collagen fibrils, thus decreasing the tensile strength of tendons (Laseter and Russell 1991) and the disproportionate loading related with increases in muscle strength (Wood *et al.* 1988).

Side effects that are prevalent amongst AAS users but not directly related to the doping agent per se include those associated with inappropriate drug administration. Needle sharing and the use of nonsterile equipment are particular issues amongst AAS users; they pose serious risks in terms of infection and the acquisition of blood-borne diseases, such as hepatitis and HIV/AIDS (Hope *et al*. 2013).

Possibly the greatest risk to AAS users are the unknown health risks associated with the use of products obtained from the illicit market. The illicit market contains drugs that are no longer licenced, those that are marketed as veterinary products, new drugs that have not been fully tested, and AAS that have not been authorised but developed as part of pharmaceutical research projects (Evans-Brown *et al*. 2012). In addition to a wide range of AAS that do not carry with them the required safety checks and information that exists with licenced products, there are real concerns relating to the sterility and authenticity of such products.

5.7. Use of anabolic androgenic steroids in sport

Whilst there is uncertainty as to who was first to use AAS in sports competition, it is suggested that the 1950s heralded the beginnings of their use in sport (Dimeo 2007). In 1954, it is alleged that Russian athletes under the influence of AAS won numerous gold medals in the World Weightlifting Championships in Vienna, Austria. Throughout the 1950s and 1960s, AAS use escalated. Whilst the International Olympic Committee introduced the first list of prohibited substances in 1967, it was not until 1976 that AAS were added to the list after the development of a reliable test for their detection in urine in 1974.

Following the reunification of Germany in 1990 it was revealed that the German Democratic Republic (GDR; the former state of East Germany) had run a systematic doping programme as part of their state-run sports programme. This programme, which was supported and financed by the state, ran from the mid-1960s through the 1980s, and it was instrumental in the success of GDR in international sports competitions throughout this period. Hundreds of scientists and physicians were involved in both researching and administering AAS and other doping agents to athletes, with the sole purpose of improving sports performance and raising the profile of a nation on a world stage (Franke and Berondonk, 1997). Particular emphasis was placed on females and their performance, where the effects of AAS are more pronounced. However, the real impact of such a programme is illustrated by the incidence of serious doping-related side effects, many of which were irreversible.

Probably one of the most well-known cases of AAS use in sport is that of the Canadian track-and-field athlete Ben Johnson at the 1988 Olympics in Seoul, South Korea. Having been crowned champion of the 100 m race, he was subsequently stripped of his medal after failing a routine postcompetition drug test. Johnson tested positive for the AAS stanozolol, and he put the issue of drug use in sport firmly in the spotlight. As a consequence, Charles Dubin, a Canadian lawyer, was charged with leading a Canadian inquiry into the use of drugs in sport, otherwise known as the Dubin Inquiry. The inquiry lasted one year and included the admission of AAS use by forty-eight athletes (including Ben Johnson). Recommendations were made to help improve doping control globally through increased and improved drug testing and stricter penalties for those that violate the rules (Moriarty *et al*. 1992).

In more recent times, designer steroids have become a particular issue in elite sport. They are designed specifically to circumvent routine anti-doping tests because their existence as doping agents is unknown. Indeed, such is the covert nature of their manufacture and use – that they only become detectable when the particular substance falls into the hands of anti-doping personnel. In the early part of this century, several international athletes, including sprinters Marion Jones, Dwain Chambers, and Kellie White, were convicted for the use of tetrahydrogestrinone (THG), a designer steroid. This case was part of what became known as the Bay Area Laboratory Cooperative (BALCO) affair, whereby a newly developed AAS was manufactured and distributed to numerous athletes from BALCO in California, led by its founder, Victor Conte (see Section 5.9).

Other than use by elite athletes and in competitive sport, there is evidence of growing, widespread use of AAS at a recreational level, including those engaged in gymnasium exercise and bodybuilding. A large extent of the bodybuilding culture is based upon the use of and experimentation with drugs, particularly AAS. Indeed, much of the information we know regarding efficacy and adverse health effects is centred upon the anecdotal evidence obtained from the bodybuilding community. The growth of AAS use within the bodybuilding community appears to have followed a similar path to the one seen in elite sport. However, with increased media focus on image and the ideal body, coupled with increased accessibility to illicit products via the internet, the market amongst recreational users seems to be burgeoning (Evans-Brown et al. 2012).

Sources, supply, and control of anabolic androgenic steroids

The use of AAS is directly associated with supply and control from a legal perspective. In the United Kingdom, AAS are controlled as Class C drugs under the Misuse of Drugs Act 1971. Whilst it is illegal to possess these drugs with the intent to supply, it is not an offence to possess them for personal use. The control measures for AAS vary between countries, with some countries legislating specifically against the use of doping agents in sport. Nevertheless, the supply of such drugs has never been greater, with the internet opening up a global market in the trade of illicit products.

The illicit market consists of products that may come from several sources. Products that are deemed to be legitimate may be manufactured in countries where the purchase of such nonprescription drugs is legal or where products have entered the market as a result of theft. Alternatively, products may be manufactured in clandestine laboratories outside of any regulatory system (Evans-Brown et al. 2009).

Trade of substandard and counterfeit products is a particular problem. Such products are a significant health concern because their quality and thus safety cannot be guaranteed. In addition to the substandard manufacturing of many products, there is a real issue concerning counterfeiting – that is, deliberately mislabelling products so there are no assurances that the alleged ingredients are present and in the correct quantity. This issue has been highlighted extensively in the research literature (Graham et al. 2009; Evans-Brown et al. 2009) and appears to be a particular issue with respect to nutritional supplements (see Chapter 21).

In a report by the UK's Advisory Council on the Misuse of Drugs (2010), recommendations were put forward to maintain the current legal classification whereby criminal prosecution is limited to those dealing, supplying, manufacturing, and trafficking AAS. In addition, improved education and harm reduction programmes should be introduced to support those engaged in nontherapeutic AAS use.

Patterns of administration

Anabolic steroids are broadly available as three types of preparation: oral, oil-based or water-based injections, or topical gels or patches. Oral preparations have a structure that is resistant to breakdown by stomach acid, can be absorbed by the gastrointestinal tract, and tends to withstand total breakdown by liver enzymes; however, they have a short half-life and require frequent dosing. Injectable oil-based preparations have a longer half-life but produce a degree of pain at the injection site; they have a slow absorption rate into the bloodstream, so that lower concentrations pass through the liver, thereby reducing liver toxicity. Injectable water-based steroids have a long half-life, although normally less than oil-based preparations; they produce less discomfort at the site of injection and can be mixed with other water-based steroids or other drugs (George and Mottram 2011). Topical gels (or creams) or patches result in low-dose administration of unmodified testosterone, which has a short half-life requiring daily application.

There are a number of administration regimes in use, known as cycling, pyramiding, and stacking. Experienced users will typically follow a combination of these regimes concurrently. Each regime is reputed to offer a particular advantage in terms of heightening the effect of a particular drug (or drugs) or limiting the potential side effects experienced. However, there is no scientific evidence to support such regimes.

Cycling is the administration of a particular drug over a period of time, followed by a period of abstinence before the administration is recommenced. Cycling patterns are typically short (i.e. 6–8 weeks of administration followed by 6–8 weeks of abstinence) or long (i.e. 6–18 weeks of administration followed by up to 12 months of abstinence). The rationale behind cycling is that the periods of abstinence may reduce the incidence of side effects.

Pyramiding is a variation of cycling whereby the dose is gradually increased during the cycle to a peak and then gradually reduced towards the end of the cycle. This regime allegedly results in fewer behavioural side effects caused by withdrawal of the drug, such as depressed mood.

Stacking is the use of more than one AAS at a time. In its simplest form, this regime might involve the simultaneous use of both an orally administered steroid and an injectable one. More sophisticated regimes involve intricate schedules of administration using many different AAS each with supposedly different pharmacological profiles. The aim of this technique is to avoid the development of tolerance to a particular drug (George and Mottram 2011). In addition to AAS, common ancillary drugs include growth hormone, clenbuterol, insulin, insulin-like growth factor-1, human chorionic gonadotrophin, ephedrine, and tamoxifen. Some of these drugs are taken for their alleged synergistic actions, whilst others are taken for their ability to combat unwanted side effects.

5.8. Prevalence of anabolic androgenic steroid use

As with all illicit drug use, it is difficult to establish an accurate indication of how prevalent AAS use is within sport. Most evidence in elite sport comes from data obtained from WADA-accredited laboratories, which highlight the annual number of positive drug tests by specific anabolic agents (Table 5.3). Whilst such data cannot provide an accurate estimate of the absolute number of individuals administering AAS, they do reveal quite clearly that AAS are still popular choices for those looking to enhance sports performance illegally. Data suggest that AAS constitute almost half of all adverse analytical findings and atypical findings reported by WADA-accredited laboratories (WADA 2013a).

Of course, these figures do not reflect the true extent of AAS use in sport, particularly at a subelite and recreational level. The use of AAS appears to be a significant problem in collegiate sport in the United States (Buckley et al. 1988; Berning et al. 2004; McCabe et al. 2007). Buckley et al. reported that 6.6 per cent of male high school seniors (17–19 years old) had used AAS; however, approximately 30 per cent of users did not participate in organised sport.

Table 5.3 Prohibited anabolic agents identified by WADA-accredited laboratories in 2012

Anabolic agent	Occurrences	Percent within class
Anabolic androgenic steroids		
Testosterone-to-epitestosterone ratio >4	1,202	55.5%
Stanozolol	240	11.1%
Nandrolone metabolites	203	9.4%
Methandienone	129	6.0%
Boldenone	63	2.9%
Dehydrochloromethyl-testosterone	49	2.3%
Drostanolone	44	2.0%
Trenbolone	43	2.0%
Metenolone	38	1.8%
Oxandrolone	27	1.2%
Others	128	5.8%
Other anabolic agents		
Clenbuterol	98	86.7%
Tibolone	10	8.8%
Selective androgen receptor modulators	5	4.4%

Source: World Anti-Doping Agency (2013a).

However, McCabe et al. were able to demonstrate that those who participated in collegiate sport were more likely to use AAS compared to their nonathletic counterparts. The structure of sport in the United States, in comparison with Europe, is such that collegiate sport is extremely popular for participants and spectators alike. Collegiate sport is regularly featured on American television, and the importance placed on success may heighten the pressure on young athletes and the likelihood that they may turn to performance-enhancing drugs (Calfee and Fadale 2006).

Anecdotal evidence would suggest that AAS use is widespread amongst those engaged in recreational sport, and numerous reports suggest that it is a developing public health issue (Evans-Brown et al. 2012). With the increased media attention on body image, there is a burgeoning market for products aimed at developing musculature and reducing body fat. This growth is also reflected amongst children, with 0.6 per cent of boys and 0.3 per cent of girls reporting having used AAS, according to a survey administered to 7,242 English school children (3,646 boys and 3,596 girls; Omole 2011). In the United States, prevalence rates appear to be higher, with 2.7 per cent of children attending middle school (9–13 years old) indicating that they had used AAS (Faigenbaum et al. 1998).

The first study to examine the extent of AAS use in the United Kingdom was by Korkia (1994). Users of twenty-one gymnasia were surveyed across five regions throughout the United Kingdom, including London, Merseyside, Edinburgh, Glasgow, and Swansea; a total of 1,669 questionnaires were returned and used in the study. Use of AAS was reported in all regions, with a total of 7.7 per cent of gymnasium users admitting to ever taking AAS, and 5 per cent of all respondents reporting current use (6 per cent of males and 1.4 per cent of females). In a more recent study in Germany, Striegel et al. (2006) reported results from a sample of 621 fitness centre visitors; a total of 13.5 per cent reported the use of 'anabolic ergogenic substances' (of which 83.6 per cent were AAS), comprising 19.2 per cent of males and 3.9 per cent of females.

Over recent years, there appears to have been an increase in the 'drive for muscularity' amongst adolescents (McCreary and Sasse, 2000) as well as the general population. This would seem to be a consequence of the way in which the media portray health and attractiveness, particularly from the perspective of the male body form. Indeed, there is evidence of increased prevalence of body dissatisfaction and low self-esteem amongst males with respect to the level of musculature, which has been termed *muscle dysmorphia* (Pope *et al.* 1997). The focus on enhanced musculature is coupled with an increase in the use of image-enhancing drugs, such as AAS (Kanayama *et al.* 2006), particularly amongst gymnasium users. Unfortunately, as with elite sport, it is difficult to establish reliable figures in terms of prevalence of AAS use.

Data from harm reduction programmes, such as needle exchange clinics, offer some indication to the extent of use. In addition to examining AAS use in gymnasia, Korkia (1994) also surveyed syringe exchange clinics. Of the eighty-eight clinics that responded, 59 per cent declared that AAS users had contact with the clinic. Later, McVeigh *et al.* (2003) revealed an increase in individuals attending syringe exchange clinics in counties in the northwest of England (Cheshire and Merseyside) for AAS-injecting equipment between the years 1991 and 2001. Such increases cannot necessarily be attributed to increased AAS use, but they clearly illustrate the success of harm reduction programmes in attracting different types of recreational drug users.

5.9. Designer steroids

The phrase *designer steroids* first became widely recognised in response to the BALCO affair in the early part of this century. Designer steroids are AAS that are developed and used specifically to evade detection by anti-doping authorities. THG, otherwise known as 'The Clear,' was supplied as a sublingual AAS preparation by BALCO, a US-based company, to athletes for the purpose of enhancing performance. Because THG was never marketed, its existence from an anti-doping perspective was unknown; therefore, it was undetectable during routine doping control analysis. Indeed, knowledge of its existence as a performance-enhancing agent was only possible because a 'whistle-blower' alerted the anti-doping authorities, who were then able to determine its molecular structure and subsequently establish a method for its detection (Catlin *et al.* 2004).

Several high-profile athletes tested positive for THG (including the British sprinter Dwain Chambers); many others were implicated in the affair (including US sprinters Marion Jones and Kelli White) and consequently received sanctions, including suspension from competition. In addition to track-and-field athletes, American football players tested positive for THG and baseball players were implicated in the affair. Several athletes were convicted of perjury under state law in the United States. Victor Conte and several coaches were convicted for their part in the distribution of AAS to athletes and received sanctions under state law, including imprisonment.

In addition to DHT, other designer steroids were identified at around the same time, including norbolethone (Catlin *et al.* 2002) and desoxymethyltestosterone (Sekera *et al.* 2005). Desoxymethyltestosterone, also known as Madol, was patented in 1961 but never approved for clinical use in human patients. Probably the first designer steroid was dehydro-chloromethyltestosterone (otherwise known as Turinabol), which was used by former-GDR athletes as part of their state-run doping programme (Parr and Schanzer 2010).

Cases involving designer steroids have led to heightened vigilance by anti-doping organisations and WADA-accredited laboratories, clearly improving the prospect of early detection. Nevertheless, the most important issue relates to the fact that, as unmarketed steroids, there is limited, if any, toxicology data and thus safety information. The use of designer steroids by athletes therefore poses a significant, yet unknown, threat to health.

5.10. Prohormones

Prohormones refer to a group of substances that are precursors to steroid hormones and are now accepted as hormones – and indeed AAS – in their own right. The prohormones andro-stenedione and DHEA are endogenous hormones produced by the gonads and adrenal gland, forming an important circulating pool of steroid hormone precursors.

Administration of exogenous prohormones is thought to enhance the circulating pool of steroid precursors and thus increase the subsequent biotransformation into testosterone. Increased circulating testosterone is then thought to positively affect skeletal muscle hyper-trophy and function. Unfortunately, the scientific literature does not confirm these hypoth-eses. Whilst there is evidence to show that the ingestion of prohormones can increase the circulating levels of DHEA and androstenedione, resultant significant elevations in the cir-culating pool of testosterone have only been demonstrated in females (Morales *et al*. 1998). This could be explained by the fact that, in females, a significant proportion (up to 100 per cent) of circulating testosterone is as a consequence of peripheral conversion of weaker androgens, namely DHEA (Labrie *et al*. 2005), as opposed to its being almost entirely based upon its production in the gonads (and to a lesser extent by the adrenal cortex), as in males (Kicman 2008).

Despite the positive outcomes in terms of increased circulating testosterone in females, there has been no indication that this might manifest itself in gains in muscle size and strength (King *et al*. 1999). The efficacy of prohormones as PIEDs is further weakened by the evidence by some scientists that they may induce a number of negative side effects. King *et al*. revealed an adverse effect on blood lipid profiles and increased levels of circulating oestrogens following the administration of 300 mg/d of androstenedione over an 8-week period.

Prohormones are commonly included as ingredients in, and marketed as, nutritional sports supplements to avoid the necessary controls required in the manufacture and sale of pharma-ceutical products. As sports supplements, they are available from sports supplements shops and via the internet, and they are used amongst the sports and fitness community. Clearly, such widespread availability poses problems in terms of both the intentional and unintentional use of AAS in elite athletes and potential failed drug tests as a consequence.

5.11. Detection of anabolic androgenic steroids

Detection of exogenous AAS is generally based upon direct quantification of a particular AAS and its metabolites in urine. However, in the case of endogenous AAS, detection is reliant on the investigation of various steroid profiles, including the ratio of testosterone to epitestosterone (T:E) for the determination of testosterone abuse. Because epitestosterone is a stable stereoisomer of endogenous testosterone, further exogenous administration of testosterone increases the T:E ratio. Accordingly, WADA states that a ratio in excess of 4:1 constitutes an adverse analytical finding and warrants further investigation. Further investigation would include confirmatory analysis of testosterone metabolites to allow for the discrimination of endogenous testosterone from that of its pharmaceutical counterpart. In addition, the quantification of epitestosterone would determine whether there has been co-administration of testosterone with its stereoisomer to ensure that a normal ratio is maintained. A urinary threshold of 200 ng/ml for epitestosterone is set, above which would constitute a doping offence. The endogenous AAS 19-norandrosterone also poses its own unique problem in that it may also be present in urine as a metabolite of the exogenous AAS 19-nortestosterone. A urinary threshold for 19-norandrosterone is therefore set as 2 ng/ml.

To further enhance the effectiveness of detecting those using endogenous AAS or other anabolic agents, such as SARMs, WADA has recently introduced profiling as part of the Athlete Biological Passport. Because there are clear individual reference ranges for endogenous AAS and their metabolites, individual steroid profiling should offer a more effective and authentic approach to the detection of doping.

Microdosing using the topical application of testosterone via dermal patches and gels is a particular concern to anti-doping personnel, particularly because of the short half-life of the drug and thus the potential to evade a positive drug test.

Clearly, the introduction of out-of-competition drug testing was in some way effective in catching those administering exogenous AAS (or in acting as a deterrent to potential users) because the use of AAS as PIED is most effective during training and in the time leading up to competition. Before the advent of out-of-competition testing, many athletes would therefore simply abstain from use leading up to a competition in order to avoid detection during an in-competition test. However, the arrival of designer steroids would prove particularly difficult because their existence as PIEDs was unknown, and therefore they would not appear on a urine drug screen. A proactive approach involving research and intelligence will no doubt help to limit the effects of such events in the future.

5.12. Selective androgen receptor modulators

Whilst the presence of SARMs on the Prohibited List suggests their potential for performance enhancement, this class of drugs remains under development; thus, they are not currently used for clinical purposes. Nevertheless, as with many doping agents, their lack of availability as therapeutic agents is typically not a barrier to their potential use as PIEDs.

SARMs may offer a possible advantage over AAS, both clinically and as PIEDs, due to their potential for tissue selectivity and in promoting anabolic rather than androgenic effects. They are also designed to be administered orally with reduced hepatotoxicity. However, despite the fact that SARMs remain under development as a therapeutic modality, their chemical characterisation and methods for their detection have been developed (Thevis *et al.* 2013b, 2014). Indeed, 2012 anti-doping testing figures confirm that SARMs have been detected in doping control samples, thus providing clear evidence of their misuse in sport (Table 5.3; WADA 2013a).

5.13. Beta-2 agonists

Several drugs classified as β_2-agonists are also included on the WADA Prohibited List as anabolic agents, namely clenbuterol and zilpaterol (Table 5.1; WADA 2013b). β_2-Agonists are typically used to combat respiratory conditions due to the stimulation of the β_2-adrenergic receptors of the bronchioles and their bronchodilatory effects (see Chapter 7). However, when administered orally, clenbuterol has been shown to possess anabolic effects in animals (Choo *et al.* 1992). Indeed, both clenbuterol and zilpaterol are used as growth promoters in livestock (Davis *et al.* 2008). Despite the evidence to support their use as anabolic agents in animals, there is limited evidence for this use in humans. Nevertheless, within the bodybuilding community, the use of β_2-agonists is relatively widespread as both an anabolic and repartitioning agent.

The consumption of meat infected with prohibited growth promoters and the impact on doping control

Given the inclusion of a number of livestock growth promoters on the WADA Prohibited List, what is the likelihood for the consumption of meat containing such agents culminating in a positive drug test? This is an obvious concern to athletes subject to doping control tests. Indeed, Parr *et al.* (2009) demonstrated that there is a real possibility of the consumption of meat from cattle given clenbuterol leading to a positive drug test. In light of this, the authors suggested that there is a need to introduce a threshold for clenbuterol in an attempt to limit the possibility of an inadvertent doping offence.

There is now concern regarding the possibility of false positives from a doping perspective as a direct consequence of improved analytical methods. The potential to detect minute traces of prohibited substances brings into question the anti-doping movement's guiding principle of strict liability, particularly as the possibility of prohibited substances entering the body unintentionally, in such small quantities, is considered significant.

During the 2011 Fédération Internationale de Football Association U17 World Cup, clenbuterol was detected in over half of the doping control samples. This was attributed to the ingestion of food contaminated with the drug, as indicated by food analysis (Thevis *et al.*, 2013a). Risk of inadvertent clenbuterol doping is deemed to be a particular risk in countries where the use of the drug in livestock is not regulated. In China, where clenbuterol use in livestock is prohibited, it remains a real risk to athletes (Guddat *et al.* 2012).

Zeranol is a synthetic compound used in some countries as a growth promoter in livestock. Whilst there have been cases of its presence in doping control samples, there is suggestion that this might be as a consequence of food contamination with a mycotoxin, zearalone (Thevis *et al.* 2011).

5.14. Tibolone

Tibolone is a synthetic steroid hormone with an affinity for oestrogen receptors. It is used for symptomatic relief in menopause and prevention of osteoporosis in women. However, whilst tibolone is indicated for its oestrogenic properties, it also has weak androgenic properties; hence, it is included in Class S1 of the WADA Prohibited List (Table 5.1; WADA 2013a).

5.15. Summary

Whilst the WADA classification of anabolic agents consists of some new and emerging drugs of abuse, AAS remain the major class of drugs misused by many who seek improvements in terms of muscle size and strength. Despite improvements in terms of drug detection and the unfolding evidence in relation to health concerns surrounding the use of AAS, there are no signs to suggest that their use is declining. Indeed, their use amongst those engaged in recreational sport or exercise, particularly gym-goers for purposes largely related to image enhancement, appears to be growing.

The scientific literature clearly supports the use of AAS as PIEDs. However, there remains some way to go before there is clear evidence to categorically link the use of AAS with serious, long-term, and even life-threatening health effects. Potentially the most disturbing issues in relation to the nontherapeutic use of anabolic agents is the availability of 'black market' products, for which there is no evidence of the products' legitimacy and thus their safety. Indeed, the use of new and emerging drugs not yet trialled, such as SARMs, offers no assurances in relation to safety.

5.16. References

Advisory Council on the Misuse of Drugs. (2010). Consideration of the anabolic steroids report. Available online at https://www.gov.uk/government/publications/advisory-council-on-the-misuse-of-drugs-consideration-of-the-anabolic-steroids--2 (accessed 31 January 2014).

Alesci, S., Koch, C. A., Bornstein, S. R., and Pacak, K. (2001). Adrenal androgens regulation and adrenopause. *Endocrine Regulations* 35(2): 95–100.

Angell, P., Chester, N., Green, D., *et al.* (2012a). Anabolic steroids and cardiovascular risk. *Sports Medicine* 42(2):119–134.

Angell, P. J., Chester, N., Green, D. J., *et al.* (2012b). Anabolic steroid use and longitudinal, radial and circumferential cardiac motion. *Medicine Science Sports and Exercise* 44(4):583–590.

Angell, P., Chester, N., Sculthorpe, N., *et al.* (2012c). Performance enhancing drug abuse and cardiovascular risk in athletes: Implications for the clinician. *British Journal of Sports Medicine* 46(Suppl 1): i78–i84.

Basaria, S., Wahlstrom, J. T., and Dobs, A. S. (2001). Anabolic-androgenic steroid therapy in the treatment of chronic diseases. *Journal of Clinical Endocrinology and Metabolism* 86(11):5108–5117.

Berning, J. M., Adams, K. J., and Stamford, B. A. (2004). Anabolic steroid usage in athletics: Facts, fiction and public relations. *Journal of Strength and Conditioning Research* 18(4):908–917.

Bhasin, S., Storer, T. W., Berman, N., *et al.* (1996). The effects of supraphysiologic doses of testosterone on muscle size and strength in normal men. *New England Journal of Medicine* 335(1):1–7.

Buckley, W. E., Yesalis, C. E., Friedl, K. E., *et al.* (1988). Estimated prevalence of anabolic steroid use among male high school seniors. *JAMA* 260(23):3441–3445.

Cabasso, A. (1994). Peliosis hepatis in a young adult bodybuilder. *Medicine Science Sports and Exercise* 26(1):2–4.

Calfee, R., and Fadale, P. (2006). Popular ergogenic drugs and supplements in young athletes. *Pediatrics* 117(3):e577–e589.

Catlin, D. H., Ahrens, B. D., and Kucherova, Y. (2002). Detection of norbolethone, an anabolic steroid never marketed, in athletes' urine. *Rapid Communications in Mass Spectrometry* 16(13):1273–1275.

Catlin, D. H., Sekera, M. H., Ahrens, B. D., *et al.* (2004). Tetrahydrogestrinone: Discovery, synthesis, and detection in urine. *Rapid Communications in Mass Spectrometry* 18(12):1245–1249.

Choo, J. J., Horan, M. A., Little, R. A., *et al.* (1992). Anabolic effects of clenbuterol on skeletal muscle are mediated by β_2-adrenoceptor activation. *American Journal of Physiology* 263(1):E50–E56.

Clark, R. V. (2009). Anabolic-androgenic steroids: Historical background, physiology, typical use and side effects. In J. L. Fourcroy (Ed.), *Pharmacology, Doping and Sports: A Scientific Guide for Athletes, Coaches, Physicians, Scientists and Administrators* (pp. 23–35). New York, NY: Routledge.

Davis, E., Loiacono, R., and Summers, R. J. (2008). The rush to adrenaline: Drugs in sport acting on the β-adrenergic system. *British Journal of Pharmacology* 154(3):584–597.

Dimeo, P. (2007). *A History of Drug Use in Sport: 1876–1976. Beyond good and evil.* Oxford, UK: Routledge.

Dunn, J. F., Nisula, B. C., and Rodbard, D. (1981). Transport of Steroid Hormones: Binding of 21 Endogenous Steroids to Both Testosterone-Binding Globulin and Corticosteroid-Binding Globulin in Human Plasma. *Journal of Clinical Endocrinology and Metabolism* 53(1):58–68.

Egner, I. M., Bruusgaard, J. C., Eftestol, E., and Gunderson, K. (2013). A cellular memory mechanism aids overload hypertrophy in muscle long after an episodic exposure to anabolic steroids. *Journal of Physiology* 591(24):6221–6230.

Elsharkawy, A. M., McPherson, S., Masson, S., *et al*. (2012). Cholestasis secondary to anabolic steroid use in young men. *British Medical Journal*, 344:e463.

Evans-Brown, M., Kimergard, A., and McVeigh, J. (2009). Elephant in the room? The methodological implications for public health research of performance-enhancing drugs derived from the illicit market. *Drug Testing and Analysis* 1(7):323–326.

Evans-Brown, M., McVeigh, J., Perkins, C., and Bellis, M. A. (2012). Human enhancement drugs: The emerging challenges to public health. Available online at http://www.cph.org.uk/publication/human-enhancement-drugs-the-emerging-challenges-to-public-health-4/ (accessed 15 July 2014).

Faigenbaum, A. D., Zaichkowsky, L. D., Gardner, D. E., and Micheli, L. J. (1998). Anabolic steroid use by male and female middle school students. *Pediatrics* 101(5):1–6.

Franke, W. W., and Berendonk, B. (1997). Hormonal doping and androgenization of athletes: A secret program of the German Democratic Republic government. *Clinical Chemistry* 43(7):1262–1279.

Freed, D. L., Banks, A. J., Longson, D., *et al*. (1975). Anabolic steroids in athletics: Crossover double-blind trial on weightlifters. *British Medical Journal* 2(5969):471–473.

George, A., and Mottram, D. R. (2011). Anabolic agents. In D. R. Mottram (Ed.), *Drugs in Sport* (5th ed., pp. 49–81). London, UK: Routledge.

Giannotti, S., Ghilardi, M., Dell'Osso, G., *et al*. (2014). Left ventricular hypertrophy and spontaneous rupture of the Achilles tendon after anabolic steroids in bodybuilder. *European Orthopaedics and Traumatology*; published online 3 January 2014.

Graham, M. R., Ryan, P., Baker, J. S., *et al*. (2009). Counterfeiting in performance and image-enhancing drugs. *Drug Test and Analysis* 1(3):135 142.

Guddat, S., Fussholler, G., Geyer, H., *et al*. (2012). Clenbuterol: Regional food contamination a possible source for inadvertent doping in sports. *Drug Testing and Analysis* 4(6):534–538.

Hickson, R. C., Czerwinski, S. M, Falduto, M. T., and Young, A. P. (1990). Glucocorticoid antagonism by exercise and androgenic-anabolic steroids. *Medicine Science Sports and Exercise* 22(3):331–340.

Hoffman, J. R., and Ratamess, N. A. (2006). Medical issues associated with anabolic steroid use: Are they exaggerated? *Journal of Sport Science and Medicine* 5(2):182–193.

Hope, V. D., McVeigh, J., Marongiu, A., *et al*. (2013). Prevalence of and risk factors for HIV, hepatitis B and C infections among men who inject image and performance enhancing drugs: A cross-sectional study. *BMJ Open* 3:e003207.

Johnson, M. D. (1990). Anabolic steroid use in adolescent athletes. *Pediatric Clinics of North America*, 37(5):1111–1123.

Kadi, F. (2008). Cellular and molecular mechanisms responsible for the action of testosterone on human skeletal muscle. A basis for illegal performance enhancement. *British Journal of Pharmacology*, 154(3):522–528.

Kanayama, G., Barry, S., Hudson, J. I., and Pope, H. G. (2006). Body image and attitudes towards male roles in anabolic-androgenic steroid users. *American Journal of Psychiatry* 163(4):697–703.

Kanayama, G., Brower, K. J., Wood, R. I., *et al*. (2009). Anabolic-androgenic steroid dependence: An emerging disorder. *Addiction* 104(12):1966–1978.

Kicman, A. T. (2008). Pharmacology of anabolic steroids. *British Journal of Pharmacology* 154(3): 502–521.

King, D. S., Sharp, R. I., Vukovich, M. D., *et al*. (1999). Effect of oral androstenedione on serum testosterone and adaptations to resistance training in young men: A randomized controlled trial. *JAMA* 281(21):2020–2028.

Korkia, P. (1994). Anabolic steroid use in Britain. *International Journal of Drug Policy* 5(1):6–10.

Kuipers, H., Wijnen, J. A. G., Hartgens, F., *et al*. (1991). Influence of anabolic steroids on body composition, blood pressure, lipid profile and liver functions in bodybuilders. *International Journal of Sports Medicine* 12(4):413–418.

Labrie, F., Luu-The, V., Belanger, A., *et al*. (2005). Is dehydroepiandrosterone a hormone? *Journal of Endocrinology* 187(2):169–196.

Lane, H. A., Grace, F., Smith, J. C., *et al*. (2006). Impaired vasoreactivity in bodybuilders using androgenic anabolic steroids. *European Journal of Clinical Investigation* 36(7):483–488.

Laseter, J. T., and Russell, J. A. (1991). Anabolic steroid-induced tendon pathology: A review of the literature. *Medicine Science Sports and Exercise* 23(1):1–3.

Lenders, J. W. M., Demacker, P. N. M., Vos, J. A., *et al.* (1988). Deleterious effects of anabolic steroids on serum lipoproteins, blood pressure and liver function in amateur body builders. *International Journal of Sports Medicine* 9(1):19–23.

Maior, A. S., Carvalho, A. R., Marques-Neto, S. R., *et al.* (2013). Cardiac autonomic dysfunction in anabolic steroid users. *Scandinavian Journal of Medicine and Science in Sports* 23(5):548–555.

McCabe, S. E., Brower, K. J., West, B. T., *et al.* (2007). Trends in non-medical use of anabolic steroids by U.S. college students: Results from four national surveys. *Drug and Alcohol Dependence* 90(2–3):243–251.

McCreary, D. R., and Sasse, D. K. (2000). An exploration of the drive for muscularity in adolescent boys and girls. *Journal of American of American College Health* 48(6):297–304.

McVeigh, J., Beynon, C., and Bellis, M. A. (2003). New challenges for agency based syringe exchange schemes: Analysis of 11 years of data (1991–2001) in Merseyside and Cheshire, United Kingdom. *International Journal of Drug Policy* 14(5):399–405.

Montisci, M., El Mazloum, R., Cecchetto, G., *et al.* (2012). Anabolic androgenic steroids abuse and cardiac death in athletes: Morphological and toxicological findings in four fatal cases. *Forensic Science International* 217(1–3):e13–e18.

Morales, A. J., Haubrich, R. H., Hwang, J. Y., *et al.* (1998). The effect of six months treatment with a 100 mg daily dose of dehydroepiandrosterone (DHEA) on circulating sex steroids, body composition and muscle strength in age-advanced men and women. *Clinical Endocrinology* 49(4):421–432.

Moriarty, D., Fairall, D., and Galasso, P. J. (1992). The Canadian Commission of Inquiry into the use of drugs and banned practices intended to increase athletic performance. *Journal of Legal Aspects of Sport* 2(1):23–31.

Nasr, J., and Ahmad, J. (2009). Severe cholestasis and renal failure associated with the use of the designer steroid Superdrol (methasteron): A case report and literature review. *Digestive Diseases and Sciences* 54(5):1144–1146.

Omole, T. (2011). Drug use. In E. Fuller (Ed.), *Smoking, drinking and drug use among young people in England in 2010* (pp. 141–179). London, UK: NHS Information Centre for Health and Social Care. Available online at http://www.esds.ac.uk/doc/6883/mrdoc/pdf/6883report_of_findings.pdf (accessed 31 January 2014).

Parr, M. K., Opfermann, G., and Schanzer, W. (2009). Analytical methods for the detection of clenbuterol. *Bioanalysis* 1(2):437–450.

Parr, M. K., and Schanzer, W. (2010). Detection of the misuse of steroids in doping control. *Journal of Steroid Biochemistry and Molecular Biology* 121(3–5):528–537.

Pope, H. G., Gruber, A. J., Choi, P. Y., *et al.* (1997). Muscle dysmorphia: An unrecognised form of body dysmorphic disorder. *Psychosomatics* 38(6):548–557.

Pope, H. G., and Katz, D. L. (1988). Affective and psychotic symptoms associated with anabolic steroid use. *American Journal of Psychiatry* 145(4):487–490.

Riebe, D., Fernhall, B., and Thompson, P. D. (1992). The blood pressure response to exercise in anabolic steroid users. *Medicine Science Sports and Exercise* 24(6):633–637.

Sachtleben, T. R., Berg, K. E., Elias, B. A., *et al.* (1993). The effects of anabolic steroids on myocardial structure and cardiovascular fitness. *Medicine Science Sports and Exercise* 25(11):1240–1245.

Salameh, W. A., Redor-Goodman, M. M., Clarke, N. J., *et al.* (2010). Validation of a total testosterone assay using high-turbulence liquid chromatography tandem mass-spectrometry: Total and free testosterone reference ranges. *Steroids* 75(2):169–175.

Sanchez-Osorio, M., Duarte-Rojo, A., Martinez-Benitez, B., *et al.* (2008). Anabolic-androgenic steroids and liver injury. *Liver International* 28(2):278–282.

Sekera, M. H., Ahrens, B. D., Chang, Y. C., *et al.* (2005). Another designer steroid: Discovery, synthesis and detection of 'madol' in urine. *Rapid Communications in Mass Spectrometry* 19(6):781–784.

Shahidi, N. T. (2001). A review of the chemistry, biological action and clinical applications of anabolic-androgenic steroids. *Clinical Therapeutics* 23(9):1355–1390.

Striegel, H., Simon, P., Frisch, S., *et al*. (2006). Anabolic ergogenic substance use in fitness-sports: A distinct group supported by health care system. *Drug and Alcohol Dependence* 81(1):11–19.

Thevis, M., Fussholler, G., and Schanzer, W. (2011). Zeranol: Doping offence or mycotoxin? A case-related study. *Drug Testing and Analysis* 3(11–12):777–783.

Thevis, M., Geyer, L., Geyer, H., *et al*. (2013a). Adverse analytical findings with clenbuterol among U-17 soccer players attributed to food contamination issues. *Drug Testing and Analysis* 5(5):372–376.

Thevis, M., Piper, T., Beuk, S., *et al*. (2013b). Expanding sports drug testing assays: Mass spectrometric characterization of the selective androgen receptor modulator drug candidates RAD140 and ACP-105. *Rapid Communications in Mass Spectrometry* 27(11):1173–1182.

Thevis, M., Kuuranne, T., Geyer, H., and Schanzer, W. (2014). Annual banned-substance review: Analytical approaches in human sports drug testing. *Drug Testing and Analysis* 6(1–2):164–184.

Thigpen, A. E., Silver, R. I., Guileyardo, J. M., *et al*. (1993). Tissue distribution and ontogeny of steroid 5α-reductase isoenzyme expression. *Journal of Clinical Investigation* 92(2):903–910.

Toth, M., and Zakar, T. (1982). Relative binding affinities of testosterone, 19-nortestosterone and their 5 alpha-reduced derivatives to the androgen receptor and to other androgen-binding proteins: A suggested role of 5 alpha-reductive steroid metabolism in the dissociation of 'myotropic' and 'androgenic' activities of 19-nortestosterone. *Journal of Steroid Biochemistry* 17(6):653–660.

Van Amsterdam, J., Opperhuizen, A., and Hartgens, F. (2010). Adverse health effects of anabolic-androgenic steroids. *Regulatory Toxicology and Pharmacology* 57(1):117–123.

Wilson, J. D. (1988). Androgen abuse by athletes. *Endocrine Reviews* 9(2):181–199.

Woerdeman, J., and de Ronde, W. (2011). Therapeutic effects of anabolic androgenic steroids on chronic disease associated with muscle wasting. *Expert Opinion on Investigational Drugs* 20(1):87–97.

Wood, T. O., Cooke, P. H., and Goodship A. E. (1988). The effect of exercise and anabolic steroids on the mechanical properties and crimp morphology of the rat tendon. *American Journal of Sports Medicine* 16(2):153–158.

World Anti-Doping Agency. (2013a). 2012 anti-doping testing figures report. Available online at https://wada-main-prod.s3.amazonaws.com/resources/files/WADA-2012-Anti-Doping-Testing-Figures-Report-EN.pdf (accessed 9 September 2014).

World Anti-Doping Agency. (2013b). The 2014 Prohibited List international standard. Available online at https://elb.wada-ama.org/en/what-we-do/prohibited-list (accessed 9 September 2014).

Yates, W. R., Perry, P., and Murray, S. (1992). Aggression and hostility in anabolic steroid users. *Biological Psychiatry* 31(12):1232–1234.

Chapter 6

Peptide hormones, growth factors, and related substances

David R. Mottram and Neil Chester

6.1. Introduction

The World Anti-Doping Agency (WADA) prohibits the use of a number of peptide hormones and related substances (Table 6.1), most of which occur naturally in the body.

6.2. Erythropoiesis-stimulating agents

Erythropoiesis-stimulating agents (ESAs) include the endogenous peptide erythropoietin (EPO), which is commercially available as recombinant EPO and the synthetically produced darbepoetin (dEPO) and methoxy polyethylene glycol-epoetin beta. In September 2014, WADA revised the 2014 Prohibited List to include hypoxia-inducible factor (HIF) activators, such as Xenon and argon, which promote the production of EPO within the body (WADA, 2014a).

Mode of action of erythropoietin

EPO increases oxygen supply to muscles, thereby increasing an athlete's endurance and performance (Elliott 2008). The effects of EPO are mediated by specific erythropoietin-sensitive receptors on the surface of the red cell progenitors. EPO works synergistically with other growth factors to cause maturation and proliferation of erythroid precursors. The net effect is an increase in the number of red blood cells (erythrocytes) that are produced and the rate at which they are released into the circulation. Therefore, EPO increases the oxygen supply for muscle tissue, allowing muscles to work longer before they build up lactic acid (Tsitsimpikou 2011).

Table 6.1 Peptide hormones, growth factors, and related substances on the WADA Prohibited List (January 2014)

1. Erythropoiesis-stimulating agents, such as erythropoietin, darbepoetin, hypoxia-inducible factor stabilizers, methoxy polyethylene glycol-epoetin beta, and peginesatide (Hematide)
2. Chorionic gonadotrophin, luteinizing hormone, and their releasing factors in males
3. Corticotrophins and their releasing factors
4. Growth hormone, its releasing factors, and insulin-like growth factor-1

In addition, the following growth factors are prohibited:
Fibroblast growth factors; hepatocyte growth factor; mechano growth factors; platelet-derived growth factors; vascular-endothelial growth factor; any other growth factor affecting muscle, tendon/ligament protein synthesis/degradation, vascularisation, energy utilization, regenerative capacity, or fibre-type switching; and other substances with similar chemical structure or similar biological effect(s).

Recombinant erythropoietin

The gene responsible for the synthesis of erythropoietin was cloned in 1985. Recombinant human erythropoietin (rHuEPO) was first patented by Amgen in 1989. There are currently three generations of rHuEPO in production: the prototype (EPO), novel erythropoiesis-stimulating protein (NESP), and continuous erythropoietin receptor activator (CERA). Because the biological activity is determined by the sialylation of the protein moiety, the therapeutic target has been to prolong the half-life of the biopharmaceutical and hence to reduce the frequency of dosing. Second-generation NESP (darbepoetin, Aranesp™) differs from EPO in having an additional eight sialic acid residues. Third-generation CERA differs in having a long polymer chain (methoxy polyethylene glycol) incorporated into the molecule. These genetically engineered modifications have increased the elimination half-lives from 8.5 to 25.3 hours (by second-gen NESP) and 142 hours (by third-gen CERA). This has decreased the frequency of initial intravenous dosing from three times weekly to once weekly and once every 2 weeks, respectively.

Adverse effects of ESAs

Because ESAs stimulate erythropoiesis, the resulting increased viscosity of the blood raises the risk of microcirculation blockage, heart failure, and stroke (Wells 2008). In addition to the health risks posed by the increase in blood viscosity and the risk of thromboembolism, there is perhaps a more sinister and long-term potential side effect of abuse of ESAs. The risks of thromboembolism will decrease with time as the haematocrit falls. However, EPO-stimulated erythropoiesis vastly augments the demands of the sportsperson for ferrous iron for the synthesis of haemoglobin (Hb). Excess iron within the body is toxic. The body can protect itself to a certain extent from increased oral intake of iron by decreasing absorption from the gastrointestinal tract (GIT). Such is the requirement engendered by EPO administration that iron must be injected, thus bypassing GIT regulation and leading to iron overload.

There is evidence from both France and Italy that elite cyclists have ferritin levels indicative of severe iron overload. Investigations in Italy revealed that a large proportion of professional cyclists had elevated ferritin levels, often in excess of 1,000 ng/ml (Cazzola 2001). A study of elite riders in France revealed a mean ferritin level of 806 ng/ml with a range of 534–1,997 ng/ml (Dine 2001). These values are equivalent to those seen in congenital haemochromatosis, a condition characterised by iron deposition in various tissues and organs leading to multiple organ failure, including cirrhosis. It also increases the risk of hepatic carcinoma. Thus, not only is EPO prohibited by WADA, but also it poses significant short- and long-term health problems to the abuser, inadvertent or not.

Detection of EPO

The first tests for EPO at the Olympic Games were introduced in Sydney in 2000. To be deemed culpable, the athlete had to test positive in both blood (Parisotto et al. 2001) and urine tests (Lasne and de Ceaurriz 2000). Blood screening was performed first, and then urine analysis was performed to confirm a positive result. In 2003, WADA's executive committee accepted the results from an independent report that urine testing alone could be used to detect the presence of recombinant EPO. Demonstration of the presence of ESAs is based upon isoelectric focusing and chemiluminescence (see Figure 6.1). These techniques may be complemented with a further technique known as sodium dodecyl sulfate polyacrylamide gel electrophoresis (SDS-PAGE; Figure 6.2). These techniques can identify not only

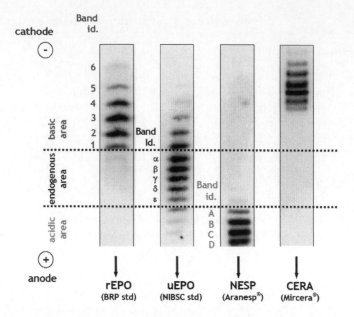

Figure 6.1 Results of the detection of erythropoiesis stimulating agents obtained using isoelectric focusing and chemiluminescence.

Source: TD2014EPO – World Anti-Doping Agency's (WADA) Technical Document on HARMONIZATION OF ANALYSIS AND REPORTING OF RECOMBINANT ERYTHROPOIETINS (i.e. EPOETINS) AND ANALOGUES (e.g. DARBEPOETIN, PEGSERPOETIN, PEGINESATIDE, EPO-Fc) BY ELECTROPHORETIC TECHNIQUES

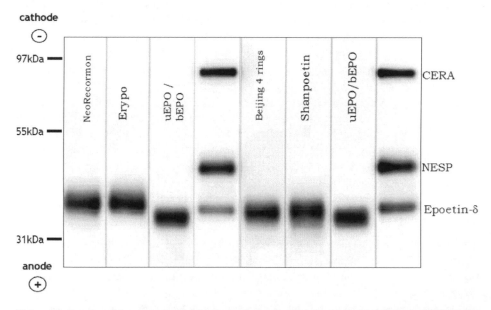

Figure 6.2 Results of the detection of erythropoiesis stimulating agents obtained using SDS-PAGE.

Source: TD2014EPO – World Anti-Doping Agency's (WADA) Technical Document on HARMONIZATION OF ANALYSIS AND REPORTING OF RECOMBINANT ERYTHROPOIETINS (i.e. EPOETINS) AND ANALOGUES (e.g. DARBEPOETIN, PEGSERPOETIN, PEGINESATIDE, EPO-Fc) BY ELECTROPHORETIC TECHNIQUES

r-HuEPO, NESP, and CERA but also biosimilars (e.g. Hemax™ and Dynepo™). Further details on the methods for detecting epoetin are described in WADA's Technical Document (WADA 2014b).

Abuse of EPO in sport

The first clinical reports of EPO were published in 1987. Amgen received a licence for r-HuEPO in 1989. Around this time, several newspaper articles linked the deaths of eighteen Belgian and Dutch cyclists with rumours of EPO abuse in the peloton (Leith 1992). At that time, it was unlikely that the magnitude of the increase in red blood cell production was accurately controlled and the haematocrit (Hct) may have been raised to dangerously high levels. Values of 60 per cent were rumoured. Indeed, one cyclist, Marco Pantani, was found to have an Hct of 60.1 per cent when admitted to hospital after an accident during a 1995 race (Rendell 2006). This concentration would cause significant increases in both systolic blood pressure and blood viscosity. In the short term, there would be an increased risk of thrombosis and stroke. In the long term, chronically elevated Hct and blood viscosity could lead to left ventricular hypertrophy and, ultimately, to left ventricular failure and death.

In 1990, the International Olympic Committee (IOC) added EPO to its list of banned substances. There was much conjecture about abuse of EPO at this time. The former professional cyclist, Paul Kimmage (1998), referred to such suspicions within the peloton. He also referred to the Donati dossier, which was a 1994 account of EPO abuse involving elite Italian cyclists. Proof of the extent of abuse of EPO did not exist until the 1998 Tour de France and what became known as the Festina Affair. Subsequent detention of the Festina team *soigneur* Willy Voet, prompted him to publish a personal account of drug abuse within the peloton (Voet 2001). He stated that provision and administration of EPO were formalized within the team and provided evidence of drugs, doses, and deductions from salaries according to drugs administered. It is difficult to imagine that other teams could compete with Festina without recourse to EPO, not least because there is undisputed evidence in sport-specific investigations of the ergogenic benefit derived from EPO (e.g. Ekblom and Berglund 1991; Birkeland *et al.* 2000). Thus, the ergogenic effects of r-HuEPO were compared to those of transfusional polycythaemia by Ekblom and Berglund (1991). These authors reported that r-HuEPO increased Hb concentration from 152 to 169 g/l and VO$_2$ max from 4.52 to 4.88 l/min. These effects did not differ significantly from those evoked by reinfusion of 1,350 ml of autologous blood. Significantly, systolic blood pressure was increased whilst cycling at 200 W from before to after r-HuEPO. In a later study, time to exhaustion was also increased from 493 ± 74 s to 567 ± 82 s following identical doses of r-HuEPO (Ekblom 1997).

There have been many examples of positive tests (adverse analytical findings) for ESAs. It is a commonly held misconception that EPO is mainly abused by cyclists, particularly by those involved in endurance events (spectacularly so in the Tour de France). On the contrary, there have been many examples from a number of different sports, including cross-country skiers, biathletes, swimmers, rowers, marathon runners, 5000-m runners, 400-m runners, and 400-m hurdlers. Confirmation that abuse of EPO is not restricted to participants in endurance events was demonstrated by US sprinters Marion Jones and Kelli White, who tested positive for EPO.

Given that there are well-defined methods for the detection of ESAs, why do athletes continue to abuse these drugs and risk sanctions? A possible explanation is that the athletes believe that they can somehow avoid detection. Various means of diluting red blood cell concentrations have been employed in the past (e.g. the use of plasma volume expanders).

Perhaps a subtler and more interesting strategy is to make combined use of the limitations of the test and the pharmacokinetics of the drug. One such strategy is to use a microdosing regime that renders EPO undetectable within a short period of administration, as demonstrated in the Lance Armstrong case (Mottram 2013). In a study involving two well-trained male athletes, Ashenden *et al.* (2006) demonstrated that a 3-week microdose regime could be utilised to maintain Hb concentrations at 164 g/l and 170 g/l (pre-EPO controls were 140 g/l and 148 g/l, respectively). Urine samples collected more than 24 hours after microdose injection typically had less than 80 per cent basic isoforms of EPO, which had been a criterion for an adverse analytical finding. An approach such as this, whilst relatively simple to conduct within a laboratory setting, requires a degree of sophistication and support well beyond the compass of the athlete alone. In the past, this has been thought to involve the coaching and medical support staff.

Cases of EPO abuse in sport

Since the first reports of EPO use in cycling, associated with the Festina Affair (Voet 2001), there have been a number of high-profile cases, particularly in cycling.

Lance Armstrong (2012)

On 24 August 2012, the United States Anti-Doping Agency (USADA) announced that it had imposed on Lance Armstrong a sanction of lifetime ineligibility and disqualification of competition results achieved since August 1998. Despite having never tested positive for a prohibited drug, USADA cited all anti-doping rule violations except those directly relating to the presence of a drug in a sample or evasion of doping tests. One of the drugs most extensively used by Armstrong and the US Postal Services Cycling Team was EPO, which Armstrong subsequently admitted to using. The evidence behind the headlines concerning the Lance Armstrong case was described by Mottram (2013).

6.3. Chorionic gonadotrophin

Chorionic gonadotrophin (CG) is produced by placental trophoblast cells during pregnancy and also by a number of different types of tumour cells. Its major physiological role is stimulation of the corpus luteum in pregnant females to maintain synthesis and secretion of the hormone progesterone during pregnancy. However, when injected into males, CG also stimulates the Leydig cells of the testes to produce testosterone and epitestosterone, so it can mimic the natural stimulation of testicular hormone produced by luteinizing hormone (LH). Administration of CG stimulates secretion of testosterone and epitestosterone in a normal ratio.

The Leydig cells of the testes possess receptors that, when stimulated by LH or CG, bring about activation of testosterone synthesis. This increase in synthesis is rapid: a 50 per cent increase in plasma testosterone concentration has been measured 2 h after intramuscular injection of 6,000 IU of CG (Kicman *et al.* 1991). Injection of CG also stimulates production of nandrolone (19-nortestosterone) metabolites, which may indicate that it can stimulate production of endogenous nandrolone itself (Reznik *et al.* 2001). An excellent review of CG has been published by Stenman *et al.* (2008).

Therapeutic use

CG is used to stimulate ovulation in conjunction with follicle-stimulating hormone in infertile women. Occasionally, CG is used to stimulate testicular hormone production when puberty is delayed.

CG Abuse in sport

CG has been used because it stimulates the secretion from the testes of both testosterone and epitestosterone. This led to the banning of CG by the IOC in 1987.

A standard doping regime for CG has been described (Brooks *et al*. 1989), in which the abuser first injects testosterone. Apart from any gains in strength or competitiveness, the testosterone causes inhibition of LH secretion from the pituitary. When testosterone is withdrawn before competition (to avoid detection), the athlete is at a disadvantage with lower than normal plasma testosterone levels. However, administration of CG stimulates testicular testosterone secretion and also that of epitestosterone.

In a small, elegant experiment, Kicman *et al*. (1991) reproduced this situation in three normal men, showing that CG can stimulate the testosterone substitution claimed by abusers and retain the testosterone/epitestosterone ratio within WADA limits. In all three cases, the CG could be detected in the urine by radioimmunoassay as long as plasma testosterone levels were raised. Brower (2000) described three separate regimes to restore endogenous testosterone secretion to normal following its suppression due to administration of testosterone or anabolic steroids. He has recorded descriptions of CG doses of 50 IU/kg producing a doubling of endogenous testosterone secretion within 3–4 days of administration.

A review by Hendelsman (2006) concluded that CG produces marked increases in blood testosterone levels in men, but the effects are negligible in women; therefore, prohibition and testing for CG should be restricted to men. Hendelsman *et al*. (2009) showed a prominent dose-dependent and sustained effect on blood and urine CG, LH, and testosterone levels after administration of recombinant CG. They further concluded that testosterone:LH ratio measurements may be a sensitive test to detect CG administration for at least 1 week after injection.

Side effects of CG in sport

The side effects of CG will be similar to those for anabolic steroids. However, the incidence of gynaecomastia may be greater as CG also stimulates oestradiol production by the Leydig cells. The increase of oestradiol may be linked to nandrolone metabolite production in the process of aromatisation (Reznik *et al*. 2001).

6.4. Luteinizing hormone and its use in sport

Luteinizing hormone is produced by the gonadotrope cells of the anterior pituitary in both males and females. In males, LH stimulates testicular sperm production and the synthesis and secretion of testosterone, whilst in females it stimulates ovulation and the production of progesterone. There are structural similarities between LH and CG; a detailed comparison was made by Kicman and Cowan (1992). LH secretion is subject to negative feedback control by testosterone; therefore, as plasma testosterone levels rise, LH secretion is reduced. A recent study on the effects of single doses of recombinant LH, up to 750 IU, had no influence on serum or urine LH or testosterone (Hendelsman *et al*. 2009).

Table 6.2 WADA statistics for the number of positive results for substances classed as peptide hormones, growth factors, and related substances (2006–2012)

	2006	2007	2008	2009	2010	2011	2012
Erythropoietin	17	22	51	56	36	43	45
Erythropoietin (active transcription factor)	–	–	–	–	–	1	–
Darbepoetin	1	2	2	4	8	5	4
Micera	–	–	5	8	1	–	–
Chorionic gonadotrophin	22	15	46	25	33	47	93
Luteinizing hormone	2	2	1	6	5	23	29
Insulins*	–	–	1	–	–	–	2
Growth hormone	–	–	–	1	3	6	8
Total	42	41	106	100	86	125	181

* Insulins were reclassified as hormone and metabolic modulators by WADA in 2014.

LH abuse is limited by its scarcity, its high costs, and its plasma half-life, which is 50 per cent less than that of CG (Kicman and Cowan 1992). 'Designer' synthesis of LH, a dual-chain peptide, is difficult owing to the complexity of its structure. Problems associated with the detection of LH were reviewed at length by Stenman *et al.* (2008). It is much more likely that LH-releasing hormone, the substance regulating LH release, will become a drug of abuse. It could be used to stimulate endogenous LH release, which will in turn stimulate the testes to secrete testosterone in males withdrawing from anabolic steroid abuse. Brower (2000) has described several LH treatment regimes, which could be used to restore testosterone secretion in males suffering anabolic steroid withdrawal syndromes or in those who need to restore normal testosterone before an event or test.

Statistics from WADA-accredited laboratories (Table 6.2) show low rates of detection for LH. It has been reported that this is possibly due to unreliable methods of detection for LH (Hendelsman *et al.* 2009).

6.5. Corticotrophins

The peptide hormone adrenocorticotropuc hormone (ACTH) is produced and secreted by the corticotrope cells of the anterior pituitary. It is a polypeptide consisting of thirty-nine amino acids, of which only the twenty-four N-terminal amino acids are necessary for its biological activity. ACTH stimulates the reticularis and fasciculata cells of the adrenal cortex to synthesise and secrete corticosteroids, such as cortisol and corticosterone.

Administration of ACTH

ACTH itself is never used for treatment or abuse. Instead, a synthetic derivative – the peptide tetracosactrin, consisting of the first twenty-four N-terminal amino acids of ACTH – is administered by injection. Tetracosactrin administration stimulates a rise in blood cortisol and corticosterone concentration within 2 hours.

Abuse of ACTH

ACTH abuse is limited to short-term boosting of plasma cortisol and corticosterone in an attempt to reduce lethargy and produce 'positive' effects on mood during training and competition. It is for this reason that it is banned by WADA, along with corticosteroids. ACTH and corticosteroids are unsuitable for chronic use because they decrease muscle protein synthesis, leading to skeletal muscle wasting.

Detection of ACTH

Tetracosactrin abuse and endogenous ACTH are difficult to detect in urine samples. In the blood, a rise in ACTH levels and therefore of corticosteroids occurs naturally during exercise. Kicman and Cowan (1992) investigated blood analysis for tetracosactrin, which should enable abuse to be detected.

6.6. Growth hormone

Growth hormone (GH) is one of the major hormones influencing growth and development in humans. The period of human growth extends from birth to the age of 20 years. A large number of hormones influence this period, producing many complex interactions. Besides GH, testosterone, oestradiol, cortisol, thyroxine, and insulin have important roles at different stages of growth and development. The exact role of GH is difficult to evaluate because of the many different developmental and metabolic processes that GH can influence. A review of GH and its abuse in sport has been published by Holt and Sonksen (2008). The regulation of muscle mass by GH and growth factors has been reviewed by Velloso (2008).

Release of growth hormone

The anterior pituitary, a small endocrine gland at the base of, but not part of, the brain, contains somatotrope cells, which secrete growth hormone. Release of GH is under the control of two hypothalamic hormones: somatostatin, which inhibits secretion, and somatocrinin, which stimulates its secretion. Oestradiol also stimulates GH secretion while testosterone has very little effect. Various brain neurotransmitter systems also influence GH secretion. This is thought to occur via a controlling influence on the hypothalamic production of somatostatin and somatocrinin, but direct effects on the somatotrope cells cannot be ruled out. The factors influencing GH secretion have been reviewed in detail by Macintyre (1987) and Muller (1987).

Daily GH secretion is episodic, with the highest levels (0.5–3.0 mg/l) occurring 60–90 min after the onset of sleep. GH is metabolised in the liver; the plasma half-life is only 12–45 min. The physiological regulation of GH release is complex. Systemic factors stimulating GH secretion include hypoglycaemia, a rise in blood amino acid concentration, stress, and exercise; conversely, GH secretion is inhibited by hyperglycaemia. Both endurance exercise and resistance training have been shown to cause an increase in GH secretion in female athletes (Consitt et al. 2002).

Growth hormone action

The most obvious action of GH is that it stimulates somatic growth in preadolescents, but it also has metabolic effects. The importance of these metabolic actions in homeostatic regulation of fuel usage and storage is unclear, as is the overall role of GH in the adult; this was discussed in detail by Macintyre (1987). Receptors for GH are present on the surface of every cell in the body (Holt 2004). GH stimulates the release (mainly from the liver) of two hormonal polypeptides, somatomedin C (or insulin-like growth factor [IGF]-1) and somatomedin A (IGF-2); a full account of this was provided by Macintyre (1987) and Kicman and Cowan (1992). Growth hormone exerts its anabolic actions through the generation of IGF-1 (Le Roith *et al.* 2001), although Sonksen (2001) expressed doubt as to whether many, if any, of the important metabolic effects of GH are mediated via IGFs. IGFs are carried in the plasma in two different forms: as ternary complexes and simpler low-molecular-weight complexes (Boisclair *et al.* 2001).

Effects on muscle

GH seems to have some effects on muscle growth, but the effect of IGF-1 is greater. This action appears to be similar to that of insulin in that it promotes amino acid uptake and stimulates protein synthesis, resulting in an increase in the length and diameter of muscle fibres in children; only the latter growth occurs in adults. This stimulation of muscle protein synthesis and growth is qualitatively different to that induced by work, because insulin is required for GH-stimulated muscle growth but not for that induced by work (Macintyre 1987). However, the action of insulin is more likely to be an anticatabolic effect on muscle protein rather than a direct stimulatory effect on muscle protein synthesis (Sonksen 2001).

Effects on bone

Both directly and via the IGFs, GH stimulates the elongation of bone in preadolescents. This is achieved by a stimulation of cartilage proliferation in the epiphyseal plates situated at each end of each long bone. Cartilage cells possess receptors for GH and IGFs.

Effects on metabolism

The actions of GH on metabolism are complex at both the cellular and organ levels and appear to be biphasic. In the first (acute) phase, which seems to involve the action of GH alone, amino acid uptake into muscle (via mobilisation of muscle membrane amino acid transporters) and liver is stimulated, and there is increased glucose uptake into muscle and adipose tissue together with reduced fat metabolism (Smith and Perry 1992). During the second (chronic) phase, mediated by the IGFs, there is increased lipolysis (triglyceride breakdown) in adipose tissue, resulting in a rise in the plasma concentration of fatty acids and increased fatty acid utilisation, thus sparing glucose.

Effects on adipose tissue

Treatment of GH-deficient adults has shown that GH can increase lean body mass by several kilograms and decrease fat mass, especially visceral fat, by an equivalent amount (Marcus and Hoffman 1998). Whether the same effect would be achieved in someone with normal GH secretion is unknown.

Treatment with GH causes a rise in blood free fatty acid levels or a rise in the blood glucose level and a reduction in the triglyceride content of adipose tissue, which contributes to a decrease in adipose tissue mass and an increase in fat-free weight (Kicman and Cowan 1992).

Effects of exercise on growth hormone

Within 20 minutes of beginning exercise to 75–90 per cent VO_2 max, GH levels rise. The intensity of the response depends on age, level of fitness, and body composition. The type of exercise undertaken also produces varying GH responses, with intermittent intense exercise claimed to result in the highest GH levels (Macintyre 1987).

Administration and supply of growth hormone

GH is a peptide that must be injected. Human GH is produced synthetically. Therapeutically, GH administration is usually recommended as either three single injections, intramuscularly or subcutaneously, or daily subcutaneous injections in the evening.

In sport, many GH supplies are known to be illicitly obtained by theft from pharmaceutical company production lines and from retail pharmacies (Sonksen 2001). The prevalence of GH use by athletes is difficult to determine because much of the evidence arises through anecdotal reports (McHugh *et al.* 2005).

Growth hormone disorders

Inadequate secretion of GH is one of the causes of the condition known as dwarfism. This disorder is usually recognised in childhood when the rate of growth is below the ninetieth percentile for that child's age, race, and sex. The treatment is regular administration of synthetic GH until the end of puberty. Treatment after adolescence is ineffective in stimulating growth in stature; by this time, the epiphyseal plates in the long bones have fused, terminating any further bone growth.

Overproduction of GH as a result of a tumour may occur in puberty and adolescence, when it gives rise to gigantism; the individual is well above average adult height for his or her age, sex, and race. The limbs and internal organs are also enlarged.

In late adulthood, a tumour of the anterior pituitary causing increased GH secretion results in the condition known as acromegaly. The affected individual does not grow any taller because the epiphyses have fused, but the internal organs enlarge (especially the heart), the fingers grow, and the skin thickens. Metabolic disorders occur, which often precipitate type 2 diabetes mellitus.

A deficiency in GH secretion in adulthood has been recognised in elderly people, some of whom have responded favourably to GH therapy (Marcus and Hoffman 1998; Gotherstrom *et al.* 2005). The investigations of this syndrome have provided interesting data on the effects of GH, but they have not indicated a universal benefit for GH treatment of the elderly.

6.7. The abuse of growth hormone in sport

There appear to be four major reasons for the abuse of GH in sport:

1   To increase muscle mass and strength
2   To increase lean body mass
3   To improve the appearance of musculature
4   To increase final adult height.

Scientific evidence from controlled trials indicating that GH increases muscle strength is controversial. There is some evidence to support the claim that GH administration may increase lean body mass. Lombardo *et al.* (1991) described experiments where GH administration has caused significant reductions in 'fat weight' and increases in fat-free weight compared to placebo.

As early as 1988, Cowart reviewed anecdotal reports by bodybuilders of increases in strength following GH administration. There are also several positive findings of increased muscle growth, strength, and protein synthesis in GH-deficient adults treated with human growth hormone (Marcus and Hoffman 1998). When Taaffe *et al.* (1996) examined the effects of growth hormone treatment on muscle strength and lean body mass in elderly men, they found no increases in strength but an increase in lean body mass and a decrease in fat mass. Similarly, when Yarasheski *et al.* (1995) examined resistance training schedules before and during GH administration in elderly men, they found that GH did not further enhance muscle strength improvements induced by exercise regimes.

In younger adult men, there is a similar picture. Sixteen healthy men, 21–34 years of age, who had not previously trained were given GH (40 mcg/kg/days) or placebo during 12 weeks of heavy resistance training. At the end of the study, lean body mass and total body water increased in the GH group compared to placebo, but there was no difference in muscle strength or limb circumference (Yarasheski *et al.* 1992). Negative results have also been obtained with seven weight-lifters who were given GH 40 mcg/kg per day over a 14-day period during which a daily resistance training programme was followed. Muscle protein synthesis did not increase and there was no change in whole-body protein breakdown (Yarasheski *et al.* 1993). When a dose of 0.09 IU/kg per day was administered to twenty-two male power athletes aged 20–28 years over a longer period (six weeks), no increases in biceps or quadriceps maximal strength occurred in the GH group compared to the placebo group (Deyssig *et al.* 1993).

The potential performance-enhancing effects of GH are still debated amongst users (Saugy *et al.* 2006). Effects may be attributed to other substances used in combination with GH. Ehrnborg *et al.* (2000) reviewed previous experiments on GH use and concluded that the studies may have been 'too short and included too few subjects.' As with early studies on anabolic steroids, the doses used may have been too low, and some of the GH abusers may also have been concurrently abusing anabolic steroids (Schnirring 2000).

It is claimed that GH administration improves the appearance of the bodybuilder, making his or her muscles more salient or 'sculpted' and more photogenic. There is no way this effect can be measured directly or objectively, but it appears to be a logical development associated with loss of fat tissue.

The desire to produce tall offspring – either for cosmetic reasons, athletic potential, or to qualify for a vocation where there is a minimum height limit – has prompted GH abuse amongst children in the United States. In addition to the ethical problems that it presents, the child may later resent his or her tallness, particularly if later he or she fails to qualify as a professional sportsperson. An apparent relentless drive for 'bigness' and 'tallness' in sport and society by selective and drug-induced means is discussed in a review by Norton and Olds (2001). Overall, there continues to be debate as to whether the adverse effects of GH outweigh the potential performance-enhancing effects (Rennie 2003).

Side effects associated with growth hormone abuse in sport

The long-term risks of GH in athletes are not well known because epidemiological data derived from users in sport are not available (Saugy *et al.* 2006).

The potential risks of GH therapy in children are clear. In the United Kingdom, the recommended standard replacement dose of GH is about 0.6 IU/kg body weight per week. It is widely assumed that athletes who abuse the drug are taking ten times this dose (Smith and Perry 1992). Major side effects include skeletal changes, enlargement of the fingers and toes, growth of the orbit, and lengthening of the jaw. The internal organs enlarge, and the cardiomegaly that is produced is often one of the causes of death associated with GH abuse. Although the skeletal muscles increase in size, there are often complaints of muscle weakness. Adverse biochemical changes include impaired glucose regulation (usually hyperglycaemia), hyperlipidaemia, and insulin resistance. These changes contribute to the prevalence of diabetes in GH abusers. Arthritis and impotence often occur after chronic GH abuse (Kicman and Cowan 1992).

A consequence of the increased protein synthesis during GH abuse is changes to the skin. This includes thickening and coarsening as the so-called 'elephant epidermis' is developed; the skin in this state is almost impenetrable by standard-gauge syringe needles (Taylor 1988). Other skin effects include activation of naevocytes and an increase in dermal viscosity (Ehrnborg *et al.* 2000). This combination of side effects – particularly the cardiomegaly, hyperlipidaemia, and hyperglycaemia – almost certainly contributes to the shortened life-span seen in those suffering from overproduction of GH (Smith and Perry 1992).

It is believed that many athletes use doses of GH that are many times higher than those used therapeutically, so it is reasonable to expect that serious side effects may develop (Holt and Sonksen 2008). It is likely that the longer-term effects of GH administration would also occur with IGF-1 (Holt and Sonksen 2008), as described in clinical trials for mecasermin rintabate (Kemp 2007).

Who abuses growth hormone and why?

The reasons for GH abuse appear to be based on some false premise that it is as effective as anabolic steroids, with fewer side effects, and is less easily detected. Abusers believe GH may protect the athlete who has abused anabolic steroids and who wishes to stop 'muscle meltdown' when anabolic steroids are withdrawn.

There are few scientific studies available on the prevalence of GH abuse in sport. In 1997, Korkia and Stimson reported that 2.7 per cent of the anabolic steroid abusers in their UK survey were also abusing GH. Evans (1997) found concordant abuse of anabolic steroids and GH in 12.7 per cent of abusers in his gymnasia survey.

Five per cent of adolescents in a survey (Rickert *et al.* 1992) admitted using GH, and 24.5 per cent claimed to know someone who was abusing it. Fifty per cent of the abusers could not name one side effect of GH. Those who abused GH were most likely to be involved in wrestling or American football and to have obtained their information about GH from another person, such as a coach. There was also some evidence of co-abuse of anabolic steroids and GH in the same adolescent sample.

Because a validated test for GH was not available until recently, reports of GH abuse have been mostly anecdotal or as observations by anti-doping agencies (Stow *et al.* 2009). On a number of occasions, athletes have confessed to using GH after testing positive for other substances. This was the case with Ben Johnson after the 1988 Seoul Olympics and a number of high-profile athletes after the Bay Area Laboratory Co-Operative affair in 2003. A review of the use of GH by athletes can be found in Holt *et al.* (2009).

Detection of growth hormone abuse

Human GH is a peptide that has a very short half-life in the blood and appears in very low concentrations in the urine. Furthermore, secretion of naturally occurring GH from the pituitary gland is pulsatile. Therefore, blood levels fluctuate significantly. Because GH secretion is affected by factors such as emotion, stress, sleep, and nutritional status, there is a high variability within individuals and between individuals (Saugy *et al.* 2006). In addition, exercise can influence GH secretion (Wallace *et al.* 2001).

Up to the 2004 Athens Olympic Games, a validated method to detect GH was not used, despite significant attempts to develop such a method. After the 1996 Atlanta Olympic Games, a research project, entitled GH-2000, was set up; it comprised a consortium of endocrinologists with expertise in growth hormone research from four European countries, with collaboration from two leading pharmaceutical companies (Holt *et al.* 2009). The project team reported their results in 1999, with a proposal for a test based on the measurement of two markers for GH, IGF-1, and type III pro-collagen (P-III-P; Powrie *et al.* 2007). Despite significant support for the proposed test, further research was recommended to ensure the test would work in ethnic groups other than Caucasians and that the test was not affected by injury. Guha *et al.* (2013) highlighted the potential increase in abuse of IGF-1 as tests for detecting GH are developed.

However, following the foundation of WADA in 1999, a second phase of research into GH testing was set up, entitled GH-2004, with significant financial support from the US Anti-Doping Agency. GH-2004 directed its efforts toward the markers approach to GH testing. At the same time, WADA focussed its funding on an isoform approach to testing (Barroso *et al.* 2009).

The direct isoform approach to GH doping detection

This approach involves immunoassays to quantify different types of GH isoforms that differentiate between naturally secreted GH and recombinant GH that has been injected by the athlete. This test was used experimentally at the Athens Olympic Games in 2004 and at the Torino Winter Olympic Games in 2006 (Saugy *et al.* 2006). To fulfil WADA requirements, two double tests were applied to serum samples. The first test quantified the 22-kDa isoform that is derived from recombinant GH. The second test measured the other isoforms derived from naturally occurring GH. When recombinant GH is administered, endogenous growth hormone secretion is inhibited; therefore, the ratio of 22 kDa to total GH increases. The ratio between these isoforms is calculated. A second double sample test was used for confirmatory purposes (Bidlingmaier and Strasburger 2000).

The direct test was also used at the 2008 Beijing Olympic Games. However, as in Athens and Torino, no positive test results were detected. This outcome may have been unsurprising because the method has a relatively short (less than 24 hour) window of opportunity. Therefore, any athlete who discontinues his or her use of GH on the day before the test would not be detected (Holt *et al.* 2009).

The indirect markers approach to GH doping detection

The indirect approach does not aim to detect GH itself but to build up a database of the normal range of a number of markers for GH. It has been suggested that this approach would not stand up in court as absolute proof of doping (Saugy *et al.* 2006). However, the results of the GH-2000 and GH-2004 studies supported the choice of IGF-1 and P-III-P as markers to detect GH in samples for several days after recombinant GH administration (Erotokritou-Mulligan *et al.* 2007).

A new test for GH was introduced for the first time at the London 2012 Olympic and Paralympic Games. This was the GH biomarker test, which detects increases in the biomarkers for GH: IGF-1 and procollagen-3 n-terminal peptide (Powrie *et al.* 2007; Erotokiritou-Mulligan *et al.* 2007). Unlike previous tests for GH, which could only detect the use of the hormone for a very short period of time, the biomarker test detects GH use for at least 1 week after it has been taken.

Two athletes at the London 2012 Paralympic Games tested positive for GH and were excluded from the Games, marking a successful introduction at a major event for the new GH biomarker test. In March 2014, WADA announced advances to the GH biomarker test, through the use of liquid chromatography-tandem mass spectrometry. This method provides increased precision for the measurement of IGF-1 (Partnership for Clean Competition 2014). Another approach that international federations are adopting is longitudinal studies on athletes' biological profiles. By regularly monitoring haematological and steroidal profiles, any abnormalities would reveal potential doping activity. This technique of Athlete Biological Passports is described in Chapter 10.

Cases of growth hormone abuse in sport

A test for GH was first introduced at the Athens 2004 Olympic Games. However, this test could only detect GH use during a very short period of time after use. A validated test with an extended detection window was introduced in 2012.

Terry Newton (2010)

Terry Newton was the first case of GH use resulting in an athlete sanction. This rugby league player was tested out of competition in November 2009, when GH was detected in a blood sample. Newton accepted the charge of doping and was banned for 2 years. Sadly, Newton committed suicide during this period; whilst not directly attributed to his positive drug test, it was clearly a factor in his tragic death. Andy Parkinson, UK Anti-Doping Chief Executive, stated that 'The positive finding was a combination of intelligence, target testing and a strong partnership with anti-doping scientific community and the Rugby Football League' (http://www.ukad.org.uk/news/article/newton-gets-two-years-for-world-first-hgh-finding).

Nikolay Marfin and Vadim Rakitin (2012)

These two Russian powerlifters tested positive for GH a week before the start of the London 2012 Paralympic Games. Before the test results were announced, Rakitin competed in the men's under-90 kg class, finishing seventh. Marfin was prevented from competing in the 100-plus kg class. Both athletes were subsequently given 2-year bans. These cases were the first successes for the newly developed biomarker test for GH, as described in this chapter.

6.8. Growth factors

In addition to IGF-1, there are a wide range of growth factors that are prohibited in sport (Table 6.1). Their prohibition is due to their role in muscle-specific signal transduction pathways involved in the growth and development of skeletal muscle. The mammalian target of rapamycin (mTOR) and myostatin pathways are the most important in terms of muscle growth.

The mTOR pathway integrates signals in response to exercise and energy levels, namely IGF-1; insulin; mechano growth factor (MGF), which is expressed in response to the stimulus of muscle stretch during exercise; dietary protein; and energy levels. The overall effect is an increase in muscle protein synthesis. The myostatin pathway unsurprisingly has a negative effect on protein synthesis and thus muscle growth. Potential pharmacological and gene therapy to inhibit myostatin would be of great interest to the unscrupulous athlete; therefore, they are discussed further in Chapters 8 and 12.

Whilst early research showed that hypertrophy in response to resistance exercise was associated with increased IGF-1 expression, it was unable to distinguish between the different types of growth factors. In fact, the increased IGF-1 reflected an increase in MGF, a local signalling molecule (i.e. an autocrine) derived from the IGF-1 gene. MGF promotes hypertrophy and repair associated with exercise-induced muscle damage by activating muscle stem cells and anabolic processes (Goldspink 2005). Although MGF has not been approved for therapeutic use, it is available on the black market (Esposito *et al*. 2012). As yet, no test has been developed for its detection.

Other growth factors that have been identified to play their part in enhancing muscle size and function include transforming growth factor-β, platelet-derived growth factor, fibroblast growth factor (FGF), epidermal growth factor, vascular endothelial growth factor (VEGF), and endothelial cell growth factor. Such growth factors are particularly important in the regenerative process following trauma as a consequence of exercise-induced muscle damage and injury.

FGF-1 is one such growth factor that has local effects in terms of promoting muscle repair angiogenesis. Whilst FGF-1 is not an approved pharmacological agent, an analysis of black market products isolated FGF-1; it was found to be slightly different from recombinant FGF-1, thus highlighting the real risk that individuals take when using unlicensed products from the black market (Walpurgis *et al*. 2011).

The practice of blood spinning has been the topic of much discussion within anti-doping circles in recent years. Blood spinning is the controversial practice of creating platelet-rich plasma (PRP) from an individual's blood by centrifugation and injecting it at a site of injury. Platelet-rich plasma is known to contain high concentrations of growth factors, which are believed to enhance the healing process. Whilst this practice in the treatment of injury is currently not prohibited, the use of growth factors *per se* is. For this reason, there are concerns as to whether the practice of intramuscular application of PRP influences systemic circulating growth factors (Schippinger *et al*. 2012). Indeed, work by Wasterlain *et al*. (2013) found that serum IGF-1, VEGF, and FGF-2 were significantly elevated after PRP administration, thus demonstrating potential ergogenic effects. Further research in this area will enable WADA to make an informed decision regarding the status of PRP administration in athletes.

Other than their potential as doping agents, the possible downside of the use of growth factors, particularly in targeting the mTOR pathway, is that by increasing protein synthesis, widespread growth (not solely in skeletal muscle) is promoted. Clearly, stimulation of growth may have negative effects in tissues. Also, because the mTOR pathway is a focus for anticancer drugs (Lui *et al*. 2009), it is conceivable that growth factors may have carcinogenic effects.

6.9. Prevalence of peptide hormone use in sport

Statistics on the number of adverse analytical findings related to peptide hormone, as recorded by WADA-accredited laboratories between 2006 and 2012, are shown in Table 6.2.

In general, there is an increasing trend toward the detection of peptide hormones, in part due to improved methods of analysis. The extension of the use of Athlete Biological Passports (see Chapter 10) will further improve rates of detection, particularly for EPO. However, Ashenden *et al.* (2011) suggested that improvements are needed to identify doping with EPO through microdosing.

6.10. Peptide hormones as potential targets for gene doping

A review by van der Gronde *et al.* (2013) highlighted peptide hormones as potential targets for gene doping because many of these hormones are being investigated for their beneficial use in gene therapy. A detailed explanation of gene doping is presented in Chapter 12.

6.11. Summary

- A number of peptide hormones that occur naturally in the body are included on the WADA Prohibited List.
- EPO increases red blood cell counts, thereby enhancing oxygen supply to muscles and other tissues.
- Illicit use of EPO can be detected in the laboratory either directly or through recording of Athlete Biological Passport markers.
- Chorionic gonadotrophin and luteinizing hormone have the potential to increase endogenous testosterone levels.
- Growth hormone has a number of significant biological effects, including an increase in muscle mass and strength. It also possesses serious potential side effects.
- The effects of GH are mediated through IGF-1, which is used to detect GH use through the biomarker test.
- Localised growth factors that are central to increased muscle size and function would appear to be infiltrating the muscle-building supplements market. The need for a validated test for their detection is therefore necessary.
- The practice of injecting platelet-rich plasma in the treatment of injury would appear to be widespread, yet the effects on the systemic circulation of growth factors would suggest that this may offer a potential performance-enhancing effect.

6.12. References

Ashenden, M., Gough, C. E., Garnham, A., *et al.* (2011). Current markers of athlete blood passport do not flag microdose EPO doping. *European Journal of Applied Physiology* 111(9): 2307–2314.

Ashenden, M., Varlet-Marie, E., Lasne, F., and Audran, M. (2006). The effects of microdose recombinant human erythropoietin regimens in athletes. *Haematologica* 91(8):1143–1144.

Barroso, O., Schamasch, P., and Rabin, O. (2009). Detection of GH abuse in sport: Past, present and future. *Growth Hormone and IGF Research* 19(4):369–374.

Bidlingmaier, M., Wu, Z., and Strasburger, C. J. (2000) Test method: GH. *Best Clinical Endocrinology and Metabolism* 14(1):99–109.

Birkeland, K. I., Stray-Gundersen, J., Hemmersbach, P., *et al.* (2000). Effect of r-HuEPO administration on serum levels of sTfR and cycling performance. *Medicine and Science in Sports and Exercise* 32(7):1238–1243.

Boisclair, Y. R., Rhoads, R. P., Ueki, I., *et al.* (2001). The acid labile subunits (ALS) of the 150 KDq IGF-binding protein complex: An important but forgotten component of the circulating IGF system. *Journal of Endocrinology* 170(1):3–70.

Brooks, R. V., Collyer, S. P., Kicman, A. T., *et al.* (1989). CG doping in sport and methods for its detection. In P. Bellot, G. Benzi, and A. Ljungavist (Eds.), *Official Proceedings of Second IAF World Symposium on Doping in Sport* (pp. 37–45). Monaco: International Athletics Foundation.

Brower, K. J. (2000). Assessment and treatment of anabolic steroid abuse, dependence and withdrawal. In C. Yesalis (Ed.), *Anabolic Steroids in Sport and Exercise* (2nd ed., pp. 305–332). Champaign, IL: Human Kinetics.

Cazzola, M. (2001). Erythropoietin pathophysiology, clinical uses of recombinant human erythropoietin, and medical risks of its abuse in sport. In *The International Society for Laboratory Hematology (ISLH) XIVth International Symposium* (p. 21). Charlottesville, VA: Carden Jennings.

Consitt, L. A., Copeland, J. L., and Tremblay, M. S. (2002). Hormonal responses to exercise in women. *Sports Medicine* 32(1):1–22.

Cowart, V. (1988). Human grown hormone: The latest ergogenic aid? *Physician and Sport Medicine* 16(3):175–175.

Deyssig, R., Firsch, H., Blum, W. F., *et al.* (1993). Effect of growth hormone treatment and hormonal parameters, body composition and strength in athletes. *Acta Endocrinologica (Copenhagen)* 128(4): 313–318.

Dine, G. (2001). Biochemical and haematological parameters in athletes. In *The International Society for Laboratory Hematology (ISLH) XIVth International Symposium* (p. 24).

Ehrnborg, C., Bengtsson, B. A., and Rosen, T. (2000). Growth hormone abuse. *Best Clinical Endocrinology and Metabolism* 14(1):71–77.

Ekblom, B. (1997). Blood doping, erythropoetin and altitude. In T. Reilly and M. Orme (Eds.), *The Clinical Pharmacology of Sport and Exercise* (pp. 199–212). Amsterdam: Elsevier.

Ekblom, B., and Berglund, B. (1991). Effect of erythropoietin administration on maximal aerobic power. *Scandinavian Journal of Medicine and Science in Sports* 1(1):88–93.

Elliott, S. (2008). Erythropoiesis-stimulating agents and other methods to enhance oxygen transport. *British Journal of Pharmacology* 154(3):529–541.

Erotokritou-Mulligan, I., Bassett, E. E., and Kniess, A. (2007). Validation of the growth hormone (GH)-dependent marker method of detecting GH abuse in sport through the use of independent data sets. *Growth Hormone and IGF Research* 17(5):416–423.

Esposito, S., Deventer, K., and Van Eenoo, P. (2012). Characterization and identification of a C-terminal amidated mechano growth factor (MGF) analogue in black market products. *Rapid Communications in Mass Spectrometry* 26(6):686–692.

Evans, N. A. (1997). Gym and tonic: A profile of 100 anabolic steroid users. *British Journal of Sports Medicine* 31(1):54–58.

Goldspink, G. (2005). Research on mechano growth factor: Its potential for optimising physical training as well as misuse in doping. *British Journal of Sports Medicine* 39(11):787–788.

Gotherstrom, G., Bengtsson, B.-A., Sunnerhagen, K. S., *et al.* (2005). The effect of five-year growth hormone replacement therapy on muscle strength in elderly hypopituitary patients. *Clinical Endocrinology* 62(1):105–113.

Guha, N., Cowan, D. A., Sonksen, P. H., *et al.* (2013). Insulin-like growth factor-1 (IGF-1) misuse in athletes and potential methods for detection. *Analytical and Bioanalytical Chemistry* 405(30):9669–9683.

Hendelsman, D. J. (2006). The rationale for banning human chorionic gonadotrophin and estrogen blockers in sport. *Journal of Clinical Endocrinology and Metabolism* 91(5):1646–1653.

Hendelsman, D. J., Goebel, C., Idan, A., *et al.* (2009). Effects of recombinant human LH and CG on serum and urine LH and androgens in man. *Clinical Endocrinology* 71(3):417–428.

Holt, R. I. G. (2004). The metabolic effects of growth hormone. *CME Bulletin of Endocrinological Diabetes* 5(1):11–17.

Holt, R. I. G., Erotokritou-Mulligan, I., and Sonksen, P. H. (2009). The history of doping and growth hormone abuse in sport. *Growth Hormone and IGF Research* 19(4):320–326.

Holt, R. I. G., and Sonksen, P. H. (2008). Growth hormone, IGF-1 and insulin and their abuse in sport. *British Journal of Pharmacology* 154(3):542–556.

Kemp, S. F. (2007). Mecasermin rinfabate. *Drugs Today* 43:149–155.

Kicman, A. T., Brooks, R. V., and Cowan, D. A. (1991). Human chorionic gonadotrophin and sport. *British Journal of Sports Medicine* 25(2):73–80.

Kicman, A. T., and Cowan, D. A. (1992). Peptide hormones and sport: Misuse and detection. *British Medical Bulletin* 48(3):496–517.

Kimmage. P. (1998). *Rough Ride*. London, UK: Yellow Jersey Press.

Korkia, P., and Stimson, G. V. (1997). Indications and prevalence, practice and effects of anabolic steroid use in Great Britain. *International Journal of Sports Medicine* 18(1):557–562.

Lasne, F., and de Ceaurriz, J. (2000). Recombinant erythropoietin in urine. *Nature* 405(6787):635.

Le Roith, D., Bondy, C., Yakar, S., et al. (2001). The somatomedin hypothesis. *Endocrinological Review* 22(1):53–74.

Leith, W. (1992, July). EPO and cycling. *Athletics* 24–26.

Lombardo, J. A., Hickson, P. C. and Lamb, D. R. (1991). Anabolic/androgenic steroids and growth hormone. In D.R. Lamb and M.H. Williams (Eds.), *Perspectives in Exercise Science and Sports Medicine, Vol. 4: Ergogenics – Enhancement of Performance in Exercise and Sport* (pp. 249–278). New York, NY: Brown & Benchmark.

Lui, Q., Thoreen, C., Wang, J., et al. (2009). mTOR mediated anti-cancer drug discovery. *Drug Discovery Today: Therapeutic Strategies* 6(2):47–55.

Macintyre, J. G. (1987). Growth hormone and athletes. *Sports Medicine* 4(2):129–142.

Marcus, R., and Hoffman, A. R. (1998). Growth hormone as therapy for older men and women. *Annual Review of Pharmacology and Toxicology* 38(1):45–61.

McHugh, C. M., Park, R. T., Sonksen, P. H., et al. (2005). Challenges in detecting the abuse of growth hormone in sport. *Clinical Chemistry* 51(9):1587–1593.

Mottram, D. R. (2013). The Lance Armstrong case: The evidence behind the headlines. *Aspetar Sports Medicine Journal* 2(1):60–65.

Muller, E. E. (1987). Neural control of somatotropic function. *Physiological Review* 67(3):962–1053.

Norton, K., and Olds, T. (2001). Morphological evolution of athletes over the 20th century. *Sports Medicine* 31(11):763–783.

Parisotto, R., Wu, M., Ashenden, M. J., et al. (2001). Detection of recombinant human erythropoietin abuse in athletes utilizing markers of altered erythropoiesis. *Haematologica* 86(2):128–137.

Partnership for Clean Competition. (2014). New discoveries by scientific working group could advance ability to detect HGH doping in sport. Available online at https://www.cleancompetition.org/news-room/press/releases/New-Discoveries-by-Scientific-Working-Group-Could-Advance-Ability-to-Detect-HGH-Doping-in-Sport) (accessed 31 March 2014).

Powrie, J. K., Bassett, E. E., Rosen, T., et al. (2007). Detection of growth hormone abuse in sport. *Growth Hormone and IGF Research* 17(3):220–226.

Rendell, M. (2006). *The Death of Marco Pantani: A Biography*. London, UK: Weidenfeld & Nicolson.

Rennie, M. J. (2003). Claims for the anabolic effects of growth hormone: A case of the emperor's new clothes? *British Journal of Sports Medicine* 37(2):100–105.

Reznik, Y., Dehennin, L., Coffin, C., et al. (2001). Urinary nandrolone metabolites of endogenous origin in man: A confirmation by output regulation under human chorionic gonadotropin stimulation. *Journal of Clinical Endocrinology and Metabolism* 86(1):146–150.

Rickert, V. I., Pawlak-Morello, C., Sheppard, V., et al. (1992). Human growth hormone: A new substance of abuse among adolescents? *Clinical Paediatrics* 31(12):723–726.

Saugy, M., Robinson, M., Saudan, C., et al. (2006). Human growth hormone doping in sport. *British Journal of Sports Medicine* 40(Suppl 1):i35–i39.

Schippinger, G., Fankhauser, F., Oettl, K., *et al.* (2012). Does single intramuscular application of autologous conditioned plasma influence systemic circulating growth factors? *Journal of Sports Science and Medicine* 11(3):551–556.

Schnirring, L. (2000). Growth hormone doping: The search for a test. *Physician and Sports Medicine* 28(1):1–6.

Smith, D. A., and Perry, P. J. (1992). The efficacy of ergogenic agents in athletic competition. Part II. Other performance enhancing agents. *Annals of Pharmacotherapy* 26(5):653–659.

Sonksen, P. (2001). Insulin growth hormone and sport. *Journal of Endocrinology* 170(1):13–15.

Stenman, U.-H., Hotakainen, K., and Alfthan, H. (2008). Gonadotrophins in doping: Pharmacological basis and detection of illicit use. *British Journal of Pharmacology* 154(3):569–583.

Stow, M. R., Wojek, N., and Marshall, J. (2009). The UK Sport perspective on detecting growth hormone abuse. *Growth Hormone and IGF Research* 19(4):375–377.

Taaffe, D. R., Jin, I. H., Vu, T. H., *et al.* (1996). Lack of effect of recombinant human growth hormone (GH) on muscle morphology and GH-insulin-like growth factor expression in resistance trained elderly men. *Journal of Clinical Endocrinology and Metabolism* 81(1):421–425.

Taylor, W. N. (1988). Synthetic human growth hormone. A call for federal control. *Physician and Sports Medicine* 16(2):189–192.

Tsitisimpikou, C., Kouretas, D., Tsarouhas, K., *et al.* (2011). Applications and biomonitoring issues of recombinant erythropoietins for doping control. *Therapeutic Drug Monitoring* 33(1):3–13.

van der Gronde, T., de Hon, O., Haisma, H. J., *et al* (2013). Gene doping: An overview and current implications for athletes. *British Journal of Sports Medicine* 47(11):670–678.

Velloso, C. P. (2008). Regulation of muscle mass by growth hormone and IGF-1. *British Journal of Pharmacology* 154(3):557–568.

Voet, W. (2001). *Breaking the Chain*. London, UK: Yellow Jersey Press.

Wallace, J. D., Cuneo, R. C., Bidlingmaier, M., *et al.* (2001). The response of molecular isoforms of growth hormone to acute exercise in trained adult males. *Journal of Clinical Endocrinology and Metabolism* 86(1):200–206.

Walpurqis, K., Thomas, A., Laussmann, T., *et al.* (2011). Identification of fibroblast growth factor 1 (FGF-1) in a black market product. *Drug Testing and Analysis* 3(11–12):791–797.

Wasterlain, A. S., Braun, H. J., Harris, A. H. S., *et al.* (2013). The systemic effects of platelet-rich plasma injection. *American Journal of Sports Medicine* 41(1):186–193.

Wells, D. J. (2008). Gene doping: The hype and the reality. *British Journal of Pharmacology* 154(3):573–574.

World Anti-Doping Agency. (2014a). The 2014 Prohibited List International Standard. Available online at https://wada-main-prod.s3.amazonaws.com/resources/files/WADA-Revised-2014-Prohibited-List-EN. PDF (accessed 11 September 2014).

World Anti-Doping Agency. (2014b). Harmonization of analysis and reporting of erythropoiesis stimulating agents (ESAs) by electrophoretic techniques. Available online at https://wada-main-prod.s3.amazonaws. com/resources/files/WADA-TD2014EPO-v1-Harmonization-of-Analysis-and-Reporting-of-ESAs-by-Electrophoretic-Techniques-EN.pdf (accessed 9 September 2014).

Yarasheski, K. E., Campbell, J. A., Smith, K., *et al.* (1992). Effect of growth hormone and resistance exercise on muscle growth in young men. *American Journal of Physiology* 262(3):E261–E267.

Yarasheski, K. E., Zachweija, J. J., Angelopoulis, T. J., *et al.* (1993). Short-term grown hormone treatment does not increase muscle protein synthesis in experienced weightlifters. *Journal of Applied Physiology* 74(6):3073–3076.

Yarasheski, K. E., Zachwieja, J. J., Campbell, J. A., and Bier, D. M. (1995). Effect of growth hormone and resistance exercise on muscle growth and strength in older men. *American Journal of Physiology* 268(2 Pt 1):E268–E276.

Chapter 7

Beta-2 agonists

Neil Chester and David R. Mottram

7.1. Introduction

Maximum performance in aerobic events, at whatever level of competition, is only achievable if respiratory function is optimal. Competitors will always be concerned about respiratory problems, be they major diseases (e.g. asthma) or minor ailments (e.g. the common cold). Respiratory function may be compromised in athletes who suffer from long-term medical conditions, such as asthma, for which one of the first-line classes of drugs is beta-2 agonists. These drugs produce their therapeutic effect through bronchodilation. Clearly, such an effect has the potential to enhance athletic performance by improving oxygen uptake. However, research in support of such performance enhancement is limited. Nonetheless, beta-2 agonists exist as a category on the World Anti-Doping Agency (WADA) Prohibited List, subject to a complex set of regulations. Because beta-2 agonists are a necessary component in the treatment regimens for patients with asthma, Therapeutic Use Exemptions (TUEs) may be requested for these athletes to allow them to compete on equal terms with fellow competitors. Some beta-2 agonists, such as clenbuterol, possess anabolic properties, although through a mechanism that is different from that produced by anabolic steroids; this is an additional reason for inclusion under the category of anabolic agents on the WADA Prohibited List.

This chapter reviews asthma and other bronchoconstriction-related conditions, as well as the types of drugs used in their treatment, with particular emphasis on beta-2 agonists. The misuse of these drugs in sport is reviewed, along with the systems in place for controlling beta-2 agonists as performance-enhancing agents whilst permitting TUEs, where appropriate.

7.2. What are beta-2 agonists?

In Chapter 1, we described how drugs interact through specific targets within the body, known as receptors. These receptors can be classified and subclassified. In the case of adrenoreceptors, through which the hormone adrenaline (epinephrine) produces its effects in the body, we reviewed the five subclasses of these receptors, including the subclass referred to as beta-2 receptors. Drugs have been developed to interact selectively on these receptors. This group of drugs is known as the beta-2 agonists.

Table 7.1 lists some of the more commonly prescribed beta-2 agonists. The table also categorises the drugs as short acting and long acting, which has a significance regarding their clinical use in the treatment of conditions such as asthma and chronic obstructive pulmonary disease.

Table 7.1 Selective beta-2 agonists

Short-acting	Long-acting
Salbutamol	Formoterol (eformoterol)
Terbutaline	Salmeterol
Bambuterol	Indacaterol

Pharmacology of beta-2 agonists

All selective beta-2 agonists are potent bronchodilators. They differ in their time to onset and duration of action. Salbutamol and terbutaline are short acting, and they are the most frequently used beta-2 agonists in the United Kingdom. There are many formulations of salbutamol and terbutaline, including tablets, slow-release tablets, elixirs, aerosols and dry powder, solutions for injection, and inhalation from a nebuliser. Inhalation is the route of choice because it is the most rapidly effective (1–2 minutes) and is associated with the fewest side effects. Tremor is the only common side effect after inhalation. However, other side effects of beta-2 agonists are common (Cockcroft 2006). This led Backer *et al.* (2007) to conclude that antiasthmatic treatment is necessary for patients with asthma, but it should not be used by nonasthmatic elite athletes due to possible systemic effects and side effects.

Side effects after oral administration include fine tremor (usually of the hands), nervous tension, and headache. Tachycardia, peripheral vasodilation, and hypokalaemia may occur after oral dosing. The duration of action of salbutamol and terbutaline after aerosol administration is approximately 4 hours. Formoterol (eformoterol) and salmeterol are the most frequently prescribed long-acting beta-2 agonists, with a duration of action of approximately 12 hours.

7.3. Clinical uses of beta-2 agonists

Asthma and its treatment

Definition

Asthma is a chronic inflammatory disorder of the airways. In susceptible individuals, this inflammation causes recurrent episodes of coughing, wheezing, chest tightness, and difficult breathing. Inflammation makes the airways sensitive to stimuli such as allergens, chemical irritants, tobacco smoke, cold air, or exercise. When exposed to these stimuli, the airways may become swollen, constricted, filled with mucus, and hyper-responsive to stimuli. The resulting airflow limitation is reversible in most patients, either spontaneously or with treatment. Adequate asthma therapy can reduce inflammation over the long term, control symptoms, and prevent most asthma-related problems (Global Initiative for Asthma 2012).

Pathophysiology

An asthma attack always consists of an early phase and frequently contains a late phase. The early phase occurs within minutes of exposure to the trigger factor, reaches a maximum in 15–20 minutes, and normally resolves within an hour. It is caused by bronchoconstriction. The late phase occurs 2–4 hours after exposure to the trigger factor and reaches a maximum after 6–8 hours. It is caused by inflammation of the airways. Appreciation of the change of emphasis from bronchoconstriction to inflammation as the cause of airway obstruction has underpinned the change in approach to the management of asthma.

Trigger factors

Numerous factors can trigger an asthma attack. The most common are allergens, which can be either inhaled (e.g. pollens, animal danders, such as hairs and feathers) or ingested (e.g. dairy produce, strawberries). Viral, but not bacterial, infection of the upper respiratory tract can trigger asthma. Indeed, the initial presenting feature of asthma may be a persistent wheeze after a self-limiting viral upper respiratory tract infection. Occupational pollution can also cause asthma. Asthma attacks also can be precipitated by emotional factors, although this should not be misinterpreted as an indication that asthma is psychosomatic. Rather, it is a reflection of neuroendocrine changes which, as yet, are poorly understood.

Certain drugs may precipitate an asthma attack, such as beta-blockers and nonsteroidal anti-inflammatory drugs (NSAIDs), particularly aspirin. Beta-blockers cause bronchoconstriction by blocking the bronchodilating beta-2 receptors on airway smooth muscle. They should not be administered to asthmatics. The mechanism by which NSAIDs evoke bronchospasm is hypothetical but may involve a shift in balance between bronchodilating and bronchoconstricting metabolites of arachidonic acid. Approximately 10 per cent of asthmatics are aspirin sensitive and will bronchoconstrict if given the drug. For this reason, aspirin and other NSAIDs should be used with caution in asthmatics. An asthmatic may be sensitive to a variety of trigger factors or to just one.

Management of asthma

Nondrug treatment of asthma involves avoidance of known trigger factors. Drug treatment of asthma is primarily directed at arresting and reversing the inflammatory process, with the emphasis shifting from the excessive and inappropriate use of beta-2 agonist bronchodilator therapy toward the earlier use of anti-inflammatory drugs. Beta-2 agonists merely relieve the symptoms of asthma without addressing the underlying inflammation. Guidelines for the treatment of chronic asthma have been prepared in several countries. They constitute a systematic approach to the treatment of increasing severity of symptoms.

Essentially, the first step involves the occasional use of short-acting inhaled beta-2 agonists to relieve the symptoms of bronchoconstriction. Thereafter, depending on the severity, more regular use of short-acting beta-2 agonists is recommended, with inhaled corticosteroids. If the symptoms are more severe, long-acting beta-2 agonists or other bronchodilators are used with inhaled corticosteroids. Corticosteroids are subject to WADA regulations, as described in Chapter 16. It must be remembered that the treatment of asthma can also be stepped down if the severity of the symptoms declines.

Exercise-induced asthma and exercise-induced bronchoconstriction

Exercise-induced asthma (EIA) can be defined as a lower airway obstruction and symptoms of cough, wheezing, or dyspnoea induced by exercise in patients with underlying asthma (Schwartz et al. 2008). The same presentation of symptoms in individuals without asthma can be defined as exercise-induced bronchoconstriction (EIB).

EIB probably includes an interplay between environmental training factors, such as allergens, temperature, humidity, air pollutants, and an athlete's personal risk factors, such as genetic and neuroimmunoendocrine determinants (Moreira *et al.* 2011).

Diagnosis of asthma and exercise-induced bronchoconstriction

A major issue with respect to ensuring the effective health care of individuals with respiratory conditions such as asthma relates to accurate diagnosis. However, there is no standardised diagnosis of asthma as a consequence of the fact that no consistent definition of the symptoms exists (British Thoracic Society 2012). Along with the clinician taking a clinical history, individuals who present with asthma symptoms will typically undertake a simple peak flow assessment. Unfortunately, a normal peak flow recorded whilst an individual is asymptomatic does not preclude a positive diagnosis of asthma.

A number of tests include the assessment of lung function before and after a bronchoprovocation challenge. A marked reduction in lung function from baseline (typically >10 per cent drop in the forced expiratory volume in 1 second) is required for an individual to test positive to a specific bronchoprovocation challenge and thus form the basis of a diagnosis of asthma or EIB. Bronchoprovocation challenges may include the administration of histamine, mannitol, metacholine, and saline or a bout of exercise.

Whilst an exercise challenge is the most ecologically valid test, it is difficult to control factors such as ventilation and environmental conditions. The Eucapnic Voluntary Hyperpnea (EVH) challenge has been established to mimic exercise in a controlled manner. The test involves an individual attaining a minute ventilation equivalent to 85 per cent of his or her predicted maximal voluntary ventilation rate for 6 minutes during which dry, CO_2-rich air (<2 per cent relative humidity and 5 per cent CO_2) is inhaled. The EVH challenge has been shown to be particularly sensitive in the assessment of EIB in athletes and has subsequently been adopted as the method of choice by the International Olympic Committee (IOC) medical commission in the diagnosis of EIB and support of subsequent prescription of inhaled beta-2 agonists (Whyte 2013).

Implementation of such tests has not only unearthed previously undiagnosed asthma but also misdiagnosis (Dickinson *et al.* 2011). In a significant number of individuals previously diagnosed with asthma, there was no confirmation following detailed assessment. In such cases, it is likely that individuals may suffer from dysfunctional breathing brought on by stressful situations during exercise. Dysfunctional breathing is a loose term, also known as hyperventilation syndrome and disproportionate breathlessness (Morgan 2002). It includes several breathing abnormalities associated with the following symptoms: breathlessness, chest tightness, chest pain, unsteady and irregular breathing, and nondiaphragmatic respiratory effort (Thomas *et al.* 2005). Whilst dysfunctional breathing commonly accompanies asthma, it may also exist in those without asthma (Thomas *et al.* 2005).

No criterion standard method of diagnosis exists. However, the Nijmegen questionnaire (van Dixhoorn and Duivenvoorden 1985) is commonly used to identify those with symptoms. Together with an objective test to diagnose asthma and EIB (involving a provocation challenge), the Nijmegan questionnaire may be used to identify those exhibiting symptoms associated with dysfunctional breathing only.

Clearly, the significance of establishing a criterion standard method of diagnosis lies in the notion that methods of treatment other than pharmacotherapy may be prescribed. Further research is needed, not only in diagnosis but in the development and application of nonpharmacological treatment, including breathing technique training.

Prevalence of exercise-induced asthma and exercise-induced bronchoconstriction in athletes

A consistent body of evidence has shown that Olympic-level athletes have an increased risk for asthma, especially those taking part in endurance sports or winter sports (Carlsen *et al.* 2008a). The incidence of asthma is reported to be more common in elite athletes than in the general population. A review of previous studies by Parsons and Mastronarde (2005) revealed that prevalence rates for bronchospasm related to exercise ranged from 11 to 50 per cent. Furthermore, up to 90 per cent of subjects with asthma will have EIA. The highest prevalence of EIA has been noted in athletes competing in the winter season, due to exposure to cold, dry air (Weiler and Ryan 2000).

The high prevalence of asthma in swimmers and other athletes training in indoor pools can be explained by exposure to chlorine and its derivatives (Langdeau and Boulet 2001). Pedersen *et al.* (2008) believe that elite swimmers do not have particularly susceptible airways when they take up competitive swimming when young but develop respiratory symptoms, airway inflammation, and airway hyperresponsiveness during their swimming careers. Similarly, Fitch (2006) reported that of the 193 athletes who met the IOC's criteria for the use of beta-2 agonists at the 2006 Winter Olympics, only 32.1 per cent had childhood asthma; 48.7 percent of the athletes reported onset at age 20 years or older. This led the authors to speculate that years of intense endurance training may be a causative factor in bronchial hyperreactivity.

The higher prevalence of airway hyperresponsiveness measured in athletes coupled with the use of subjective methods to diagnose asthma may mean that the prevalence of respiratory problems in athletes is underdiagnosed (Langdeau and Boulet 2003). A review by Carlsen *et al.* (2008a) confirmed the view that the prevalence of asthma and bronchial hyperresponsiveness is markedly increased in athletes, especially within endurance sports, and that environmental factors often contribute to this increase. These authors provided recommendations for the diagnosis of asthma in athletes. A review by Fitch (2012) concluded that asthma is the commonest chronic medical condition experienced by Olympic athletes, and that years of endurance training may be a contributory factor. The increased exposure through sporting activity to environmental agents, such as cold dry air in skiers and chlorine compounds in swimmers, increases symptoms and signs of asthma and bronchial hyperresponsiveness, either worsening an existing asthma or leading to a novel disease in a previously healthy athlete (Carlsen *et al.* 2011).

Management of exercise-induced asthma and exercise-induced bronchoconstriction

The management of EIB should involve preventative/nonpharmacological measures as well as treatment with drugs, such as beta-2 agonists (Schumacher *et al.* 2011; Anderson and Kippelen 2012; Ansley *et al.* 2013).

Nondrug treatment

Fitness does not prevent EIA. However, aerobic fitness does improve lung function, retards deterioration in lung function with age (in nonasthmatics), and enables asthmatics to exercise with less EIA. There is no evidence to suggest that aerobic training is deleterious to asthmatics, provided that their treatment is optimal and that they have a satisfactory management plan, which includes access to appropriate bronchodilator therapy if required.

Minimisation of the cooling and drying of the airways can be achieved by nasal breathing, whenever possible. Susceptible individuals should seek to avoid exercising in a cold, dry environment. If this is unavoidable, then a face mask may reduce cooling and drying of the airways.

The inhalation of particulate matter, a key component of air pollution, may have a detrimental effect on exercising athletes. Cutrufello *et al.* (2012) provided some useful advice for athletes on how to avoid the inhalation of particulate matter during exercise.

Drug treatment for exercise-induced asthma and exercise-induced bronchoconstriction with beta-2 agonists

A review by Carlsen *et al.* (2008a) of the treatment of EIA concluded that it should be treated in athletes along the same principles as for nonathletes because there is little evidence for improvement in athletic performance by inhaled beta-2 agonists.

Beta-2 agonists are the most effective prophylactic treatment of EIA. Short-acting beta-2 agonists (Table 7.1) should be administered 15–30 minutes before commencing exercise (Rupp 1996; Lacroix 1999). They induce bronchodilation within 5 minutes and afford protection against EIA for approximately 3–6 hours. They also prevent asthma symptoms in 90 per cent of patients (Lacroix 1999).

Beta-2 agonists should be available to the athlete for rapid relief of symptoms should they develop despite pre-exercise treatment. Salmeterol, a long-acting beta-2 agonist, should be taken 30 minutes before exercise; it is effective for up to 9 hours (Nelson *et al.* 1998). Because of its slower onset of action, salmeterol should not be used as a rescue medication to relieve symptoms of an asthma attack.

7.4. The illicit use of beta-2 agonists in sport

Prevalence of beta-2 agonists in sport

Beta-2 agonists have been a target for athletes for many years. They have appeared in large numbers on the WADA annual statistics for adverse analytical findings (Table 7.2). These annual

Table 7.2 WADA statistics for the number of adverse analytical findings for substances classed as beta-2 agonists (2005–2012)

	2005	2006	2007	2008	2009	2010	2011	2012
Salbutamol	357	391	60	56	29	9	6	6
Terbutaline	171	175	182	163	157	111	130	117
Formoterol	18	42	107	91	84	78	84	–
Salmeterol	4	16	37	30	23	6	1	3
Fenoterol	3	5	11	10	5	5	2	5
Reproterol	4	2	2	–	3	–	1	–
Bitodrine	–	–	–	–	1	–	–	–
Pirbuterol	–	–	–	–	1	–	–	–
Bambuterol	–	–	–	–	–	–	1	–
Clenbuterol*	52	53	53	73	67	116	129	98
Total	609	684	452	423	370	325	354	229

Results on beta-2 agonists include adverse findings for which the athlete may have been granted a Therapeutic Use Exemption under WADA regulations.
* Recorded under Anabolic Agents from 2006.

figures for positive test results for beta-2 agonists include cases where athletes have received permission to use the drugs for therapeutic purposes. However, it has been acknowledged that there has been a marked increase in applications to use short-acting beta-2 agonists (Fitch *et al.* 2008).

Figures for the percentage of all athletes applying to inhale beta-2 agonists at Summer Olympic Games show 3.6 per cent at Atlanta in 1996, 5.7 per cent at Sydney in 2000, and 4.6 per cent at Athens in 2004 (Carlsen *et al.* 2008a). The equivalent figures for the Winter Olympic Games were higher, with 5.6 per cent at Nagano in 1998, 6.3 per cent at Salt Lake City in 2002, and 8.3 per cent at Torino in 2006 (Carlsen *et al.* 2008a), perhaps reflecting the higher incidence of EIA in cold conditions.

Cases involving beta-2 agonists

There are few high-profile cases involving drugs commonly used to combat the symptoms of asthma. However, in response to a case involving the detection of high levels of salbutamol in a rugby league player, there has been renewed interest in the possible misuse of such drugs.

Ian Sibbit (2009)

Despite holding a TUE for the use of salbutamol, Ian Sibbit, a Rugby Football League player, was accused of misusing the drug and not following prescription guidelines. However, confusion exists because it is typically prescribed on an as-needed basis or *pro re nata*. This can be misunderstood and viewed as permission to use the drug as many times as required, which may ultimately lead to the administration of doses in excess of the recommended maximal therapeutic doses (400 µg up to four times daily) by individuals with poorly controlled asthma. The player was eventually acquitted following appeal and advised on how to manage his condition more effectively.

Most high-profile cases involve the use of clenbuterol, which is misused typically for its anabolic effects.

The Festina Affair (1998)

Clenbuterol was one of the frequently used drugs cited by Willy Voet in his account of the notorious Festina Affair in the 1998 Tour de France cycle race (Voet 2001).

Jessica Hardy (2008)

Jessica Hardy was dropped from the US Olympic team 1 month before the 2008 Beijing Olympic Games after testing positive for clenbuterol. She claimed that she had accidentally ingested the banned substance when taking a nutritional supplement. The Arbitration Panel for Sport accepted her claim and reduced her suspension from 2 years to 1 year.

Alberto Contador (2010)

The Spanish professional cyclist Albert Contador tested positive for clenbuterol during the 2010 Tour de France, an event which he won. His victory was subsequently annulled and he received a 2-year suspension from competition. Contador's defence included the claim that his positive test was as a consequence of contaminated meat in his diet (see Chapter 5).

Do beta-2 agonists enhance performance?

Several studies have investigated the effects of inhaled beta-2 agonists, both in asthmatic and in healthy athletes. Few studies have reported an increase in exercise performance following inhaled treatment (Signorile *et al.* 1992; van Baak *et al.* 2004). The majority of studies failed to show an ergogenic effect (Morton and Fitch 1992; Norris *et al.* 1996; Larsson *et al.* 2005; Carlsen *et al.* 2008b; Kippelen *et al.* 2012). Inhaled salbutamol, even in high doses, did not have a significant effect on endurance performance in nonasthmatic, highly trained cyclists (Goubault *et al.* 2001). These authors did note that salbutamol had a slight but significant bronchodilator effect, which may be sufficient to improve respiratory adaptation at the beginning of exercise. However, they further concluded that it is unlikely that the widespread use of salbutamol by athletes is driven by the weak effects of the inhaled drug.

A study by Elers *et al.* (2012a) concluded that no ergogenic effect of a high dose of salbutamol on aerobic capacity was found in healthy trained men. In a review of twenty randomised, placebo-controlled studies, only three studies reported a performance-enhancing effect of inhaled beta-2 agonists (Kindermann and Meyer 2006), although methodological shortcomings were cited as being factors in the findings. These authors concluded that there is no ergogenic potential of inhaled beta-2 agonists in nonasthmatic athletes and questioned the inclusion of inhaled beta-2 agonists on the list of WADA prohibited substances.

In cold environments, where athletes with EIA are more likely to experience symptoms of the condition, inhaled formoterol did not improve endurance performance in healthy, well-trained male athletes (Tjørhom *et al.* 2007). The authors therefore concluded that formoterol can be used in competitive sports without fear of a possible performance-enhancing effect.

Fitch (2012) reported that Olympic athletes with asthma and airway hyperresponsiveness have consistently outperformed their peers, which research suggests is not due to their treatment-enhancing sports performance. Although studies using inhaled beta-2 agonists have generally failed to show improved performance, a review by Collomp *et al.* (2010) reported that almost all research trials after acute or short-term oral administration at therapeutic dosage levels demonstrated significant improved performance, whatever the exercise intensity.

Anabolic effects of beta-2 agonists

Beta-2 agonists possess anabolic activity, although the extent of this varies between drugs. The anabolic effects of oral beta-2 agonists have been clearly demonstrated in animals (Ryall *et al.* 2006). Clenbuterol is a long-acting beta-2 agonist, which is licensed for the treatment of asthma in some countries. It is not licensed for human use in either the United Kingdom or the United States. It is licensed for veterinary use (Ventopulmin, Boehringer Ingelheim) in horses for the treatment of bronchoconstriction caused by several equine respiratory diseases.

As with any drug, clenbuterol has side effects. It is a beta-2 agonist and has side effects that are typical of this group of drugs – tremor, restlessness, agitation, headache, increased blood pressure, and palpitations. These side effects are dose-related and purported to decrease after 8–10 days. This is due to a decrease (i.e. downregulation) of beta-2 receptors, a consequence of which is also a decrease in the anabolic effects of the drug. Other potential adverse, dose-dependent effects include tissue desensitization and cell necrosis in the heart and slow-twitch soleus muscle, as demonstrated in an animal model (Burniston *et al.* 2005).

Zilpaterol, like clenbuterol, was introduced as a growth promoter in cattle. It has a similar pharmacological profile to clenbuterol (Davies *et al.* 2008). It has a reputation as an anabolic agent with bodybuilders, despite little published work on its efficacy in this respect.

With respect to the anabolic effects of beta-2 agonists, it is dependent on the receptor density of muscles (Beerman 2002). Because chronic administration of beta-2 agonists produces downregulation of receptors (Johnson 2006), this may limit the effectiveness and therefore the value of beta-2 agonists as anabolic agents (Davies *et al.* 2008).

7.5. Beta-2 agonists and the WADA Prohibited List

From an anti-doping perspective, the status of inhaled beta-2 agonists has changed over recent years. Whilst terbutaline remains prohibited in competition, several other commonly inhaled beta-2 agonists, such as salbutamol, salmeterol, and formoterol, are permitted for therapeutic use. The WADA Prohibited List regulations relating to beta-2 agonists are shown in Table 7.3.

Clearly, athletes who require treatment with beta-2 agonists have recourse, under WADA regulations, to use salbutamol, formoterol, or salmeterol. However, the WADA regulations are designed to ensure that athletes who require bronchodilation with these drugs limit their use to recommended therapeutic dose regimes. Other beta-2 agonists, such as terbutaline, are subject to TUE regulations. Similarly, the administration of salbutamol, formoterol, or salmeterol by routes other than inhalation is also subject to TUE regulation.

In an attempt to differentiate between misuse and recommended therapeutic use, urinary thresholds have been introduced for salbutamol and formoterol. Any athlete exceeding the threshold or the decision limit (a concentration set above the recognised WADA threshold) will be asked to perform a controlled pharmacokinetic study in an attempt to establish

Table 7.3 WADA Prohibited List regulations relating to beta-2 agonists

All beta-2 agonists, including all optical isomers where relevant, are prohibited except:

- Inhaled salbutamol (maximum 1,600 µg over 24 hours)
- Inhaled formoterol (maximum delivered dose 54 µg over 24 hours)
- Salmeterol when taken by inhalation in accordance with the manufacturers' recommended therapeutic regimen

The presence in urine of salbutamol in excess of 1,000 ng/mL or formoterol in excess of 40 ng/mL is presumed not to be an intended therapeutic use of the substance and will be considered an adverse analytical finding unless the athlete proves, through controlled pharmacokinetic study, that the abnormal result was the consequence of the use of the therapeutic inhaled dose up to the maximum indicated above.

Source: World Anti-Doping Agency. (2014). The 2014 Prohibited List international standard. Available online at https://elb.wada-ama.org/en/resources/science-medicine/prohibited-list#.VAmEt8sg83F (accessed 4 September 2014).

whether the positive test was as a consequence of administering the drug up to a maximal therapeutic dose. Unfortunately, there is evidence to suggest that high interindividual variation exists in terms of urinary drug levels following the inhalation of therapeutic doses of beta-2 agonists, to the extent that exceeding the thresholds in such circumstances is likely (Elers *et al.* 2012b; Dickinson *et al.* 2014). This likelihood is increased further through poor management of respiratory conditions and the prescribing of many short-acting beta-2 agonists *pro re nata*. As a prophylactic and when used by those with poorly controlled asthma, doses may exceed recommended maximal daily doses and thus risk an anti-doping rule violation. Whilst this may be deemed misuse, it does not necessarily constitute intentional doping.

McKenzie and Fitch (2011) have proposed that there is no pharmacological difference between permitted and prohibited beta-2 agonists; therefore, asthmatic athletes are being managed differently, based on a WADA directive that has no foundation in pharmacological science or in clinical practice.

Beta-2 agonists such as clenbuterol, zeranol, and zilpaterol appear on the WADA Prohibited List under *anabolic agents* (subsection *other anabolic agents*), reflecting their potential anabolic properties.

7.6. Summary

- Beta-2 agonists are first-line drugs in the treatment of asthma and other obstructive airways diseases because of their bronchodilatory activity.
- Exercise-induced asthma and bronchoconstriction are particularly troublesome for athletes; therefore, beta-2 agonists may be required for therapeutic use in athletes.
- Beta-2 agonists are included on the WADA Prohibited List.
- The performance-enhancing potential for beta-2 agonists is dependent on the dose and route of administration of the drugs. This is reflected in WADA's regulations concerning the prohibition of this class of drugs.
- The beta-2 agonists salbutamol, formoterol, and salmeterol are permitted for use by athletes, provided they are taken by inhalation and in accordance with the manufacturers' recommended therapeutic regimen. All other beta-2 agonists require a TUE to be used in sport.
- Certain beta-2 agonists, such as clenbuterol, possess anabolic effects, as well as bronchodilatory activity. They are classified on the WADA Prohibited List under anabolic agents.

7.7. References

Anderson, S. D., and Kippelen, P. (2012). Assesment and prevention of exercise-induced bronchoconstriction. *British Journal of Sports Medicine* 46(6):391–396.

Ansley, L., Rea, G., and Hull, J. H. (2013). Practical approach to exercise-induced bronchoconstriction in athletes. *Primary Care Respiratory Journal* 22(1):122–125.

Backer, V., Lund, T., and Pedersen, L. (2007). Pharmaceutical treatment of asthma symptoms in elite athletes – doping or therapy? *Scandinavian Journal of Medicine and Science in Sports* 17(6):615–622.

Beerman, D. H. (2002). β-Adrenergic receptor agonist modulation of skeletal muscle growth. *Journal of Animal Science* 80E(Suppl 1):E18–E23.

British Thoracic Society. (2012). British guideline on the management of asthma. Available online at http://www.sign.ac.uk/pdf/sign101.pdf (accessed 1 July 2013).

Burniston, J. G., Chester, N., Clark, W. A., *et al.* (2005). Dose-dependent apoptotic and necrotic myocyte death induced by the β_2-adrenergic receptor agonist, clenbuterol. *Muscle Nerve* 32(6):767–774.

Carlsen, K. H., Anderson, S. D., Bjermer, L., *et al.* (2008a). Exercise induced asthma, respiratory and allergic disorders in elite athletes: Part I of the report from the Joint Task Force of European Respiratory Society (ERS) and European Academy of Allergy and Clinical Immunology (EAACI) in cooperation with GA²LEN. *Allergy* 63(4):387–403.

Carlsen, K. H., Anderson, S. D., Bjermer, L., *et al.* (2008b). Treatment of exercise induced asthma, respiratory and allergic disorders in sports and the relationship to doping: Part II of the report from the Joint Task Force of European Respiratory Society (ERS) and European Academy of Allergy and Clinical Immunology (EAACI) in cooperation with GA²LEN. *Allergy* 63(5):492–505.

Carlsen, K. H., Hem, E., and Stensrud, T. (2011). Asthma in adolescent athletes. *British Journal of Sports Medicine* 45(16):1266–1271.

Cockcroft, D. W. (2006). Clinical concerns with β_2-agonists: Adult asthma. *Clinical Reviews in Allergy and Immunology* 31(2–3):197–207.

Collomp, K., Le Panse, B., Candau, R., *et al.* (2010). Beta-2 agonists and exercise performance in humans. *Science and Sports* 25(6):281–290.

Cutrufello, P. T., Smoliga, J. M., and Rundell, K. W. (2012). Small things make a big difference. Particulate matter and exercise. *Sports Medicine* 42(12):1041–1058.

Davies, E., Loiacono, R., and Summers, R. J. (2008). The rush to adrenaline: Drugs in sport acting on the β-adrenergic system. *British Journal of Pharmacology* 154(3):584–597.

Dickinson, J., Chester, N., Hu, J., *et al.* (2014). The impact of ethnicity, gender and dehydration on the urinary excretion of inhaled salbutamol with respect to doping control. *Clinical Journal of Sports Medicine* Feb 10 [Epub ahead of print].

Dickinson, J., McConnell, A., and Whyte, G. (2011). Diagnosis of exercise-induced bronchoconstriction: Eucapnic voluntary hyperpnoea challenges identify previously undiagnosed elite athletes with exercise-induced bronchoconstriction. *British Journal of Sports Medicine* 45(14):1126–1131.

Elers, J., Morkeberg, J., Jansen, T., *et al.* (2012a). High-dose inhaled salbutamol has no acute effects in aerobic capacity or oxygen uptake kinetics in healthy trained men. *Journal of Medical Science in Sports* 22(2):232–239.

Elers, J., Pedersen, L., Henninge, J., *et al.* (2012b). The pharmacokinetic profile of inhaled and oral salbutamol in elite athletes with asthma and non-asthmatic subjects. *Clinical Journal of Sports Medicine* 22(2):140–145.

Fitch, K. (2006). β_2-agonists at the Olympic Games. *Clinical Reviews in Allergy and Immunology* 31(2–3):259–268.

Fitch, K. (2012). An overview of asthma and airway hyper-responsiveness in Olympic athletes. *British Journal of Sports Medicine* 46(6):413–416.

Fitch, K., Sue-Chu, M., Anderson, S., *et al.* (2008). Asthma and the elite athlete: Summary of the International Olympic Committee's Consensus Conference, Lausanne, Switzerland, January 22–24, 2008. *Journal of Allergy and Clinical Immunology* 122(2):254–260.

Global Initiative for Asthma. (2012). Pocket guide for asthma management and prevention. Available online at http://www.ginasthma.org/local/uploads/files/GINA_Pocket_2014_Jun11.pdf (accessed 16 July 2014).

Goubault, C., Perault, M.-C., Leleu, E., *et al.* (2001). Effects of inhaled salbutamol in exercising non-asthmatic athletes. *Thorax* 56(9):675–679.

Johnson, M. (2006). Molecular mechanisms of β_2-adrenergic receptor function, response and regulation. *Journal of Allergy and Clinical Immunology* 117(1):18–24.

Kindermann, W., and Meyer, T. (2006). Inhaled β_2 agonists and performance in competitive athletes. *British Journal of Sports Medicine* 40(Suppl 1):i43–i47.

Kippelen, P., Fitch, K. D., Anderson, S. D., *et al.* (2012). Respiratory health of elite athletes – Preventing airway injury: A critical review. *British Journal of Sports Medicine* 46(7):471–476.

Lacroix, V. J. (1999). Exercise-induced asthma. *The Physician and Sportsmedicine* 27(12):75–92.

Langdeau, J.-B., and Boulet, L.-P. (2001). Prevalence and mechanisms of development of asthma and airway hyperresponsiveness in athletes. *Sports Medicine* 31(8):601–616.

Langdeau, J.-B., and Boulet, L.-P. (2003). Is asthma over- or under-diagnosed in athletes? *Respiratory Medicine* 97(2):109–114.

Larsson, K., Carlsen, K. H., and Bonini, S. (2005). Anti-asthmatic drugs: Treatment of athletes and exercise-induced bronchoconstriction. *European Respiratory Monthly* 33(1):73–88.

McKenzie, D. C., and Fitch, K. D. (2011). The asthmatic athlete: Inhaled beta-2 agonists and doping. *Clinical Journal of Sports Medicine* 21(1):46–50.

Moreira, A., Delgado, L., and Carlsen, K. H. (2011). Exercise-induced asthma: Why is it so frequent in Olympic athletes? *Expert Review of Respiratory Medicine* 5(1):1–3.

Morgan, M.D.L. (2002) Dysfunctional breathing in asthma: Is it common, identifiable and correctable? *Thorax* 57(Suppl II):ii31–ii35.

Morton, A. R., and Fitch, K. D. (1992). Asthmatic drugs and competitive sport. An update. *Sports Medicine* 14(4):228–242.

Nelson, J. A., Strauss, L., Skowronski, M., *et al.* (1998). Effect of long-term salmeterol treatment on exercise-induced asthma. *New England Journal of Medicine* 339(3):141–146.

Norris, S. R., Petersen, S. R., and Jones, R. L. (1996). The effects of salbutamol on performance in endurance cyclists. *European Journal of Applied Physiology and Occupational Physiology* 73(3–4): 364–368.

Parsons, J. P., and Mastronarde, J. G. (2005). Exercise-induced bronchoconstriction in athletes. *Chest* 128(6):3966–3974.

Pedersen, L., Lund, T. K., Barnes, P. J., *et al.* (2008). Airway responsiveness and inflammation in adolescent elite swimmers. *Journal of Allergy and Clinical Immunology* 122(2):322–327.

Rupp, N. T. (1996). Diagnosis and management of exercise-induced asthma. *The Physician and Sportsmedicine* 24(1):77–87.

Ryall, J. G., Sillence, M. N., and Lynch, G. S. (2006). Systemic administration of β_2-adrenoceptor agonists, formoterol and salmeterol, elicit skeletal muscle hypertrophy in rats at micromolar doses. *British Journal of Pharmacology* 147(6):587–595.

Schumacher, Y. O., Pottgeisser, T., and Dickhuth, H. (2011). Exercise-induced bronchoconstriction: Asthma in athletes. *International Sports Medicine Journal* 12(4):145–149.

Schwartz, L. B., Delgado, L., Craig, T., *et al.* (2008). Exercise-induced hypersensitivity syndromes in recreational and competitive athletes: A PRACTALL consensus report. *Allergy* 63(8): 953–961.

Signorile, J. F., Kaplan, T. A., Applegate, B., *et al.* (1992). Effects of acute inhalation of the bronchodilator, albuterol, on power output. *Medicine and Science in Sports and Exercise* 24(6):638–642.

Thomas, M., McKinley, R. K., Freeman, E., Foy, C., and Price, D. (2005). The prevalence of dysfunctional breathing in adults in the community with and without asthma. *Primary Care Respiratory Journal* 14(1):78–82.

Tjørhom, A., Riiser, A., and Carlsen, K. H. (2007). Effects of formoterol on endurance performance in athletes at an ambient temperature of −20°C. *Scandinavian Journal of Medicine and Science in Sports* 17(6):628–635.

Van Baak, M. A., de Hon, O. M., Hartgens, F., *et al.* (2004). Inhaled salbutamol and endurance cycling performance in non-asthmatic athletes. *International Journal of Sports Medicine* 25(7):533–538.

Van Dixhoorn, J., and Duivenvoorden, H. J. (1985). Efficacy of Nijmegan questionnaire in recognition of the hyperventilation syndrome. *Journal of Psychosomatic Research* 29(2):199–206.

Voet, W. (2001). *Breaking the Chain*. London, UK: Yellow Jersey Press.

Weiler, J. M., and Ryan, E. J., III. (2000). Asthma in United States Olympic athletes who participated in the 1998 Olympic winter games. *Journal of Allergy and Clinical Immunology* 106(2):267–271.

Whyte, G. (2013). Asthma, EIB and the athlete – diagnosis, prevalence, treatment and anti-doping. *Aspetar Sports Medicine Journal* 2(3):334–338.

Chapter 8

Hormone and metabolic modulators

Neil Chester

8.1. Introduction

According to the World Anti-Doping Agency (WADA) Prohibited List, the S1 and S2 classes of doping agents are composed of, by and large, naturally occurring hormones and their synthetic derivatives (WADA 2014). The S4 class of hormone and metabolic modulators (Table 8.1) contains several groups of synthetic compounds, which act by modulating various endogenous hormonal pathways and local muscle-specific transduction pathways. In most cases, the aim of such modulators is to enhance exercise performance; however, in the case of aromatase inhibitors, selective oestrogen receptor modulators (SERMs), or other anti-oestrogenic substances, the aim may be to counteract the unwanted side effects of anabolic androgenic steroid (AAS) administration.

8.2. Hormone and metabolic modulators and the WADA Prohibited List

The class of doping agents categorised as Hormone and Metabolic Modulators is prohibited at all times, both within competition and out of competition. As a class, these substances were grouped together in 2013. Previously, all of these drugs, except for the metabolic modulators and insulins, were classified as Hormone Antagonists and Modulators after their introduction

Table 8.1 Class S4 of the 2014 WADA List of Prohibited Substances and Methods

S4. HORMONE AND METABOLIC MODULATORS

1. Aromatase inhibitors, including but not limited to aminoglutethimide, anastrozole, androsta-1,4,6-triene-3,17-dione (androstatrienedione), 4-androstene-3,6,17 trione (6-oxo), exemestane, formestane, letrozole, and testolactone
2. Selective estrogen receptor modulators, including but not limited to raloxifene, tamoxifen, and toremifene
3. Other antiestrogenic substances, including but not limited to clomiphene, cyclofenil, and fulvestrant
4. Agents modifying myostatin function(s), including but not limited to myostatin inhibitors
5. Metabolic modulators:
   a. Insulins
   b. Peroxisome proliferator activated receptor δ (PPAR-δ) agonists (e.g. GW 1516) and PPAR-δ-AMP-activated protein kinase axis agonists (e.g. AICAR)

Source: World Anti-Doping Agency (2014).

Table 8.2 Prohibited hormone and metabolic modulators identified by WADA-accredited
laboratories in 2012

Hormone and metabolic modulator	Occurrences	Percent within class
Aromatase inhibitors		
Letrozole	7	9.5%
Anastrozole	6	8.1%
Androstatrienedione	5	6.8%
Formestane	4	5.4%
Androstene-3,6,17 trione (6-oxo)	1	1.4%
Selective estrogen receptor modulators		
Tamoxifen	38	51%
Other antioestrogenic substances		
Clomiphene	12	16.2%
Agents modifying myostatin function(s)	–	–
Metabolic modulators		
Insulins	–	–
PPAR-δ and AMPK agonists	1	1.4%

Source: World Anti-Doping Agency (2013).

to the WADA Prohibited List in 2008. Prior to 2008, many of these substances were classified as agents with antiestrogenic activity. The number of positive drug tests attributed to the use of substances within this class is relatively low. The exception is the SERM tamoxifen, which accounted for more than half of the total number of adverse analytical findings attributed to hormone and metabolic modulators in 2012, as reported by WADA-accredited laboratories (WADA 2013; Table 8.2).

8.3. Aromatase inhibitors

Androgens are readily converted to oestrogens by the enzyme aromatase. Aromatase inhibitors limit this conversion by binding to aromatase and rendering it inactive. As doping agents, aromatase inhibitors are only of potential benefit to males. They are typically used in an attempt to elevate testosterone levels and to combat some of the unwanted side effects attributed to the use of AAS.

Clinical use of aromatase inhibitors

Aromatase inhibitors have been used in the treatment of breast tumours, particularly in postmenopausal women. Because oestrogens have been implicated in the development and progression of such tumours, the objective of treatment is to deprive the tumour of oestrogens. This can be accomplished by inhibiting aromatase, the enzyme that catalyses the final step in the biosynthesis of oestrogen (Njar and Brodie 1999). Postmenopausal women tend to have tumours that are positive for oestrogen receptors and are therefore more responsive to treatment involving hormone antagonism.

Aromatase inhibitors include both steroidal and nonsteroidal mechanism-based inhibitors. The steroidal agents are mostly analogues of androstenedione, including testolactone, formestane, exemestane, and atamestane. The nonsteroidal analogues include fadrozole, letrozole, anastrozole, vorozole, and finrazole (Handelsman 2006).

Use of aromatase inhibitors in sport

Natural androgens, such as testosterone and androstenedione, are the precursors of the principal oestrogen, estradiol; this conversion is achieved by the enzyme aromatase. Clearly, the inhibition of aromatase will lead to elevated levels of the endogenous androgens, testosterone, and androstenedione, thereby increasing potential anabolic effects. The most potent natural androgen, dihydrotestosterone, cannot be aromatized and cannot therefore be converted to an oestrogen (Handelsman 2008).

Aromatase inhibitors may also be used by AAS users in an attempt to treat the development of breast tissue (gynaecomastia), a common side effect associated with androgen use in men, although the clinical efficacy for this is debatable (Handelsman 2008).

8.4. Selective oestrogen receptor modulators

SERMs are particularly attractive antioestrogen drugs because they target specific tissues without affecting other organs. Tamoxifen is by far the most common SERM, being misused by elite athletes subject to doping control measures (Table 8.2) and gymnasium users alike.

Clinical use of SERMs

The first drugs to be used clinically as blockers of oestrogen receptors were nonsteroidal drugs, such as clomiphene and tamoxifen. Newer antioestrogens such as raloxifene, toremifene, droloxifene, and lasoxifene have been developed. These drugs also possess partial agonist activity and are now described by the term SERM. Tamoxifen and other SERMs have been the most widely prescribed antioestrogens in the management of hormone-receptor positive breast cancer in postmenopausal women. Tamoxifen has both an antagonist and a partial agonist effect on oestrogen receptors. As a result, long-term use has been associated with an increased risk of endometrial cancer. The partial agonist effect of tamoxifen has also been associated with the development of tamoxifen resistence, in which the drug ceases to inhibit tumour growth and appears to promote it (Bundred and Howell 2002).

Use of SERMs in sport

As antioestrogens, SERMs have the potential to elevate testosterone levels through competitive binding of oestrogen hypothalamic and pituitary receptors, thus blocking the negative feedback loop and stimulating follicle-stimulating hormone and luteinising hormone release (Mazzarino *et al.* 2011). Nevertheless, this is only evident in males. In females, circulating testosterone is derived largely from the adrenal cortex and peripheral conversion of circulating androgens and is not controlled by homeostatic feedback (Handelsman 2006).

Despite the potential effects on testosterone, the use of SERMs as performance- and image-enhancing drugs has tended to centre on the treatment of adverse side effects attributed to AAS use. Indeed, tamoxifen is widely used in the treatment of gynecomastia and was attributed to widespread use in a survey of recreational gymnasium users in South Wales (Baker *et al.* 2006). Indeed, 22 per cent of respondents who reported AAS use also reported using tamoxifen.

8.5. Other antioestrogenic substances

As previously mentioned, antioestrogens are drugs that act as oestrogen receptor antagonists to block the action of oestrogen. Whilst SERMs are selective in terms of their target tissue, traditional antioestrogens are nonselective; these include clomiphene, cyclofenil, and fulvestrant.

Clinical use of antioestrogenic substances

This subclass of drugs is used primarily for the treatment of breast cancer in postmenopausal women. Fulvestrant is an oestrogen receptor antagonist that competitively binds to the receptors with an affinity similar to that of oestradiol but higher than that of tamoxifen (McKeage et al. 2004). The binding of fulvestrant to the oestrogen receptor sets off a series of changes to downregulate receptor function. Unlike tamoxifen, fulvestrant has no partial oestrogen receptor agonist activity and therefore has fewer side effects.

Use of antioestrogenic substances in sport

Synthetic anabolic steroids are used by athletes, primarily for their anabolic effects. However, most have some androgenic effects that inhibit the release of gonadotropin-releasing hormone from the hypothalamus and follicle-stimulating hormone and luteinising hormone from the anterior pituitary gland. With prolonged use, the resulting hypogonadotropic state results in testicular atrophy. This decreases serum testosterone levels, causing impotence and decreased libido. Clomiphene has been reported to be used to treat these conditions by an antioestrogen effect on the hypothalamus, resulting in increased gonadotropin-releasing hormone release and oestrogen-like effects on the pituitary, thus increasing the sensitivity to gonadotropin-releasing hormone (Bickelman et al. 1995).

In women, it has been argued that there is no convincing evidence that oestrogen blockers cause any consistent, biologically significant increase in blood testosterone concentrations (Handelsman 2008). Furthermore, Handelsman suggested that oestrogen blockade poses no unusual medical risks to female athletes, and there is therefore no basis to ban oestrogen blockade in female athletes.

8.6. Agents modifying myostatin function(s)

As introduced in Chapter 6, the myostatin signalling pathway is important in the regulation of skeletal muscle growth. As its name suggests, myostatin is involved in the inhibition of muscle growth, opposing the mammalian target of rapamycin pathway. In a healthy individual, there is a balance between both pathways to ensure that normal muscle growth is maintained. As a local signalling molecule, myostatin initiates protein breakdown through its binding with a membrane-bound receptor on skeletal muscle. As demonstrated in animals such as thoroughbred horses, myostatin deficiency manifests itself in muscle hypertrophy and heightened physical performance (Hill et al. 2010). Therefore, the myostatin gene is the focus of much attention with regards to gene therapy and doping; however, the focus in this chapter relates to agents with the potential to inhibit myostatin function.

Clinical uses of agents modifying myostatin function

Myostatin is a member of the transforming growth factor-β group of proteins that regulates muscle growth during embryogenesis (Matsakas et al. 2005). Myostatin contributes to muscle development during growth and then negatively regulates muscle growth in adulthood. Myostatin is upregulated in disease states and during prolonged bed rest where muscle wasting is symptomatic (Han and Mitch 2011). It is also present in relatively high levels in the muscle of aging individuals (Yarasheski *et al.* 2002). It therefore follows that inhibition of myostatin would have a huge potential in promoting health.

The clinical applications for the development of myostatin-based medicines include muscular dystrophy, cachexia (muscular atrophy associated with acquired immunodeficiency syndrome and other chronic diseases), myopathies resulting from inflammation, and sarcopenia, the loss of muscle associated with increasing age (Wagner 2005). However, drugs that manipulate myostatin signalling are also being considered as lifestyle drugs in antiaging therapies and for their potential to enhance physical performance in athletes (Matsakas and Diel 2005). Therapies for inhibiting myostatin function are under clinical investigation; however, as yet there are no reliable treatments available (Han and Mitch 2011).

Use of agents modifying myostatin in sport

In humans, resistance or endurance training has been shown to suppress myostatin expression (Raue *et al.* 2006). This allows muscle to grow in size. It is not surprising, therefore, that suppression of myostatin function is deemed to be a potential method for increasing the growth response to training, or even to stimulate muscle growth independently of training. It is for this reason that WADA introduced agents modifying myostatin function(s) to the Prohibited List in January 2008, despite there being no therapeutic agents at present.

8.7. Metabolic modulators

As the name suggests, metabolic modulators are concerned with controlling metabolic processes and pathways. The metabolic modulators comprise two distinct groups – namely, insulins and peroxisome proliferator activated receptor delta (PPAR-δ) agonists and PPAR-δ-5′ adenosine monophosphate-activated protein kinase (AMPK) axis agonists. The former were classified under category S2 of the WADA Prohibited List (Peptide Hormones, Growth Factors, and Related Substances) until 2013, whereas the latter were classified in category M3 (Gene Doping) until 2012.

Clinical use of metabolic modulators

Insulin is a commonly used therapy for millions of individuals worldwide who suffer from diabetes mellitus. Insulin therapy can take several forms and is typically based upon an individual's type of diabetes. Type 1 diabetes, often termed *insulin-dependent diabetes*, requires regular daily insulin injections to combat the body's inability to produce insulin. Therapeutic approaches to type 2 diabetes may vary based on the condition of the patient. In mild cases, alternative strategies to drug therapy might be considered, such as lifestyle changes including exercise and weight loss. However, drug therapy, including insulin, is usually prescribed. Insulin is administered subcutaneously via injection or an infusion pump.

Whilst insulin was exclusively derived from animals in the past (i.e. bovine and porcine pancreases), it now tends to be human insulin produced by recombinant DNA technology. Analogues of insulin are also manufactured to modify the action of insulin in terms of its onset and duration of action.

According to the International Diabetes Federation (2012), there are four general types of insulin:

1 Long acting (onset of action: 6–14 h; duration of action: 24–36 h)
2 Intermediate acting (onset of action: 90 min; duration of action: 3–6 h)
3 Short acting (onset of action: 30–60 min; duration of action: 3–6 h)
4 Rapid acting (onset of action: 15 min; duration of action: 3–4 h)

Both PPAR-δ and AMPK agonists are relatively new drugs whose capabilities as therapeutic agents (and otherwise) are currently being developed. PPAR-δ agonists are a class of drugs that have the potential to treat both cardiovascular and metabolic diseases. These drugs show great promise, although they are not without their problems. For example, clinical trials of the PPAR-δ agonist GW501516, which was developed by GlaxoSmithKline, were stopped due to concerns over potential carcinogenic effects (Geiger *et al.* 2009). However, this has not prevented its availability and illicit use as a performance- and image-enhancing drug.

The AMPK agonist, 5-amino-4-imidazolecarbamide ribonuleoside (aminomidazole carboxamide ribonucleotide; AICAR) has undergone clinical trials for the treatment of ischemia-reperfusion injury during heart surgery (Alkhulaifi and Pugsley 1995). It has also been considered as a possible treatment for a wide range of diseases, including diabetes mellitus (Pold *et al.* 2005) and cancer (Jose *et al.* 2011).

Use of metabolic modulators in sport

Although insulins are essential in the pharmacotherapy of diabetes mellitus, they are thought to have huge potential as performance-enhancing agents. Sonksen (2001) outlined ways by which insulin might enhance exercise performance:

1 Increased glucose uptake by skeletal muscle as a consequence of elevated insulin levels would lead to augmented glycogen storage, which would be advantageous in prolonged exercise and the recovery between training or competition.
2 The inhibition of protein breakdown by insulin would limit the catabolic effects associated with heavy training and further enhance the effectiveness of resistance training in increasing muscle bulk. Insulin would therefore appear to work in synergy with other anabolic agents, such as AAS, growth hormone, and insulin-like growth factor-1.

The use of insulin as anabolic agents was reported by Dawson and Harrison (1997) amongst patients at a needle exchange and support clinic in the United Kingdom. Also, it was reported by Rich *et al.* (1998) that 25 per cent of AAS users were using insulin concurrently. One investigation reported that, of 41 nondiabetic insulin users, 95 per cent also administered AAS (Ip *et al.* 2012). Bodybuilders are a group that is particularly prone to using insulin to increase muscle mass, and there is a particular risk of hypoglycaemia associated with competitive bodybuilders who may be using insulin with concurrent fasting prior to a competition. Indeed, there are reports of individuals suffering from hypoglycaemic coma (Evans and Lynch 2003).

Insulin was added to the list of prohibited substances by the International Olympic Committee after concerns regarding its possible misuse at the Nagano Olympics in 1998 (Sonksen 2001). Of course, athletes with diabetes may use insulin with a valid Therapeutic

Use Exemption. From a drug-testing perspective, it is difficult to differentiate between the endogenous hormone and that which might be administered exogenously. In addition, the pulsatile nature of insulin release coupled with its short half-life makes doping control extremely challenging.

PPAR-δ agonists are important regulators of substrate utilisation and are involved in the regulation of muscle fibre type (Wang *et al.* 2004). Whilst research examining the effect of a PPAR agonist, namely GW501516, in an animal model resulted in a shift from carbohydrate to fat utilisation in skeletal muscle, no improvement in endurance performance was found in sedentary mice. However, endurance performance was improved when exercise training was combined with GW501516 (Narkar *et al.* 2008). The same research study also demonstrated the effectiveness of the AMPK-agonist AICAR on enhanced endurance running in mice (Narkar *et al.* 2008).

AMPK is often described as the master metabolic regulator due to its effect on lipid and glucose metabolism. It is activated in response to changes in energy levels (i.e. low adenosine triphosphate levels) that occur during stress (e.g. exercise). Drugs that target AMPK (and indeed PPAR-δ) have been termed *exercise mimetics* because of their ability to activate numerous signalling pathways and regulate the expression of particular genes in a similar way to exercise. It is for this reason that such drugs have become attractive to individuals looking to enhance sports performance.

From a drug-testing perspective, the first case of GW501516 use was in cycling, coinciding with the development of a test for its detection by Thevis *et al.* (2013). The cyclist in question was a Russian, Valery Kaykov, who won the gold medal in the European Track Championship team pursuit in 2012. AICAR is a naturally occurring AMPK agonist that is readily detected in urine; therefore, quantitative analysis and the implementation of a suitable threshold is likely to determine its misuse (Thevis *et al.* 2009).

8.8. Summary

Hormone and metabolic modulators are a diverse group of substances with a diverse range of therapeutic uses. As performance- and image-enhancing drugs, they have the potential to boost skeletal muscle growth and function by increasing the availability of testosterone or limiting protein breakdown and increase endurance capacity via PPAR-δ and AMPK agonists. In addition, by modulating oestrogen and its receptors, the side effects attributed to androgen use may be tackled.

According to WADA-accredited laboratory data, other than antioestrogens (particularly SERMs), this group of substances is not widely used for performance and image enhancement. Nevertheless, these drugs represent a group of emerging drugs that, in many cases, remain under development and therefore may prove attractive to athletes in the future.

8.9. References

Alkhulaifi, A. M., and Pugsley, W. B. (1995). Role of acadesine in clinical myocardial protection. *British Heart Journal* 73(4):304–305.

Baker, J. S., Graham, M. R., and Davies, B. (2006). Steroid and prescription medicine abuse in the health and fitness community. A regional study. *European Journal of Internal Medicine* 17(7):479–484.

Bickelman, C., Ferries, L., and Eaton, R. P. (1995). Impotence related to anabolic steroid use in a body builder. Response to clomiphene citrate. *Western Journal of Medicine* 162(2):158–160.

Bundred, N., and Howell, A. (2002). Fulvestrant (Faslodex): Current status in the therapy of breast cancer. *Expert Review in Anticancer Therapy* 2(2):151–160.

Dawson, R. T., and Harrison, M. W. (1997). Use of insulin as an anabolic agent. *British Journal of Sports Medicine* 31(3):259.

Evans, P. J., and Lynch, R. M. (2003). Insulin as a drug of abuse in body building. *British Journal of Sports Medicine* 37(4):356–357.

Geiger, L. E., Dunsford, W. S., Lewis, D. J., *et al*. (2009). Rat carcinogenicity study with GW501516, a PPAR delta agonist. *The Toxicologist* 108(1):Abstract 895.

Han, H. Q., and Mitch, W. E. (2011). Targeting the myostatin signalling pathway to treat muscle wasting diseases. *Current Opinion in Supportive and Palliative Care* 5(4):334–341.

Handelsman, D. J. (2006). The rationale for banning human chorionic gonadotropin and estrogen blockers in sport. *Journal of Clinical Endocrinology and Metabolism* 91(5):1646–1653.

Handelsman, D. J. (2008). Indirect androgen doping by oestrogen blockade in sports. *British Journal of Pharmacology* 154(3):598–605.

Hill, E. W., Gu, J., Eivers, S. S., *et al*. (2010). A sequence of polymorphism in MSTN predicts sprinting ability and racing stamina in thoroughbred horses. *PLoS One* 5(1):e8645.

International Diabetes Federation. (2012). About insulin. Available online at http://www.idf.org/node/1056 (accessed 4 September 2014).

Ip, E. J., Barnett, M. J., Tenerowicz, M. J., and Perry, P. J. (2012). Weightlifting's risky new trend: A case of 41 insulin users. *Current Sports Medicine Reports* 11(4):176–179.

Jose, C., Hebert-Chatelain, E., Bellance, N., *et al*. (2011). AICAR inhibits cancer cell growth and triggers cell-type distinct effects on OXPHOS biogenesis, oxidative stress and Akt activation. *Biochimica et Biophysica Acta* 1807(6):707–718.

Matsakas, A., and Diel, P. (2005). The growth factor myostatin, a key regulator in skeletal muscle growth and homeostasis. *International Journal of Sports Medicine* 26(2):83–89.

Mazzarino, M., Bragano, M. C., de la Torre, X. *et al*. (2011). Relevance of the selective oestrogen receptor modulators tamoxifen, toremifene and clomiphene in doping field: Endogenous steroids urinary profile after multiple oral doses. *Steroids* 76(12):1400–1406.

McKeage, K., Curran, M. P., and Plosker, G.L. (2004). Fulvestrant. A review of its use in hormone receptor-positive metastatic breast cancer in postmenopausal women with disease progression following antiestrogen therapy. *Drugs* 64(6):633–648.

Narkar, V. A., Downes, M., Yu, R. T., *et al*. (2008). AMPK and PPARδ agonists are exercise mimetics. *Cell* 134(3):405–415.

Njar, V. C. O., and Brodie A. M. H. (1999). Comprehensive pharmacology and clinical efficacy of aromatase inhibitors. *Drugs* 58(2):233–256.

Pold, R., Jensen, L. S., Buhl, E. S., *et al*. (2005). Long-term AICAR administration and exercise prevents diabetes in ZDF rats. *Diabetes* 54(4):928–934.

Raue, U., Slivka, D., Jemiolo, B., *et al*. (2006). Myogenic gene expression at rest and after a bout of resistance exercise in young (18–30 yr) and old (80–89 yr) women. *Journal of Applied Physiology* 101(1):53–59.

Rich, J. D., Dinkinson, B. P., and Merriman, N. A. (1998). Insulin use in bodybuilders. *JAMA* 270(20):1613–1614.

Sonksen, P. H. (2001). Insulin, growth hormone, and sport. *Journal of Endocrinology* 170(1):13–25.

Thevis, M., Moller, I., Beuck, S., and Schanzer, W. (2013). Synthesis, mass spectrometric characterization and analysis of the PPARδ agonist QW1516 and its major human metabolites: Targets in sports drug testing. *Methods in Molecular Biology* 952:301–312.

Thevis, M., Thomas, A., Kohler, M., *et al*. (2009). Emerging drugs: Mechanism of action, mass spectrometry and doping control analysis. *Journal of Mass Spectrometry* 44(4):442–460.

Wagner, K. R. (2005). Muscle regeneration through myostatin inhibition. *Current Opinions in Rheumatology* 17(6):720–724.

Wang, Y. W., Zhang, C. L., Tu, R. T., *et al*. (2004). Regulation of muscle fibre type and running endurance by PPARδ. *PLoS Biology* 2(10):e294.

World Anti-Doping Agency. (2013). 2012 anti-doping testing figures report. Available online at https://wada-main-prod.s3.amazonaws.com/resources/files/WADA-2012-Anti-Doping-Testing-Figures-Report-EN.pdf (accessed 1 October 2013).

World Anti-Doping Agency. (2014). The 2014 Prohibited List international standard. Available online at https://www.wada-ama.org/en/what-we-do/prohibited-list (accessed 9 September 2014).

Yarasheski, K. E., Bhasin, S., Sinha-Hikim, I., *et al*. (2002). Serum myostatin-immunoreactive protein is increased in 60–92 year old women and men with muscle wasting. *Journal of Nutrition, Health and Aging* 6(5):343–348.

Chapter 9

Diuretics and other masking agents

David R. Mottram

9.1. Introduction

Diuretics are drugs that act on the kidneys to increase the rate of urine flow. They have a number of important clinical uses, particularly in the treatment of cardiovascular disorders. However, they are also widely misused in sport, as their pharmacological action has led some athletes to believe that increased urine excretion will mask the use of other prohibited substances. Furthermore, diuretics have been misused to temporarily reduce weight in sports where weight categories apply. In this chapter, the use of diuretics, and other agents that may be used to mask prohibited drug use, will be reviewed along with the World Anti-Doping Agency (WADA) regulations to prohibit their use.

9.2. What are diuretics?

The main function of the kidneys is to maintain a constant interior environment of the body by regulating the volume, electrolyte content, and pH of extracellular fluid in response to variations in diet and fluctuations in external environmental conditions. The kidneys are also responsible for eliminating waste and noxious products from the body. Within the kidneys, fluid salts and low-molecular-weight constituents of the plasma are extracted from the blood and mostly reabsorbed, leaving excess water, ions, and foreign chemicals to be excreted within the urine so produced.

Diuretics are drugs that act on the kidneys to increase the rate of urine flow and the excretion of ions, particularly sodium (Na^+). They therefore adjust the volume and composition of body fluids. There are different types of diuretics, which are classified according to their mode of action (Table 9.1). Diuretics can also be classified according to their chemical structure. This does not pose a problem with respect to doping analysis (Deventer *et al*. 2002; Morra *et al*. 2006). The major clinical uses of diuretics are presented in Table 9.1.

9.3. Action and use of diuretics in sport

Diuretics as masking agents

One of the principal reasons for athletes' use of diuretics is for their masking effects through the production of copious volumes of urine. This attempt at disguising other drugs being excreted is highly unlikely to succeed, considering the levels of sensitivity and accuracy exhibited by modern analytical testing regimens. Some diuretics can alter urinary pH and inhibit the passive excretion of acidic and basic drugs in urine (Cadwallader *et al*. 2010).

Table 9.1 Classification of diuretics and their major clinical uses

Class of diuretics	Examples	Major clinical uses
Loop diuretics	Furosemide Bumetanide Torasemide	Chronic heart failure Renal failure
Thiazide and related diuretics	Bendroflumethazide Hydrochlorothiazide Chlortalidone Indapamide Metolazone Chlorothiazide Cyclopenthiazide Xipamide	Hypertension Oedema
Potassium-sparing diuretics	Amiloride Triamterene	In conjunction with loop or thiazide diuretics to maintain potassium balance
Aldosterone antagonists (also potassium sparing)	Spironolactone Eplerenone Canrenone	Primary hyperaldosteronism Cirrhosis of the liver
Carbonic anhydrase Inhibitors	Acetazolamide Dorzolamide Brinzolamide	Rarely used except orally (Acetazolamide) or topically to treat glaucoma
Osmotic diuretics	Mannitol	Cerebral oedema

Diuretics in sports requiring weight limitations or categorisation

A number of sports require weight categorisation to ensure some degree of equivalence between competitors. Most of these sports involve physical contact, such as boxing, judo, and wrestling, or they compare the ability to lift weights. Such sports require a weigh-in prior to competition. Athletes must ensure that they meet the limits of their respective weight categories and often need to resort to weight-lowering strategies to achieve that objective. These strategies have sometimes included the use of diuretics. In a Brazilian study of methods used to reduce body mass by competitive combat sport athletes, it was found that around one third used diuretics or laxatives (Brito *et al.* 2012).

Another sport in which weight is of prime importance is professional horse racing, in which jockeys are required to maintain very low body weight and precise weight control. All jockeys routinely adopt practices of restricting food intake and sauna-induced sweating. However, a study in which professional jockeys in Australia were questioned on their weight management revealed that 22 per cent of subjects frequently resorted to diuretics for rapid weight loss (Moore *et al.* 2002). This practice is widespread and reports date back many years (Price 1973).

Sports federations within which weight control is a factor reserve the right to administer anti-doping tests at the time of the weigh-in as well as at the time of competing, because the weigh-in may take place some period of time before the competition.

Diuretic use with other prohibited substances

Diuretics have been shown to have a widespread appeal as part of the culture of polydrug use in activities such as bodybuilding (Delbeke *et al.* 1995). In this context, the principal function of diuretics is to counter the fluid-retentive properties of anabolic steroids. In the case of bodybuilders, this is an essential property to attain the required 'cut' look. A similar result was found in gymnasium users, where polypharmacy was practiced by over 80 per cent of steroid users, with 22 per cent using diuretics as part of their regime (Evans 1997).

Other uses of diuretics associated with sport

Acetazolamide is a weak diuretic, but it has been used for prophylaxis against mountain sickness in skiers and mountain climbers (Cadwallader *et al.* 2010) – an indication for which it is not licensed. However, it is not suitable for altitude acclimatisation. A study into the effects of acetazolamide on exercise performance and muscle mass at high altitude concluded that the subjects taking acetazolamide had fewer symptoms of acute mountain sickness than controls, although the difference was not statistically significant (Bradwell *et al.* 1986). The authors also showed that weight loss, including muscle mass, was greater in controls; this correlated with a decrease in exercise performance, leading to the conclusion that acetazolamide is useful for climbers and trekkers who are acclimatised to high altitudes and that the drug could be most useful at extreme altitudes. There is no published evidence for benefits of acetazolamide at altitudes where most sports are undertaken.

Diuretics have been used for weight loss in sports other than those where weight categories apply. In a study by Martin *et al.* (1998), the use of diuretics by female basketball, softball, and volleyball players was investigated. Volleyball players (23.6 per cent), in particular, used diuretics for weight loss purposes, but in 79.6 per cent of cases this was specifically for appearance enhancement.

Interrelationship between exercise and diuretics

Diuretics can have a variety of effects on exercise physiology, including effects on metabolism (thermoregulation and potassium homeostasis) and the cardiovascular and respiratory systems, mostly as a consequence of fluid volume depletion and electrolyte imbalance and depletion (Cadwallader *et al.* 2010). These authors also reviewed the significant variety of ways that exercise can affect the pharmacological actions of diuretics, with associated serious side effects.

9.4. Action and uses of other masking agents in sport

Probenecid

Probenecid is an inhibitor of renal tubular transport mechanisms. Because it inhibits the resorption of uric acid, it increases the elimination of urate through the kidneys. Therefore, it reduces plasma uric acid and the likelihood of this substance crystallising out in joints and soft tissue, the effects of which lead to the painful symptoms of gout.

Probenecid has an opposite effect on the elimination of other drugs, such as penicillins, for which it inhibits urinary excretion, leading to increased plasma concentrations. This has been used to a therapeutic advantage in the case of penicillins, which are otherwise rapidly excreted, leading to the necessity for frequent dosing in order to maintain therapeutically effective plasma levels of the drug.

Probenecid has also been shown to inhibit the urinary excretion of other drugs, including anabolic steroids and their metabolites, and has therefore been used as a masking agent (Ventura and Segura 2010). However, the urinary excretion of anabolic steroids and their metabolites is not completely inhibited by probenecid; therefore, athletes would still record an adverse analytical finding during drug testing. It is therefore not surprising to find that probenecid has, in recent years, rarely appeared in WADA's laboratory statistics (see Table 9.2).

Desmopressin

Desmopressin (1-desamino-8-D-arginine-vasopressin) is a synthetic analogue of the posterior pituitary hormone vasopressin (antidiuretic hormone). It is used clinically in the treatment of pituitary ('cranial') diabetes insipidus (Kim *et al*. 2004). It has a more potent diuretic effect than vasopressin. Desmopressin works by limiting the amount of water that is eliminated in urine by binding to V2 receptors in renal collecting ducts, thereby increasing water resorption.

A landmark study was conducted by Sanchis-Gomar *et al*. (2010) to test whether desmopressin-induced haemodilution would alter the concentration of haematological parameters used to detect blood doping in sports. After treatment with desmopressin, they found a significant decrease in the haematocrit, haemoglobin, and the OFF Hr-Score (a method based on the calculation of erythropoietic response; Gore *et al*. 2003; Sanchis-Gomar *et al*. 2011) values. The authors concluded that desmopressin has a very significant haemodilution effect and recommended that desmopressin should be included on the WADA Prohibited List. WADA introduced desmopressin in the 2011 List of Prohibited Substances and Methods.

In 2011, Sanchis-Gomar *et al*. tested desmopressin-induced haemodilution after the administration of recombinant human erythropoietin (rHuEPO) to subjects. Analysis of blood parameters indicated that desmopressin has a very effective haemodilution effect after rHuEPO administration. It significantly modifies the haematological values measured by the anti-doping authorities to detect blood doping as part of the WADA Athlete Biological Passport scheme (Gilbert 2010).

Plasma volume expanders

Plasma volume expanders contain large molecules that, when administered by intravenous infusion, do not readily leave the blood vessels. Within blood vessels, they exert osmotic pressure and hold extra fluid in the blood, thereby elevating plasma volume and total blood volume. This can disguise elevated red blood cell levels. This property of plasma expanders was exploited by athletes using erythropoietin (EPO) prior to the validated test for EPO that was introduced in 2000. Before the introduction of this test, evidence for EPO use relied on blood tests showing elevated haematocrit levels (Ventura and Segura 2010).

Albumin is an endogenous plasma protein. Its concentration in the plasma can be increased through intravenous infusion of albumin solution, derived by extraction from whole blood that has had most other constituents removed. Albumin also has the potential to bind drugs, thereby delaying their excretion via the urine. There are a number of side effects associated with albumin infusion, the most serious of which is the risk of hypersensitivity reactions leading to anaphylaxis.

Other plasma expanders include the plasma substitutes dextran, gelatin, and hydroxyethyl starch (HES). They expand and maintain increased blood volume and are only slowly metabolised. They also expose the user to the risk of hypersensitivity reactions. HES was added to the Prohibited List in 2000 after reports of its use by athletes. This led to the search for a validated method to identify this substance in urine (Thevis *et al*. 2000). Rapid screening techniques for HES and dextran are now available (Guddat *et al*. 2008).

9.5. History of diuretics and other masking agents in sport

Masking agents are drugs that do not possess performance-enhancing properties but are taken in an attempt to disguise the fact that other prohibited substances are being used. Athletes quickly realised the potential for this type of subterfuge; therefore, these drugs have been used for as long as athletes have been subject to drug testing.

The International Olympic Committee (IOC) and then WADA have classified and reclassified diuretics and masking agents in a variety of ways. Diuretics were first added to the IOC Prohibited List, as a class of doping substances, in 1985. From 1985 to 2003, diuretics were listed as a class of drugs alongside other major classes of drugs, such as anabolic agents and stimulants. In 2004, they were reclassified under substances prohibited in certain sports. In 1987, probenecid and other masking agents were added under Doping Methods as part of the class referred to as Pharmacological Chemical and Physical Manipulation. In 2005, WADA combined diuretics with other masking agents as substances and methods that are prohibited at all times (both in- and out-of-competition), where they have remained to the current time (2014 WADA Prohibited List).

The principal reason for these variations in classification lies in the fact that diuretics have been used over the years not only as masking agents but also as drugs to produce short-term weight loss in sports where weight categories apply. These sports include boxing, wrestling, and horse racing, in which jockeys are required to attain specific weight levels. The extent to which diuretics and other masking agents have been used in sport can be gauged by Table 9.2.

Table 9.2 WADA statistics for the number of positive results for substances classified as diuretics and other masking agents (2006–2012)

	2006	2007	2008	2009	2010	2011	2012
Diuretics							
Furosemide	90	111	104	92	152	123	127
Hydrochlorothiazide	88	103	137	90	120	123	101
Canrenone	8	15	15	21	27	29	24
Triamterene	7	15	7	10	8	10	7
Amiloride	10	10	6	8	13	12	6
Chlorothiazide	1	7	27	12	25	36	24
Indapamide	5	4	12	14	7	4	8
Acetazolamide	2	4	6	8	12	8	8
Others	18	20	27	10	23	19	13
Alpha reductase inhibitors*							
Finasteride	44	53	84				
Epitestosterone[+]	15	14	8				
Probenecid	2	3	3	7	2	3	4
Hydroxyethyl starch	–	–	–	1	7	1	–
Total	290	359	436	273	396	368	322

* Alpha reductase inhibitors were removed from the WADA Prohibited List in 2009.
[+] Epitestosterone was reclassified by WADA in 2009 to Anabolic Agents.

During the period from 2006 to 2012, diuretics and other masking agents represented between 5.4 per cent and 7.9 per cent of the adverse analytical findings (AAFs) reported by WADA laboratories. This is a significant proportion of AAFs, considering that anabolic agents accounted for approximately 50 per cent of the AAFs in each of those years. The most frequently abused diuretics are furosemide and hydrochlorothiazide, perhaps because they have a short half-life and can be difficult to detect if urine samples are not collected within 24–48 hours after the last administration (Cadwallader *et al.* 2010).

The statistics in Table 9.2 include alpha-reductase inhibitors and epitestosterone; however, WADA removed both of these groups of drugs from the class of Diuretics and Masking Agents in 2009. Alpha-reductase inhibitors were removed completely from the Prohibited List, whilst epitestosterone was reclassified under Anabolic Agents.

Case studies involving diuretics and other masking agents

There have been a number of high-profile cases involving this class of substances. Masking agents can act in a variety of ways, but their presence generally indicates that the athlete was taking another prohibited substance. The Pedro Delgado case was therefore of interest.

Pedro Delgado (1988)

In 1988, the professional road race cyclist Pedro Delgado tested positive for the masking agent probenecid whilst leading the twelfth stage of the Tour de France cycle race. Probenecid was included on the IOC Prohibited List at that time; however, the governing body for cycling, Union Cycliste International, did not prohibit the drug. Pedro Delgado was therefore allowed to continue the race, which he eventually won. Remarkably little comment ensued, despite the fact that probenecid possesses no performance-enhancing properties itself but had been used solely as a masking agent. This should have raised the question as to what the cyclist was trying to mask. This case was a classic example of the lack of harmonization that existed in international doping control at that time – a position that would not be rectified until the establishment of WADA more than 10 years later.

Some cases involve collusion between team members.

Eighth Swimming World Championships, Australia (1998)

These championships were marred by a number of doping-related events surrounding the Chinese swimming team. In addition to the discovery of vials of human growth hormone by Australian Customs officials prior to the games, out-of-competition pretesting at the games resulted in adverse analytical findings for the diuretic, triamterene, in four members of the Chinese squad.

In addition to the athletes themselves, some cases involving the use of masking agents have involved collaboration with team supporters, including medical practitioners.

World Nordic Skiing Championships, Finland (2001)

At the time before a validated test for EPO had been widely adopted by laboratories, the International Ski Federation had reduced the acceptable 'safe' haemoglobin limit in blood to 17.5 mg/dl for men in an attempt to control the use of EPO. Some athletes realised that by combining EPO with plasma volume expanders, they could elevate haemoglobin and total blood volume while holding haemoglobin below the legal limit. At the World Nordic Skiing Championships in 2001, six Finnish skiers tested positive for hydroxyl ethyl starch, not having realised that the WADA laboratories had devised a detection method for HES without generally announcing its availability (Seiler 2001). In this case, it was further revealed that the use of EPO along with the intravenous administration of HES had been undertaken systematically with the collusion of the head coach and two national team doctors. It served as a reminder that such personnel can be implicated as accessories to athlete doping.

At least one case has involved an athlete whose adverse analytical finding resulted from the use of a prohibited substance that was later removed from the Prohibited List.

Zach Lund (2006)

In February 2006, skeleton sled racer Zach Lund was banned from competition for 1 year after testing positive for finasteride (a constituent in his hair growth stimulant) on the eve of the Winter Olympic Games in Torino, Italy. The 1-year ban was a reduction from the 2-year ban recommended by WADA because the Court of Arbitration for Sport had determined that Lund 'bears no significant fault or negligence.' Finasteride was removed from the WADA Prohibited List in January 2009.

9.6. Current WADA classification of diuretics and masking agents

The substances that are included under Diuretics and Other Masking Agents in the 2014 WADA Prohibited List are shown in Table 9.3. The list describes the masking agents that are prohibited, with examples where appropriate.

In 2013, WADA decided that the potential masking effect of felypressin, an anaesthetic used in dental practice, did not warrant its inclusion as a prohibited substance when administered locally.

Four diuretics are not prohibited by WADA. Drospirenone is an analogue of the aldosterone antagonist diuretic spironolactone, and it has weak diuretic effects. However, its principal pharmacological effect lies in the fact that it is a progestin, a synthetic version of the hormone progestogen. As such, it is used clinically in combined oral contraceptive pills. The diuretic effect of drospirenone was therefore deemed insufficient by WADA to warrant its prohibition as a masking agent. Similarly, WADA does not prohibit the carbonic anhydrase inhibitors dorzolamide and brinzolamide when used topically, such as in eyedrop preparations for the treatment of glaucoma, because they will not be absorbed into the systemic circulation in sufficient quantities to act as masking agents. Pamabrom is a weak diuretic that is widely

Table 9.3 List of substances included under diuretics and other masking agents in the WADA Prohibited List

---

Masking agents are prohibited, including:

Diuretics, desmopressin, plasma expanders (e.g. glycerol, intravenous administration of albumin, dextran, hydroxyethyl starch, mannitol), probenecid, and other substances with similar biological effect(s)

Local administration of felylpressin in dental anaesthesia is not prohibited.

Diuretics include:

Acetazolamide, amiloride, bumetanide, canrenone, chlorthalidone, ethacrynic acid, furosemide, indapamide, metolazone, spironolactone, thiazides (e.g. bendroflumethazide, chlorothiazide, hydrochlorothiazide), triamterene, vaptans (e.g. tolvaptan), and other substances with a similar chemical structure or similar biological effect(s) (except drosperinone, pamabrom, and topical dorzolamine and brinzolamide, which are not prohibited)

The use of in- and out-of-competition, as applicable, of any quantity of a substance subject to threshold limit (i.e. formoterol, salbutamol, cathine, ephedrine, methylephedrine, pseudoephedrine) in conjunction with a diuretic or other masking agent requires the deliverance of a specific Therapeutic Use Exemption for that substance in addition to one granted for the diuretic or other masking agent.

Source: World Anti-Doping Agency. (2014). The 2014 Prohibited List international standard. Available online at https://elb.wada-ama.org/en/resources/science-medicine/prohibited-list#.VAmEt8sg83F (accessed 4 September 2014).

available as a combined over-the-counter medication for premenstrual/menstrual symptoms and therefore is not prohibited by WADA.

Diuretics have a number of important clinical uses (see Table 9.1), and therefore athletes may apply for Therapeutic Use Exemptions (TUEs) when appropriate (WADA 2011). The WADA Prohibited List pays particular attention to the use of TUEs with diuretics and other masking agents. An athlete may apply for and be granted a TUE for a diuretic or masking agent alone. However, if that diuretic or other masking agent is used with another drug that is subject to a WADA threshold limit (see Table 9.3), the athlete must apply for a TUE for this other drug, regardless of the quantity that is prescribed or whether the drug is taken in-competition or out-of-competition.

Common conditions for which TUEs are applied for in sport include spironolactone for polycystic ovary syndrome in women, hypertension, and renal disorders. A TUE for a diuretic will never be approved for an athlete in a sport with weight categories (Fitch 2012).

9.7. Summary

- Diuretics act on the kidneys to increase urine flow.
- Diuretics may be misused by athletes to mask the use of other prohibited substances, but they may also be taken to temporarily reduce weight in sports where weight categories apply.
- A number of nondiuretic drugs, such as probenecid, desmopressin, and plasma volume expanders, may also be used to attempt to mask prohibited drug use.
- Diuretics are used extensively by athletes who use illegal performance-enhancing drugs, as gauged by WADA's annual laboratory statistics.
- Specific criteria apply with regard to Therapeutic Use Exemptions for diuretics. Exceptions are not permitted in sports where weight categories apply.

9.8. References

Bradwell, A. R., Coote, J. H., Milles, J. J., *et al*. (1986). Effect of acetazolamine on exercise performance and muscle mass at high altitude. *Lancet* 327(8488):1001–1005.

Brito, C. J., Roas, A. F. C. M., Brito, I. S. S., *et al*. (2012). Methods of body-mass reduction by combat sport athletes. *International Journal of Sport Nutrition and Exercise Metabolism* 22(2):89–97.

Cadwallader, A. B., de la Torre, X., Tieri, A., *et al*. (2010). The abuse of diuretics as performance enhancing drugs and masking agents in sport doping: Pharmacology, toxicology and analysis. *British Journal of Pharmacology* 161(1):1–16.

Delbeke, F. T., Desmet, N., and Debackere, M. (1995). The abuse of doping agents in competing body builders in Flanders (1988–1993). *International Journal of Sports Medicine* 16(1):66–70.

Deventer, K., Delbeke, F. T., Roels, K., *et al*. (2002). Screening for 18 diuretics and probenecid in doping analysis by liquid chromatography-tandem mass spectrometry. *Biomedical Chromatography* 16(8):529–535.

Evans, N. A. (1997). Gym and tonic: A profile of 100 male steroid users. *British Journal of Sports Medicine* 31(1):54–58.

Fitch, K. (2012). Proscribed drugs at the Olympic Games: Permitted use and misuse (doping) by athletes. *Clinical Medicine* 12(3):257–260.

Gilbert, S. (2010). The biological passport. *Hastings Central Report* 40(5):18–19.

Gore, C. J., Parisotto, R., Ashenden, M. J., *et al*. (2003). Second-generation blood tests to detect erythropoietin abuse by athletes. *Haematologica* 88(9):333–344.

Guddat, S., Thevis, M., Thomas, A. *et al*. (2008). Rapid screening of polysaccharide-based plasma volume expanders dextran and hydroxyethyl starch in human urine by liquid chromatography-tandem mass spectrometry. *Biomedical Chromatography* 22(7):695–701.

Kim, R. J., Malattia, C., Allen, M., *et al*. (2004). Vasopressin and desmopressin in central diabetes insipidus: Adverse effects and clinical considerations. *Pediatric Endocrinology Review* 2(Suppl. 1): 115–123.

Martin, M., Schlaback, G., and Shibinski, K. (1998). The use of non-prescription weight loss products among female basketball, softball and volleyball athletes from NCAA Division 1 Institutions: Issues and concerns. *Journal of Athletic Training* 33(1):41–44.

Moore, J. M., Timperio, A. F., Crawford, D. A., *et al*. (2002). Weight management and weight loss strategies of professional jockeys. *International Journal of Sports Nutrition* 12(1):1–13.

Morra, V., Davit, P., Capra, P., *et al*. (2006). Fast gas chromatographic/mass spectrometric determination of diuretics and masking agents in human urine. Development and validation of a productive screening protocol for antidoping analysis. *Journal of Chromatography A* 1135(2):219–229.

Price, D. (1973). Abuse of diuretics by jockeys. *British Medical Journal* 1(5856):804.

Sanchis-Gomar, F., Martinez-Bello, V. E., Nascimento, A. L., *et al*. (2010). Desmopressin and hemodilution: Implications in doping. *International Journal of Sports Medicine* 31(1):5–9.

Sanchis-Gomar, F., Martinez-Bello, V. E., Debre, F., *et al*. (2011). Rapid hemodilution induced by desmopressin after erythropoietin administration in humans. *Journal of Human Sport and Exercise* 6(2):315–322.

Seiler, S. (2001). Doping disaster for Finnish Ski Team: A turning point for drug testing? *Sportscience* 5(1):1–3.

Thevis, M., Opfermann, G., and Schanzer, W. (2000). Detection of plasma volume expander hydroxyethyl starch in human urine. *Journal of Chromatography B – Analytical Technologies in the Biomedical and Life Sciences* 744(2):345–350.

Ventura, R., and Segura, J. (2010). Masking and manipulation. *Handbook of Experimental Pharmacology* 195:327–354.

World Anti-Doping Agency. (2011). International standard for Therapeutic Use Exemptions. Available online at https://www.wada-ama.org/en/resources/science-medicine/international-standard-for-therapeutic-use-exemptions-istue#.VA9VCssg_X4 (accessed 9 September 2014).

Chapter 10

Manipulation of blood and blood components and the Athlete Biological Passport

Yorck Olaf Schumacher and David Armstrong

10.1. Introduction

In sports events or strenuous exercise lasting more than 1 minute, the predominant mode of energy production is aerobic. Performance is limited by the oxygen that is delivered to and used by the active muscles. Genetic factors aside, the level of performance is determined by the nature of training, which can affect both central and peripheral physiological factors. In most cases, the limiting factors for maximal oxygen uptake are cardiac output and the oxygen-carrying capacity of the blood.

The oxygen-carrying capacity of the blood is determined by the haemoglobin content, which helps bind oxygen within the red blood cells. It is the total body haemoglobin rather than its relative concentration, which is correlated with the maximal oxygen uptake. When the total haemoglobin level falls, exercise performance is impaired. Various ways have been devised to augment the oxygen-carrying capacity of the blood of athletes. These methods include the so-called procedures of blood doping.

The World Anti-Doping Agency (WADA) Prohibited List of Substances and Methods differentiates between the substances used to enhance oxygen transport (erythropoiesis stimulating agents, ESAs) and the methods that are subclassified into blood doping as artificially enhancing the uptake, transport, and delivery of oxygen. The misuse of erythropoietin (EPO) is described in Chapter 6. The WADA regulations for the manipulation of blood and blood components, as published in the WADA Prohibited List, are shown in Table 10.1

Table 10.1 WADA Prohibited List regulations relating to manipulation of blood and blood components

The following are prohibited:
1. The administration or reintroduction of any quantity of autologous, allogeneic (homologous), or heterologous blood or red blood cell products of any origin into the circulatory system
2. Artificially enhancing the uptake, transport, or delivery of oxygen, including, but not limited to, perfluorochemicals, efaproxiral (RSR13), and modified haemoglobin products (e.g. haemoglobin-based blood substitutes, microencapsulated haemoglobin products), excluding supplemental oxygen
3. Any form of intravascular manipulation of the blood or blood components by physical or chemical means

Source: World Anti-Doping Agency. (2014). The 2014 Prohibited List international standard. Available online at https://elb.wada-ama.org/en/what-we-do/prohibited-list (accessed 4 September 2014).

10.2. Blood doping

Blood transfusion

There are two forms of transfusional polycythaemia: autologous and homologous. Autologous blood doping is the transfusion of one's own blood, which has been stored (refrigerated or frozen) until needed. Homologous blood doping is the transfusion of blood that has been taken from another person with the same blood type. The improved performance capability is achieved virtually overnight. The athlete is left with supranormal red blood cell count, haemoglobin concentration, total body haemoglobin, and hence oxygen-carrying capacity of the blood. This will ultimately increase the athlete's aerobic capacity, conferring a positive ergogenic benefit in both training and competition.

The period from 1972 to 1984 marked the heyday of blood doping, and there are numerous reports of allegations and admissions (e.g. Leigh-Smith 2004; Eichner 1987, 2007) involving athletes from a variety of countries (including Finland, Italy, the United States, Russia, East Germany) participating in a variety of different sports (e.g. long-distance running, cycling, skiing). The infusion of one's own blood was not officially banned until 1986. The practice of blood doping was largely superseded in the late 1980s by abuse of EPO, which removed the risks associated with homologous transfusions and the inconvenience of autologous transfusions.

Methods of blood doping

The original method of autologous blood doping involved withdrawing 1–4 units of blood (500–1,500 ml) from an athlete. The blood was then treated further, and the packed red blood cells (RBCs) were stored at 4 °C. The athlete then required 8–12 weeks to replenish the RBCs that had been withdrawn. The blood was then reinfused prior to important competitions.

The advent of glycerol freezing of RBCs at −80 °C permitted storage for up to 10 years with only 10–15 per cent haemolysis. Nevertheless, this process is not applied routinely and only available in very few transfusion centres. Of course, before reinfusion, the RBCs had to be thawed, washed, and resuspended in physiological saline. Detection of residual contaminants of the process has been proposed as a basis for testing for autologous transfusion.

Testing for blood doping

The history of testing for blood doping reflects concerns both for the ethics of sport and the health of participants. The International Olympic Committee (IOC) added blood doping to its banned procedures in 1986. In 1988, the Federation Internationale de Ski (FIS) classified EPO as a doping substance. The FIS made the first attempts to introduce blood sampling for the detection of heterologous/homologous erythrocyte infusions in 1989. Samples were analysed for blood groups, EPO, and haemoglobin (Hb) concentration. Erythropoietin was banned by the IOC in 1990. In 1997, the Union Cycliste Internationale (UCI) and the FIS accepted random blood testing before competition and fixed maximum haematocrit and haemoglobin levels. These tests were instigated, in part, for the benefit of the riders and skiers. Indeed, they were called health checks.

A test for blood doping using a homologous transfusion was introduced in the 2004 Summer Olympic Games in Athens. Detection is based upon a technique known as fluorescence-activated cell sorting (Nelson *et al.* 2003). However, there is currently no method of detecting blood doping through the administration of an autologous transfusion. WADA is funding several scientific studies designed to address this shortcoming. This has led to the development of the Athlete Biological Passport, as described in Section 10.4.

10.3. Blood substitutes

Due to problems with the availability of blood for transfusions and the associated risk of infections (e.g. hepatitis C virus, variant Creutzfeldt-Jakob disease) from transfusions, there has been much research into blood substitutes and into drugs that can increase tissue oxygenation. There are two major types of blood substitutes: haemoglobin-based oxygen carriers (HBOCs) and perfluorocarbons (PFCs).

Haemoglobin-based oxygen carriers

Free Hb is simple to prepare and purify but is unstable, dysfunctional, and ultimately toxic. Even autologous Hb, if infused, will dissociate into dimers, which will impair the function of the blood vessels by inducing vasoconstriction (narrowing of the vessels). The dimers are filtered by the kidney and cause renal tubule necrosis, chronic renal failure, and death.

Numerous techniques have been developed to overcome these problems. Haemoglobin has been polymerised, cross-linked, conjugated, and even encapsulated in attempts to mimic the RBC. The first-generation HBOCs caused vasoconstriction because native Hb binds to the endogenous vasodilator, nitric oxide (NO), in the so-called NO-scavenging effect. Moreover, Hb is readily oxidised and causes a perturbation of the oxidant/antioxidant balance within the vasculature. Second-generation HBOCs incorporated antioxidants (e.g. catalase-superoxide dismutase) into the Hb molecule, but again these were not protected by a red cell membrane mimic. Third-generation HBOCs have incorporated Hb and red cell enzymes into membranes, initially into liposomes and latterly into biodegradable polylactic acid nanoparticles. HBOCs are approved for veterinary use and have been found in possession of athletes, although there is no study that confirms their beneficial effect on performance.

Perfluorocarbons

The PFCs are synthetic, highly fluorinated, inert organic compounds that can dissolve oxygen and other respiratory gases (Lowe 2001). There is no chemical interaction between oxygen and the PFC. The amount of oxygen dissolved in the PFC particles is directly proportional to the partial pressure of oxygen. Thus, the PFC will dissolve oxygen in the lungs, then release it in exchange for carbon dioxide when it passes through the tissues. This process will be repeated for the time that the PFC remains in the body.

First-generation PFCs (e.g. Perftoran) had a long half-life (65 days) but a low capacity to dissolve oxygen (5 ml/dl at a pO_2 of 500 mmHg). Second-generation PFCs (e.g. perflubron) have a shorter half-life (4–6 hrs) and a higher capacity to dissolve oxygen (16 ml/dl at a pO_2 of 500 mmHg). This is comparable to the oxygen-carrying capacity of whole blood. More significantly, because of the linear relationship between the partial pressure of oxygen and the amount of oxygen dissolved in the PFC, 12 ml/dl of oxygen will come out of solution in the tissues, which is greater than that released from whole blood under standard conditions of temperature and pressure (Gaudard *et al.* 2003). The obvious drawback for the athlete wishing to abuse a PFC is that the latter functions best when the subject is inhaling oxygen at greater than ambient partial pressures.

PFCs, as inert organic chemicals, are immiscible in water and must be infused as an emulsion. The droplets are removed from the circulation by phagocytosis by the cells of the reticuloendothelial system. They are not metabolised but are gradually released back into the circulation and excreted in the expired air. They can be detected in both blood and expired air, either by gas chromatography or by a combination of gas chromatography and mass spectrometry. Although these methods exist, they are not applied routinely but only under special circumstances (e.g. when requested by the sporting federation; Gaudard *et al.* 2003).

There have been no published reports of studies of PFCs in humans performing exercise. Neither have there been any confirmed reports of abuse of PFCs in sport. However, they are mentioned specifically in the 2014 WADA Prohibited List.

Haemoglobin modifiers

Another approach to increasing oxygen delivery to the tissues is to decrease the oxygen affinity of Hb (i.e. shifting the oxyhaemoglobin dissociation curve to the right). This is achieved physiologically by increases in $[H^+]$, pCO_2, temperature, and 2,3-bisphosphoglyceric acid (2,3-BPG).

Efaproxiral (RSR13) is a drug that mimics the effects of 2,3-BPG and decreases the oxygen affinity of Hb by binding allosterically to the Hb tetramer. Unlike the naturally occurring 2,3-BPG, RSR13 binds to the α-subunits and not into the cleft between the β-subunits (Gaudard *et al.* 2003). Therefore, it has the potential to be used synergistically to augment the action of the endogenous allosteric inhibitor 2,3-BPG.

One study demonstrated a dose-dependent shift in p50, which is the partial pressure of oxygen at which Hb is 50 per cent saturated. The peak pharmacological effect occurs immediately at the end of the infusion and lasts for 3–6 hours. The drug, which must be given by slow intravenous infusion, was in clinical trials in Canada and the United States as a radiosensitizing agent in cancer therapy. However, it failed to meet a primary endpoint in a phase 3 clinical trial and development has been suspended (Elliott 2008). The drug did have obvious potential for abuse in sport but, to date, this abuse has not materialised.

There have been no adverse analytical findings for RSR13. There has been one media report of an elite Italian cyclist being in possession of RSR13 in 2001. The manufacturer, Allos Therapeutics (Denver, CO) reported that sensitive and validated methods of detection exist for both human blood and urine (Paranka 2001). Breidbach and Catlin (2001) developed a detection method using gas chromatography and mass spectrometry.

10.4. The Athlete Biological Passport

Historical perspective

Since the first introduction of doping controls in sport in the 1960s, doping testing was associated with the direct detection of forbidden substances in a biological sample of urine or blood. The key element in the detection was the fact that the forbidden substance was usually foreign to the human organism and could thus readily be isolated and identified by appropriate analytical methods. With the ever-accelerating technological progress, new treatments for many diseases and new therapeutic substances are emerging every day, many of which potentially enhance athletic performance. A large number of these substances are identical to body components because they are aimed at replacing a lack of production of these components in the diseased human organism. Typical examples are the hormones insulin and EPO, which are nowadays produced through genetically modified cells, providing molecules that are nearly identical to the endogenous hormones. Therefore, the detection of these substances in conventional doping tests is virtually impossible.

The production of recombinant human erythropoietin (rhEPO) was one of the major drug discoveries of the 1980s, and the substance has since been one of the commercially most successful drugs that have ever been marketed. In all endurance sports, the commercial introduction of rhEPO has radically changed the landscape of performance. The substance is believed to have entered the arena of world sports shortly after its commercial introduction in 1989. Several scientific studies show its massive impact on endurance capacity, which is best illustrated by a quote from multiple Tour de France winner and cycling world champion Greg LeMond, who recalled the 1991 Tour de France:

> I was the fittest I had ever been, my split times in spring training rides were the fastest of my career.... But something was different in the 1991 Tour. There were riders from previous years who could not stay on my wheel which were now dropping me on even modest climbs.

This description is matched by the development in performances during that time that were visible in many sports, such as long-distance running and speed skating.

A first attempt at indirect doping detection: Threshold values for blood markers

To tackle the phenomenon of rampant, undetectable rhEPO abuse in the 1990s, sporting federations implemented a new approach of doping detection – so-called indirect doping detection. In contrast to conventional tests that aim at detecting the forbidden substance directly in a sample, the effects of the substance on the organism are investigated in indirect doping detection. Blood manipulation aims at increasing the number of oxygen-carrying red cells in the human organism; the laboratory marker that describes the red cell mass of the organism is haemoglobin concentration, which can easily be measured in any blood sample. Thus, the first approach of indirect detection of blood manipulation through rhEPO abuse was, in 1997, the definition of threshold levels for haemoglobin concentration or haematocrit (a measure that describes the percentage of cellular elements in the blood, closely related to haemoglobin concentration): Male cyclists who presented with haemoglobin values above 17 g/dl or haematocrit readings above 50 per cent at precompetition blood tests were not allowed to start the race, officially for health reasons because this indirect approach could not, at that time, be defined as a doping test as no forbidden substance was detected.

Given that approximately 3 per cent of the healthy male population have haemoglobin values above 17 g/dl or haematocrits above 50 per cent, it quickly became clear that these measures were unsuitable to continue any further in the fight against doping, due to a lack of specificity and poor sensitivity.

Second-generation blood tests: A combination of markers

The second generation of blood tests for the detection of blood manipulation in sports used combinations of several blood markers related to the RBC production: The most commonly used combination is the so-called OFF score, which is calculated from the aforementioned haemoglobin concentration and the percentage of young RBCs (reticulocytes). The name 'OFF score' stems from the fact that this approach is most sensitive to discontinuation of erythropoietic substances; thus, it will flag individuals who have stopped taking rhEPO shortly before the test. The score can be related to a likelihood of finding such result in a healthy, undoped population of athletes. Threshold values of this OFF score were soon established, in addition to the existing simple haemoglobin or haematocrit cut-off values.

An individual approach: The longitudinal monitoring of biomarkers

One of the main criticisms of the first- and second-generation approaches based on fixed thresholds was the fact that athletes with naturally low haemoglobin values could use rhEPO until they reach a level close to the defined thresholds without ever raising suspicion, whereas athletes with higher natural levels had no option to manipulate. This gave birth to the idea of individual, longitudinal monitoring of certain biological markers to identify doping-specific patterns. The ideal marker for longitudinal monitoring is a marker with small intraindividual variability but large interindividual variability (Harris 1974). Another condition is a standardised analytical procedure to reduce the analytical variation, which might also affect any longitudinal monitoring.

Several mathematical approaches have been developed to formally evaluate longitudinal data. These algorithms compare the biological marker to a reference collective and the previous data from the athlete. To describe the variance of each marker, variance estimates from large reference collectives are used, assuming a universal individual variance that is the same for each athlete. The mathematical algorithms thus define individual limits (upper and lower) for each variable, taking into account the previous data of each athlete individually.

The range of these individual limits is predefined by the desired specificity of the analysis. For example, a typical specificity would be 99.9 per cent, which would define an individual range that is only exceeded in one of 1,000 cases of undoped athletes. (The mathematically interested reader is referred to Sharpe et al. (2006) and Sottas et al. (2006, 2010a) for details of the calculations for the different approaches.) A typical profile analysis is illustrated in Figure 10.1, where the measured haemoglobin values of the athlete are shown in the centre, and the individually calculated limits are presented on either side.

The Athlete Biological Passport procedure

If a value is found outside the individually calculated reference ranges, it must be emphasized that this does not automatically mean the anomaly is caused by doping. To identify potential causes for such abnormalities, the profile is then examined by a dual-layer system of experts, who determine one of the following:

1   The observed abnormality is an extreme of natural variation and can therefore be considered as normal.
2   The observed abnormality is caused by a pathology.
3   The observed abnormality is indicative of doping, but further testing is required to confirm the suspicion.
4   The observed abnormality and the profile bear clear features of doping and do not need any further tests.

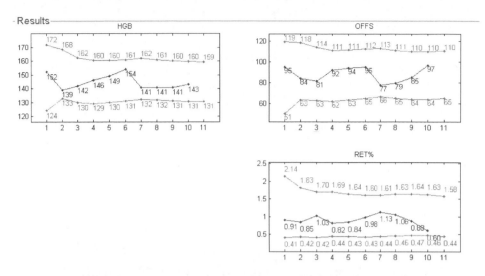

Figure 10.1 Normal haematological profile depicting the haematological markers of haemoglobin concentration (*top left*), reticulocytes (*bottom right*), and OFF score (*top right*). The horizontal axis shows the blood samples of the athlete (ten in this case). The vertical axis shows the unit (g/l for haemoglobin concentration, per cent for reticulocytes).

A first expert evaluates the profile and renders one of the four opinions mentioned above. If he deems it typical for doping, it is then independently evaluated by two further experts under the same criteria. For their evaluation, they can ask for additional information, such as the athlete's whereabouts or competition schedule. One of the key elements in their evaluation is the identification of a doping scenario (i.e. a likely manipulation strategy), which is necessary to take legal action in order to prevail in court. If all three experts independently conclude from the available data that the profile is highly likely to be caused by doping and unlikely by any other cause, the athlete is contacted to provide explanations regarding his or her profile. These explanations are again anonymously evaluated by the experts, who will reassess their previous opinion in light of the explanations of the athlete. If they confirm their suspicion, a disciplinary procedure will be engaged against the athlete.

An example of an ABP profile indicating likely abuse of an erythropoietic stimulant is presented in Figure 10.3. The process of evaluation of the data of the Athlete Biological Passport is illustrated in Figure 10.2.

Implementation

The first sporting federation to implement the Athlete Biological Passport was UCI in 2008. In their passport program, approximately 800 athletes are followed on a regular basis. Since 2008, the program has had a significant success. Not only were a number of athletes convicted based solely on their passport data, but other athletes were also found to be positive for forbidden substances in targeted, traditional doping tests scheduled based on information from the athlete's blood passport. Epidemiological data show that the prevalence of abnormal blood values in the collective of cyclists submitted to the longitudinal monitoring has heavily decreased since the introduction of the Athlete Biological Passport (Zorzoli and Rossi 2010).

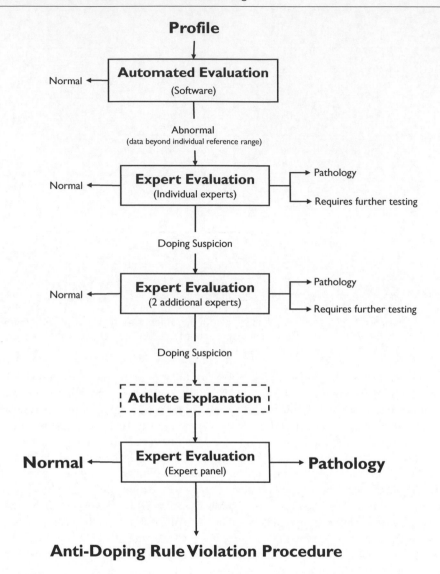

Figure 10.2 Flowchart of the evaluation process for the assessment of blood profiles in the Athlete Biological Passport. (Adapted from Schumacher *et al.* 2012.)

Since then, a large number of national and international anti-doping stakeholders have implemented the Athlete Biological Passport program, which is now under the supervision of WADA. The organisation publishes and updates the guidelines for the Athlete Biological Passport on a regular basis (WADA 2012).

Other applications

Unlike conventional anti-doping samples, data from the tests conducted for the Athlete Biological Passport contain valuable information that can be used for a multitude of purposes

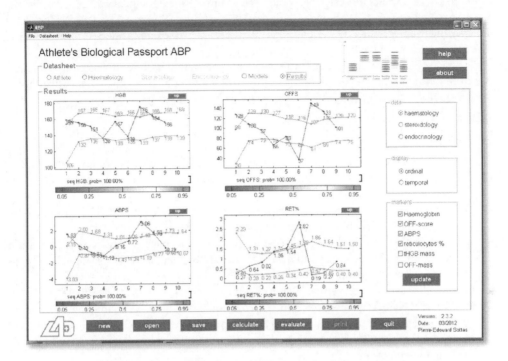

Figure 10.3 Example of a blood passport indicating the abuse of an erythropoietic stimulant. A stimulation/withdrawal phase (*arrows*) can clearly be identified in the reticulocyte panel. Sample 6 shows a stimulation. In samples 7 and 8, the haemoglobin concentration is increased and the reticulocytes are suppressed. Other examples can be found in Zorzoli and Rossi (2012).

in the fight against doping. First, testing a large number of competitors at a given race allows the calculation of the prevalence of doping in the examined collective at the given race. Through comparison of the distribution of the passport markers in the tested collective with the data of an undoped reference group, the prevalence can be estimated (Sottas *et al.* 2011). As mentioned, the scrutiny of passport data also allows the identification of new doping trends through changes in an athlete's profiles for certain variables (Zorzoli and Rossi 2010). Finally, the Athlete Biological Passport and its targeted testing have a considerable deterrent effect. Athletes who are tested will know that, unlike in conventional doping tests with a borderline result, the data from the Athlete Biological Passport will remain with them over their entire career.

Future developments

The current passport application, with its haematological module, aims at detecting blood doping with erythropoietic stimulants or blood transfusions. New modules for the detection of steroid and growth hormone abuse are under development. For the steroidal module, several metabolites in the testosterone metabolism are analysed and traced over time, adhering to the same principles as described for the haematological variables: the testosterone-epitestosterone ratio, the testosterone:androsterone ratio, the androsterone:atiocholanolone ratio, and the 5α-androstane-3α,17β-diol:5β-androstane-3α,17β-diol ratio (Sottas *et al.* 2010b). The steroidal module was introduced on 1 January 2014 and now runs alongside the haematological module as part of the ABP.

The endocrinological module for growth hormone detection is currently under development. It will likely include the main mediators of growth hormone in the body, namely insulin-like growth factor 1 and procollagen type III, as the primary markers.

10.5. Summary

•   The Athlete Biological Passport is a longitudinal collection of biological data obtained from an athlete to detect doping indirectly through the effect of the doping substances on certain biological markers.
•   It is currently used for the detection of blood doping. The key biological markers in this context are haemoglobin concentration and reticulocytes.
•   The evaluation procedure consists of a formal, software-based analysis of the data of the athlete and a subsequent qualitative analysis of suspicious patterns identified by the software through a panel of experts.
•   Other applications derived from the information obtained from the Athlete Biological Passport include improved targeting of conventional doping tests, the detection of new doping trends, and the calculation of doping prevalence.
•   New developments are passport modules for the indirect detection of doping with steroids and growth hormone.

10.6. References

Breidbach, A., and Catlin, D. H. (2001). RSR13, a potential athletic performance enhancement agent: Detection in urine by gas chromatography/mass spectrometry. *Rapid Communications in Mass Spectrometry* 15(24):2378–2382.

Eichner, E. R. (1987). Blood doping: Results and consequences from the laboratory and the field. *Physician and Sportsmedicine* 15(7):121–129.

Eichner, E. R. (2007). Blood doping: Infusions, erythropoietin and artificial blood. *Sports Medicine* 37(4–5):389–391.

Elliott, S. (2008). Erythropoiesis-stimulating agents and other methods to enhance oxygen transport. *British Journal of Pharmacology* 154(3):529–541.

Gaudard, A., Varlet-Marie, E., Bressolle, F., *et al.* (2003). Drugs for increasing oxygen transport and their potential use in doping. *Sports Medicine* 33(3):187–212.

Harris, E. K. (1974). Effects of intra-and interindividual variation on the appropriate use of normal ranges. *Clinical Chemistry* 20(12):1535.

Leigh-Smith, S. (2004). Blood boosting: A review. *British Journal of Sports Medicine* 38(1):99–101.

Lowe, K. C. (2001). Fluorinated blood substitutes and oxygen carriers. *Journal of Fluoride Chemistry* 109(1):59–65.

Nelson, M., Popp, H., Sharpe, K., and Ashenden, M. (2003). Proof of homologous blood transfusion through quantification of blood group antigens. *Haematologica* 88(11):1284–1295.

Paranka, N. (2001). Haemoglobin modifiers: Is RSR 13 the next aerobic enhancer? In the *International Society for Laboratory Hematology (ISLH) XIVth International Symposium* (p. 23). Glenview, IL: International Society for Laboratory Hematology.

Schumacher, Y. O., and d'Onofrio, G. (2012). Scientific expertise and the athlete's biological passport: 3 years of experience. *Clinical Chemistry* 58(6):979–985.

Sharpe, K., Ashenden, M. J., and Schumacher, Y. O. (2006). A third generation approach to detect erythropoietin abuse in athletes. *Haematologica* 91(3):356.

Sottas, P.-E., Robinson, N., Fischetto, G., Dollé, G., Alonso, J. M., and Saugy, M. (2011). Prevalence of blood doping in samples collected from elite track and field athletes. *Clinical Chemistry* 57(5):762–769.

Sottas, P.-E., Robinson, N., Giraud, S., Taroni, F., Kamber, M., Mangin, P., *et al.* (2006). Statistical classification of abnormal blood profiles in athletes. *International Journal of Biostatistics* 2(1):3.

Sottas, P.-E., Robinson, N., and Saugy, M. (2010a). The athlete's biological passport and indirect markers of blood doping. *Handbook of Experimental Pharmacology* 195:305–326.

Sottas, P.-E., Saugy, M., and Saudan, C. (2010b). Endogenous steroid profiling in the Athlete Biological Passport. *Endocrinological Metabolism Clinics North America* 39(1):59–73.

World Anti-Doping Agency. (2012). Athlete Biological Passport operating guidelines v. 3.1. Available online at https://wada-main-prod.s3.amazonaws.com/resources/files/WADA-ABP-Operating-Guidelines_v3.1-EN.pdf (accessed 9 September 2014).

Zorzoli, M., and Rossi, F. (2010). Implementation of the biological passport: The experience of the International Cycling Union. *Drug Testing Analysis* 2(11–12):542–547.

Zorzoli, M., and Rossi, F. (2012). Case studies on ESA-doping as revealed by the Biological Passport. *Drug Testing Analysis* 4(11):854–858.

Chapter 11

Chemical and physical manipulation

David R. Mottram

11.1. Introduction

Athletes are liable for both targeted and randomised, no-notice drug testing, both in competition and out of competition. Those athletes who use prohibited substances and methods are keen to avoid detection. Procedures that are used for this subterfuge are classified by the World Anti-Doping Agency (WADA) as chemical and physical manipulation and are subject to anti-doping rule violation regulations. This chapter outlines some of the techniques that have been used by athletes in attempts to avoid detection and the methods by which such abuse is monitored and controlled.

11.2. The 2014 WADA regulations on chemical and physical manipulation

The 2014 WADA regulations related to the prohibited methods involving chemical and physical manipulation are shown in Table 11.1. Clearly, there are significant legitimate circumstances where an athlete may require intravenous infusions. WADA therefore provides clarification with respect to these regulations as follows (WADA 2011):

> By definition, an [intravenous] infusion is the supply of fluids or other liquid substrates via the insertion of a specialized needle into a vein and infusing fluids at a predetermined rate from a reservoir usually situated above the level of the body. An intravenous injection is the supply of fluid or medication by means of a syringe with a standard or butterfly needle, directly into a vein. Infusions or injections are permitted if the infused/injected substance is not on the Prohibited List [and] the volume of intravenous fluid administered does not exceed 50 mL per 6-hour period. Intravenous infusions are prohibited and thus require Therapeutic Use Exemption except in the management of surgical procedures, medical emergencies or clinical investigations.

Table 11.1 WADA Prohibited List regulations related to chemical and physical manipulation

The following are prohibited:
1. Tampering or attempting to tamper in order to alter the integrity and validity of samples collected during doping control. These include, but are not limited to, urine substitution and/or adulteration (e.g. proteases).
2. Intravenous infusions and/or injections of more than 50 mL per 6-hour period, except for those legitimately received in the course of hospital admissions or clinical investigations.

Source: World Anti-Doping Agency. (2014). The 2014 Prohibited List international standard. Available online at https://elb.wada-ama.org/en/what-we-do/prohibited-list (accessed 4 September 2014).

Table 11.2 Positive test results related to chemical and physical manipulation from WADA statistics (2003–2012)

Year	Number of adverse analytical findings
2003	2
2004	–
2005	–
2006	4
2007	3
2008	–
2009	5
2010	6
2011	3
2012	1

It is difficult to anticipate the varied and imaginative ways in which athletes may undertake chemical and physical manipulation to avoid detection of prohibited drug use. In 2007, Jaffee *et al.* reported that adulterants and urine substitutes that are designed to defeat doping control tests are readily available over the internet, along with data on their efficacy. However, the authors concluded that vigilant precautions will be able to detect most instances of tampering. The next section provides illustrative case studies in which various methods have been used.

11.3. Prevalence of chemical and physical manipulation in sport

WADA statistics related to chemical and physical manipulation

Table 11.2 shows the number of positive test results from WADA-accredited laboratories related to chemical and physical manipulation since 2003. It is clear that few instances have been identified. To what extent this reflects athletes' disinclination to use such techniques or an inability on behalf of the laboratories to identify such practices is difficult to establish.

Case studies of attempted chemical and physical manipulation

Athletes have attempted to avoid detection of prohibited substances and methods for many years using a wide variety of methods, either alone or in collaboration with others.

Katrina Krabbe (1992)

Katrina Krabbe won three gold medals at the 1990 European Athletic Championships, the last time East Germany competed in track-and-field athletics under its own flag. She won two gold medals for the unified German team in the 100- and 200-m events at the 1991 World Championships in Tokyo. Prior to the 1992 Olympic Games, Katrina Krabbe and her teammates, Grit Breuer and Silke Moeller, provided allegedly identical urine samples during a test at a training camp in South Africa. All three athletes were suspended from racing, although the suspension was lifted 4 months later on a technicality associated with the test. Katrina Krabbe and Grit Breuer received subsequent suspensions after testing positive for clenbuterol prior to the 1992 Barcelona Olympic Games.

At the 1996 Atlanta Olympic Games, Michelle de Bruin won three gold medals in swimming events – somewhat unexpectedly, in the minds of many observers. Her trainer had been her husband, Eric de Bruin, a former Dutch discus thrower who had served a 4-year suspension for failing a drug test for testosterone.

Michelle de Bruin (1998)

Following the 1996 Atlanta Olympic Games, Michelle de Bruin missed at least one out-of-competition drug test and received a warning from her governing body, Fédération Internationale de Natation (FINA). In January 1998, she was asked to provide a urine sample at her home in Dublin during an unannounced out-of-competition drug test administered by FINA. The sample was analysed at the International Olympic Committee Accredited Laboratory in Barcelona and was found to have unequivocal signs of adulteration, according to the laboratory report.

The report stated that the concentration of alcohol present 'is in no way compatible with human consumption' and that the sample showed 'a very strong whiskey odor.' A second test on the urine B sample was performed in May 1998; the results were compatible with the January findings. At a hearing in July 1998, a FINA doping panel found that the sample had been manipulated in an uncertain manner by de Bruin.

Michelle de Bruin was banned from national and international competition for 4 years. She appealed the decision at the Court of Arbitration for Sport (CAS). The hearing revealed that traces of a metabolic precursor of testosterone had been found in three samples from the swimmer during tests taken between November 1997 and March 1998. The CAS upheld the ban.

A number of cases have involved athletes sharing urine samples with other athletes.

Galabin Boevski (2003)

The Bulgarian weightlifters Galabin Boevski, Zlatan Vanev, and Georgi Markov were suspended from competition after it was alleged that they provided identical urine samples derived from one person when tested at the World Championships in Vancouver in 2003. Zlatan Vanev and Georgi Markov, both world champions, were given 18-month suspensions. Galabin Boevski, who won a gold medal at the 2000 Olympic Games in Sydney, was given an 8-year suspension because it was his second adverse analytical finding since 1995.

Rebecca Gusmao (2007)

A Brazilian swimmer, Rebecca Gusmao, underwent a doping control test at the 2007 Pan American Games in Rio de Janeiro, Brazil. The WADA-accredited laboratory at Rio reported the test to be negative. However, the games were attended by a WADA independent observer (IO) team, whose role was randomly to monitor and report on all phases of the doping control and results management processes in a neutral and unbiased fashion.

The IO team reported to the international swimming federation, FINA, that Gusmao had been tested on multiple occasions prior to and over the course of the games, and that these tests had yielded some suspicious results suggestive of possible manipulation. Upon review of the steroid profiles for the swimmer, it appeared that the samples were from two different people because the endogenous steroid profile was very different.

The urine samples were retested to compare genotypes. It was confirmed that they belonged to different donators. Gusmao denied having tampered with the samples and, furthermore, claimed invalidity of the follow-up tests. The FINA Doping Panel rejected her claims and instituted a lifetime ban because Gusmao had already received a previous suspension from FINA.

Other cases have involved substitution of urine samples at the time of testing.

Olga Yegorova (2008)

Olga Yegorova, along with seven other leading Russian track-and-field athletes, was suspended by the International Association of Athletics Federations (IAAF) after being charged with manipulating urine samples. The athletes were accused of urine substitution when samples taken at the world championships in Osaka did not match samples taken in out-of-competition tests in May 2007.

Yegorova had previously tested positive for erythropoietin at the 2001 world championships in Edmonton, but her suspension for that offence was lifted because incomplete testing procedures had taken place.

Miscellaneous cases of chemical and physical manipulation

Thevis *et al*. (2012) described a number of selected cases of suspected urine manipulation. In one case, an athlete substituted a urine sample with nonalcoholic beer, as identified through the presence of saccharides in the sample, accompanied by hordenine and Serpine-Z4; no endogenous steroids were detected, as would be expected within a normal urine sample.

In other cases, unusual colouration of the urine samples was observed (Thevis *et al*. 2012). The red colouration in some urine samples may be produced through the presence of betacyanins, betanin, and isobetanin; these are natural constituents of urine following the consumption of beetroot juice, which is sometimes used as a dietary nitrate supplement, and they do not indicate a doping offence. An unusual case involving green colouration of urine was attributed to the presence of methylene blue, a rarely used therapeutic agent; again, no doping violation had occurred in this case.

Finally, Thevis *et al*. (2012) described the case of four urine specimens that returned similar steroid profiles. The results of an investigation into this, using DNA analysis, revealed that a doping control officer had filled the urine collection containers with her own urine. All of these cases led Thevis and co-workers to urge doping control laboratories to follow up suspicious results that might indicate tampering.

11.4. Techniques for identifying chemical and physical manipulation

The most common method of manipulation used by athletes, as determined from WADA laboratory results, has involved the sharing of urine samples between fellow athletes or from other individuals. In recent years, it has been possible to individualize urine specimens using steroid and metabolic profiling. An athlete steroid profile is made by recording ratios of various urinary steroid components repeatedly, each time the athlete is tested. The steroidal ratios recorded include testosterone:epitestosterone, andresterone:etiocholanolone, 5α-androstane-3α,17β-diol:5β-androstane-3α,17β-diol, and androstane/testosterone (Mareck *et al*. 2008). The successful detection of manipulation by three weightlifters was described by Thevis *et al*. (2007a), who employed steroid profiling along with common drug testing approaches, including chromatographic and mass spectrometric assays as well as DNA typing.

Adulteration of urine samples with highly oxidative chemicals that produce changes in endogenous steroid profile parameters has been reported (Kuzhiumparambil and Fu 2013). Athletes have reportedly introduced protease granules into the urethra. When flushed out into the urine sample, protease enzymes digest urinary proteins, such as erythropoietin and insulins, without affecting other urinary parameters. Testing regimes can detect increased levels of protease enzymes in the urine and also detect the absence of proteins normally excreted in the urine, such as albumin (Thevis *et al*. 2008). It is for this reason that WADA includes proteases as prohibited urine adulterants (see Table 11.1). Effective analytical procedures are available to detect the use of proteases (Thevis *et al*. 2007b). Such strategies for combating drug misuse and sample manipulation require comprehensive out-of-competition testing and intelligent targeting of athletes.

In addition to biochemical laboratory urine testing, blood sampling, and longitudinal monitoring of steroid profiles, a further refinement involves performance profiling (Schumacher *et al*. 2009). Although sudden increases in performance can be induced by many factors, including improved training methods and nutrition regimes, performance profiling can identify suspicious athletes.

11.5. Summary

- Athletes who use prohibited substances and methods are keen to avoid detection of such practices at the time of testing.
- WADA classifies these methods as chemical and physical manipulation.
- Although infrequently detected, diverse methods have been attempted by athletes to avoid detection, either alone or in collaboration with other athletes.
- Effective techniques for identifying manipulation have been developed.

11.6. References

Jaffee, W. B., Trucco, E., Levy, S., *et al*. (2007). Is this urine really negative? A systematic review of tampering methods in urine drug screening and testing. *Journal of Substance Abuse Treatment* 33(1):33–42.

Kuzhiumparambil, U., and Fu, S. (2013). Effect of oxidising adulterants on human urinary steroid profiles. *Steroids* 78(2):288–296.

Mareck, U., Geyer, H., Opfermann, G., *et al*. (2008). Factors influencing the steroid profile in doping control analysis. *Journal of Mass Spectrometry* 43(7):877–891.

Schumacher, Y. O., and Pottgiesser, T. (2009). Performance profiling: A role for sport science in the fight against doping? *International Journal of Sports Physiology and Performance* 4(1):129–133.

Thevis, M., Geyer, H., and Mareck, U. (2007a). Detection of manipulation in doping control urine sample collection: A multidisciplinary approach to determine identical urine samples. *Analytical and Bioanalytical Chemistry* 388(7):1539–1543.

Thevis, M., Geyer, H., Sigmund, G., *et al*. (2012). Sports drug testing: Analytical aspects of selected cases of suspected, purported and proven urine manipulation. *Journal of Pharmaceutical and Biomedical Analysis* 57:26–32.

Thevis, M., Kohler, M., and Schanzer, W. (2008). New drugs and methods of doping and manipulation. *Drug Discovery Today* 13(1/2):59–66.

Thevis, M., Maurer, J., Kohler, M., *et al*. (2007b). Proteases in doping control analysis. *International Journal of Sports Medicine* 28(7):545–549.

World Anti-Doping Agency. (2011). Medical information to support the decisions of TUECs intravenous infusions. Available online at https://www.wada-ama.org/en/resources/science-medicine/medical-information-to-support-the-decisions-of-tuecs-intravenous#.VA9a18sg_X4 (accessed 9 September).

Chapter 12

Gene doping

Dominic J. Wells

12.1. Introduction

Genetic manipulation is now a standard tool for biologists interested in understanding gene function in health and disease. This can take the form of adding genetic material to an organism (a transgene) or modifying the expression of endogenous genes (knockout or knock-in experiments). The majority of such studies involves the modification of cells in culture or the modification of the reproductive cells of animals, mostly mice, so that the modification is expressed in all of the cells of a tissue (e.g. muscle) and the modification is heritable. However, it is also possible to modify nonreproductive (somatic) tissues in the mature animal. The latter technology, which is mostly intended for genetic therapies of inherited or acquired disease, raises the possibility of genetic manipulation for increased sporting performance (gene doping).

The vast majority of drug treatments are given on an intermittent basis by mouth or by injection, such as weekly, daily, or twice daily. Because all drugs are removed from the body by metabolism or excretion, it is necessary to administer a large dose to maintain concentrations at or above the minimum effective dose in the target tissue(s) until the time of the next administration of drug. In the case of doping for increased athletic performance, these large doses increase the possibility of detection of the prohibited drug. In contrast, gene transfer generally leads to a continuous steady-state expression that avoids the need for intermittent large doses. This is likely to make detection harder because the protein may only be close to the minimum therapeutic level. Secondly, because the protein is made within the body of the treated individual, it is more likely to be indistinguishable from the normal endogenous protein. Finally, in many cases, the gene and its product may remain within the treated tissue (e.g. skeletal muscle) and thus are less likely to be detected by assays using urine or blood. Consequently, gene doping may be harder to detect than conventional drug doping. It therefore may be more likely to be adopted by athletes who are seeking to gain an unfair competitive advantage.

Detection of gene doping is likely to prove challenging and requires different methodologies compared to current strategies for detection of doping. The main targets, methods, and detection of gene doping are reviewed in the following sections.

12.2. What is gene doping?

The potential of gene doping was first raised by experiments in mice showing that increased expression of insulin-like growth factor 1 (IGF-1) could aid repair and increase the performance of muscle. The key experiment was reported in 1998 when Barton-Davis *et al.* demonstrated that viral vector delivery of IGF-1 to the skeletal muscles of mice increased muscle mass and strength in both young and old mice. This was an important finding because it showed that it was possible to genetically enhance muscle in an adult animal by somatic gene transfer – a technology that should be applicable to humans. The same group went on to demonstrate that gene transfer of IGF-1 can act synergistically with training to enhance muscle strength in rats (Lee *et al.* 2004). Others have noted that IGF-1 can improve the rate of muscle repair (Schertzer and Lynch 2006), which further adds to the attractiveness of this form of performance enhancement.

There are now a large number of candidate genes that might be chosen for gene doping. Particularly important are genes that increase muscle mass, modify the metabolic properties of muscle, or improve the performance of the cardiovascular system, either by increasing cardiac output or by increasing the carriage of oxygen in the blood. Well-known examples of genetic mutations conferring increased strength or endurance are the marked muscle hypertrophy reported in a myostatin-null infant (Schuelke *et al.* 2004) and the Finnish cross-country skier Eero Mäntyranta, whose natural mutation in his erythropoietin (Epo) receptor gene led to high haemoglobin levels and thus high endurance (de la Chapelle *et al.* 1993).

A number of genetic manipulations conferring increased athletic performance have been tested only in laboratory animals; it is the results of these studies that have concerned the regulatory authorities. These include experiments in which the myostatin gene was removed or repressed. Myostatin is a negative regulator of muscle growth, acting to reduce muscle mass when the physical demand on the muscle is reduced. Mice lacking the myostatin gene (knockout) have muscles with both a greater number of muscle fibres (hyperplasia) and larger fibres (hypertrophy) than normal mice (McPherron *et al.* 1997). A number of natural myostatin mutants have been identified in dogs, cattle, and sheep (Grobet *et al.* 1997; Mosher *et al.* 2007; Boman *et al.* 2009) and the human example quoted previously (Schuelke *et al.* 2004). Although the complete knockout of myostatin in mice has been linked to a decrease in specific force (Amthor *et al.* 2007), partial knockdown of myostatin due to a heterozygous genetic mutation has been clearly linked to improved muscle performance in the whippet (Mosher *et al.* 2007).

A number of studies have shown that a partial knockdown of myostatin can be performed in normal animals using a variety of approaches, including antibody blockade (Whittemore *et al.* 2003), blockade by use of a mutant propeptide (Qiao *et al.* 2008), and antagonism using follistatin or molecules derived from follistatin (Iezzi *et al.* 2004; Nakatani *et al.* 2008). Myostatin polymorphisms in racehorses have been linked to improved athletic performance at different distances (Hill *et al.* 2010). Studies have shown that bone morphogenetic protein signalling, acting through Smad1, Smad5, and Smad8 (Smad1/5/8), is the fundamental hypertrophic signal in mice (Sartori *et al.* 2013). This finding opens up additional potential routes to try to induce muscle hypertrophy through gene doping.

Our increasing understanding of the regulation of energy balance and fibre-type determination in skeletal muscle has revealed a number of additional targets. Transgenic mice expressing peroxisome-proliferator-activated receptor-gamma (PPAR-γ) have been shown to have double the running endurance compared to wild-type mice (Wang *et al.* 2004). Gene transfer of PPAR-γ into rat muscle by plasmid electroporation increased IIa and decreased IIb fibres following acute gene transfer (Lunde *et al.*, 2007). Transgenic mice expressing the PPAR-γ co-activator alpha (PGC-1α) develop muscles comprised mostly of type I; they demonstrated a high fatigue resistance (Lin *et al.* 2002) and improved aerobic performance

(Calvo *et al.* 2008). Similar mice expressing PGC-1β develop muscles with a high proportion of type IIX fibres and have increased endurance at high workloads (Arany *et al.* 2007). Finally, transgenic mice expressing phosphoenolpyruvate carboxykinase show a substantially enhanced aerobic capacity (Hakimi *et al.* 2007). These findings correlate with observations in elite human athletes; for example, mRNA expression of PPAR-α, PPAR-δ, PPAR-η, PGC-1-α, and PGC-1β is naturally increased in elite human cyclists, with an increased proportion of type I slow-twitch, oxidative fibres, when compared with normally active subjects (Krämer *et al.*, 2006).

It should be noted that, apart from the study by Lunde *et al.* (2007), all the other experimental animal studies were performed in transgenic mice; therefore, it is not certain that the same responses will follow gene transfer in the adult. In addition, some studies of transgenic mice show conflicting results. Although two reports showed improved performance in PGC-1α transgenic mice, Miura *et al.* (2006) found that overexpression of PGC-1α leads to muscle atrophy. Choi *et al.* (2008) reported PGC-1α transgenics that showed fat-induced insulin resistance in muscle, similar to type 2 diabetics. In contrast, the PPAR-δ agonist GW 1516 raised endurance levels by 75 per cent in normal exercising mice and the PPAR-δ-AMP-activated protein kinase (AMPK) agonist AICAR improved exercise performance by 44 per cent after 4 weeks of treatment without any training (Narkar *et al.* 2008), which demonstrates that these pathways can be effectively manipulated. Indeed, such molecules are specified on the World Anti-Doping Agency (WADA) Prohibited List.

A significant limitation to endurance in high-performance athletes is the rate of delivery of oxygen to the muscle. This can be improved by increasing the proportion of red blood cells (haematocrit), and hence the oxygen-carrying haemoglobin, in the blood. Red blood cell production is governed by the hormone erythropoietin (Epo), which is produced in the kidney. Recombinant Epo has a long history of abuse in endurance events, such as cross-country skiing and cycling, and a number of studies in animals have demonstrated the potential of gene transfer to boost circulating levels of Epo. For example, electroporation of plasmid encoding Epo into mouse and nonhuman primate muscle resulted in a raised haematocrit (Fattori *et al.* 2005). In addition, drug-regulated expression of Epo has been demonstrated following intramuscular delivery of adeno-associated viruses (AAV) encoding Epo into muscles of nonhuman primates (Rivera *et al.* 2005). In the latter study, the haematocrit could be controlled by the administration of rapamycin, thus avoiding the dangers associated with an excessively high haematocrit.

Finally, Schuler *et al.* (2014) recently described the role that alpha-calcitonin-gene-related peptide (aCGRP) plays in cardiac hypertrophy. Cardiac hypertrophy occurs in response to exercise in order to be able to increase blood delivery to the skeletal muscle; this is mediated by the release of aCGRP from contracting skeletal muscles. Thus, it is technically possible to accelerate cardiac hypertrophy through administration of aCGRP, either from an exogenous source or from gene transfer into muscle. However, although this would initially be beneficial for delivery of oxygen to the muscle, it is uncertain what the health consequences of long-term exposure to elevated levels of aCGRP might be.

12.3. Clinical uses of gene therapy

There is concern that methods developed for genetic approaches to human disease (gene therapy) may be used for athletic enhancement (Fischetto and Bermon 2013). Although there have been 1,892 human gene therapy trials approved worldwide between 1989 and 2013

(*Journal of Gene Medicine* 2014), very few have shown clear efficacy. Only one therapy (for lipoprotein lipase deficiency) has been licensed in Europe for human use (Kastelein *et al.* 2013) and two viral products for the treatment of cancer have been licensed in China (Kim *et al.* 2008).

Genetic manipulation of the early embryo can be used to produce transgenic animals in which additional gene(s) are added or where specific genes are inactivated in all cells of the body or in all cells of a specific cell type, such as skeletal muscle cells. The technology for this early manipulation is relatively inefficient and is thus not suitable for use in humans, even if such modifications were ever considered to be ethically acceptable. However, in animals, particularly the mouse, the effects of such manipulations can be used to understand gene function and the potential consequences of genetic manipulation at the whole body level. This technology can be used to look at the ability of different forms of a therapeutic protein to prevent disease in a mouse model of human disease, such as testing different forms of dystrophin in the *mdx* mouse model of the lethal muscle wasting disease Duchenne muscular dystrophy (Wells *et al.* 1995; Phelps *et al.* 1995).

Genetic material can be delivered to cells both *in vitro* (cell culture) and *in vivo* (whole animal) using transfer systems called vectors. Modified viruses are the most common form of vectors; during evolution, viruses developed highly efficient systems for introducing their genomes into cells in order to complete their life cycle and generate more viruses. By deleting part or all of the viral genes from the modified viruses, they can be rendered replication deficient; therefore, the introduction of genetic material into the cell is not followed by the normal cell damage associated with viral replication. Not only does this help to prevent cell damage, but it also ensures that the spread of such modified viruses is limited. The production of replication-deficient viral vectors is accomplished in specific cell lines where the genes for viral replication are introduced in a form that allows viral replication but does not allow these genes to be packaged into the viruses that are produced by the cells. The removal of viral genes from the virus also provides space for introduction of the gene(s) of choice together with the regulatory elements controlling their expression. The latter can be used to ensure that the genes are only expressed in the correct tissue, such as skeletal muscle.

A large number of viruses have been developed as viral vectors, including adenoviruses, AAV, herpesviruses, retroviruses (including lentiviruses), and alphaviruses (e.g. Semliki forest virus). The retroviruses have the particular property of inserting their genomes into the host genome, which leads to a permanent modification of the host cell. In contrast, most of the other viruses exist as nonintegrated episomes within the nucleus and can be lost with successive rounds of cell division. All viruses have viral proteins on their surface; these determine the cell types that the viruses are able to enter. This tropism can be modified by altering the viral proteins, either by selecting different serotypes or by pseudotyping with proteins from other viruses. Advances in understanding AAV serotypes have identified minor changes in capsid protein sequences that dramatically alter the tissue targeting of the specific serotypes; these can be used to increase the efficiency and specificity of tissue targeting (Gao *et al.* 2002; Vandenberghe *et al.* 2009).

Preclinical studies have shown that AAV is the viral vector of choice, particularly for targeting skeletal muscle. A number of studies have shown that it is possible to achieve bodywide genetic modification of skeletal muscle in rodents and larger species using AAV vectors of several different serotypes (e.g. Gregorevic *et al.* 2004; Zhu *et al.* 2005; Denti *et al.* 2006; Yue *et al.* 2008; Vitiello *et al.* 2009). However, a significant drawback with the use of viral vectors is that the presence of viral proteins on the surface leads to interaction with the acquired immune system, which can neutralize and thus block any effects of repeated administration. In people exposed to the wild-type virus, such antibodies can effectively block the initial administration. Indeed, approximately 60 per cent of healthy people in France have neutralizing antibodies to the most common form of AAV (Boutin *et al.* 2010). While it appears possible to use immunosuppression to modify the interaction with the immune system, this increases the risks associated with gene transfer. Recently, plasmapheresis, which temporarily removes antibodies from the blood, has been used to allow successful administration of an AAV vector in nonhuman primates with preexisting immunity to AAV (Chicoine *et al.* 2014). Removal of the antibodies causes a temporary immunosuppression, but levels are restored rapidly.

An alternative to using viral vectors is to use plasmid DNA grown in bacteria. Plasmids are circular forms of DNA that replicate in bacteria separately from the bacterial genome. These can be isolated and highly purified so that the product is plasmid DNA without any protein contamination. When administered to animals, the plasmid does not provoke an acquired immune response nor does it generate an autoimmune response. However, it does activate the innate immune response, which produces an inflammatory reaction to DNA of bacterial origin. This inflammatory response can cause local swelling and transient, nonspecific flu-like symptoms, but these do not prevent repeated administration of plasmid. Thus, it is possible to top up the effects of previous treatments.

The biggest problem with this approach is that the efficiency of cell entry is very poor, although it can be improved by two methods. The first is to condense the plasmid, which protects the DNA from degradation and enhances uptake by the cell. Specific ligands can be added to enhance cell uptake via receptor-mediated pathways. This approach can work very efficiently in cell culture and moderately efficiently for some tissues *in vivo* (e.g. Midoux *et al.* 2008), but it is not effective in skeletal muscle. The alternative method of enhanced delivery is to use a physical force to drive the plasmid across the cell membrane and into the cell, mostly commonly through transient micropores. This can be achieved using high volume and high pressure (hydrodynamic approach; reviewed by Herweijer and Wolff 2007), a set of electrical pulses (electroporation; reviewed by Trollet *et al.* 2008), firing the DNA into the cell/tissue (ballistic approach; reviewed by Wells 2004), or ultrasound, commonly in conjunction with contrast microbubbles (reviewed by Newman and Bettinger 2007). It is therefore not feasible to consider efficient whole-body treatment with nonviral vectors; these systems are better suited to local or regional treatment, such as a limb.

An alternative to the use of viral or nonviral vectors *in vivo* is to use cells modified *in vitro*. For example, genetically modified cells can be used to aid the repair of damaged muscle or may be used as a platform for secreting proteins. In the latter case, it is possible to encapsulate the cells in an inert capsule that can prevent the immune rejection of the cells. This has the advantage that such implants can be readily removed if they fail to express the protein of interest at appropriate levels, and the coating means that the cells do not need to be those of the recipient (Ponce *et al.* 2006).

With all of the above techniques, it is important to consider the regulation of gene expression. When cells have been modified *ex vivo*, they can be assessed for the level of expression of the transferred gene prior to implantation. However, for *in vivo* gene transfer, the efficiency of gene transfer and hence the level of expression will be variable. In some cases, excess expression carries significant health risks and may decrease performance. There are a range of drug-inducible systems that would allow athletes to regulate the amount of gene expression. These include tetracycline-, rapamycin-, and tamoxifen-regulated systems (e.g. Nordstrom 2003; Rivera *et al.* 2005; Stieger *et al.* 2009). These not only allow control over any harm associated with excessive levels of expression, but they may also provide a method for avoiding doping detection in the case of systemically secreted proteins.

Temporary genetic modification can also be performed with the use of antisense sequences, either to reduce the expression of a specific gene, most commonly using small interfering RNAs, or by steric block oligonucleotides to inhibit translation or modify splicing of the primary transcript. The latter have been extensively studied in the context of restoring the open reading frame Duchenne muscular dystrophy and are in clinical trials at present. By preventing an exon from being spliced into the mature mRNA, the reading frame can also be disrupted; this approach could conceivably be used to eliminate the open reading frame and thus prevent gene expression. A number of chemical modifications are available for oligonucleotide chemistry; such molecules can be highly gene specific and may be difficult to identify unless the testing authorities suspect they are being used.

Finally, there are a number of small-molecule drugs that are more or less gene specific and can be used to increase gene expression, such as by stabilising the mRNA or allowing the ribosomal apparatus to read through premature stop mutations (e.g. PTC 124; Welch *et al.* 2007). This list can be expanded to include agonists or antagonists that act on the expression and function of specific genes, such as GW 1516, an agonist of PPAR-δ, and AICAR, an agonist of AMPK (Narkar *et al.* 2008).

12.4. History of gene doping in sport

Gene doping was first added to the International Olympic Committee/WADA list in 2003. In 2004, gene doping was included in the WADA Prohibited List with the following definition: 'Gene or cell doping is defined as the non-therapeutic use of genes, genetic elements and/or cells that have the capacity to enhance athletic performance' (Fischetto and Bermon, 2013). To date, there have been no recorded incidents of gene doping. However, anecdotal accounts exist of an attempt to procure gene doping and of one laboratory reportedly offering gene doping services (Friedmann *et al.* 2010).

12.5. Action and use of gene doping in sport

Many of the impressive studies showing an increased athletic performance in experimental animals were performed with transgenic mice, in which the genetic modification is made to the very early embryo. This is highly unlikely to be undertaken in humans due to the low efficiency of the procedures, let alone the major ethical concerns that such manipulations raise. Relatively few of the genes in question have been modified by the somatic gene transfer in adult animals, and most examples are in laboratory rodents. In these models, a single intramuscular injection is often sufficient to modify most, if not all, of one muscle. However, in larger animals, the diffusion of gene transfer vectors from the site of treatment is very limited (O'Hara *et al.* 2001); thus, multiple intramuscular injections would be needed to modify human muscle. Systemic administration of AAV vectors have been effective in treating all muscles in mice, but such high efficiencies have not been noted with studies in larger animals such as dogs, except after neonatal administration (Yue *et al.* 2008). However, regional perfusion in a limb temporarily isolated from the general circulation by a tourniquet has been quite successful in adult dogs (Arruda *et al.* 2005; Qiao *et al.* 2009). Plasmid DNA can also be delivered hydrodynamically to the temporarily isolated limb, although probably with a lower gene transfer efficiency than AAV (Hagstrom *et al.* 2004).

Intramuscular injection of either AAV or plasmid delivered by electroporation would probably be sufficient to boost the circulating Epo levels and would be quite practical using current technology. More risky but essentially feasible would be the perfusion of a limb with AAV or plasmid. Although it would not be possible to target all of the muscle fibres in a limb, transfer of genes whose products work in an autocrine or paracrine fashion, such as IGF-1, might be sufficient to marginally improve performance. The production of plasmid DNA free of major contaminants, although not at a clinical grade acceptable for legal use in humans, is relatively easy and would be within the capabilities of a small illegal laboratory. The production of large quantities of AAV is more difficult and currently would require specialist skills. However, as the methodologies continue to be refined, it is becoming a more practical possibility for a well-equipped laboratory.

There are clear dangers associated with gene doping. Administration of large quantities of viral vectors or plasmids risks activating the innate immune system; in one trial in 1999 using an adenoviral vector, this led to disseminated intravascular coagulation, organ failure, and death (Raper et al. 2003). Plasmid DNA can also activate the innate immune system via specific sequences that are recognised as bacterial, which leads to inflammation and fever. However, developments in nonviral vector design have largely removed these sequences, which significantly reduces the interaction with the innate immune system and increases the longevity of expression. The use of integrating viral vectors has been associated with oncogenesis in human clinical trials (Hacein-Bey-Abina et al. 2008). However, the vectors that are more likely to be used for gene doping, AAV and plasmid, do not integrate at a significant rate, so this oncogenesis risk is relatively small.

Overexpression of genes may have harmful consequences. Excess Epo leads to polycythaemia, an excess of red blood cells that makes the blood more viscous and thus puts a greater load on the heart. This in turn can lead to blockage of the microcirculation, including stroke and heart failure. In addition, the production of Epo following gene transfer has been reported to cause autoimmune anaemia in macaques (Chenuaud et al. 2004; Gao et al. 2004). Overexpression of PGC-1a has been linked to a tendency toward muscle atrophy and type 2 diabetes in some of the transgenic mouse studies (Miura et al. 2006; Choi et al. 2008). IGF-1 is a potent mitogen and has anti-apoptotic effects. Consequently, overexpression following gene transfer would imply an increased risk of oncogenesis (reviewed by Perry et al. 2006).

12.6. Gene doping and the WADA Prohibited List

WADA (2014) currently defines gene doping as

- The transfer of polymers of nucleic acids or nucleic acid analogues
- The use of normal or genetically modified cells.

Although there is no evidence to date that athletes have practised gene doping, the threat of gene doping has led to many laboratories to work toward developing systems to detect any possible gene doping.

Doping controls were originally developed to detect approved drugs and known methods of performance enhancement, such as blood doping. However, there is increasing evidence of the use of nonclinically approved or designer drugs, such as the anabolic steroid tetrahydrogestrinone. Emerging drugs under development that could be used for doping have been reviewed by Thevis et al. (2009). The problems posed by designer drugs are more difficult.

Screening for a type of action rather than the specific drug will become an important part of the methodology, such as screening for androgenic activity in a mammalian cell bioassay (Houtman *et al.* 2009). The diagnostic challenge posed by gene therapy may be even greater. Doping detection relies on urine and blood samples, and it is not currently possible to take the solid tissues that are most likely to give clear evidence of genetic manipulation. Fortunately, products of gene doping that are secreted following gene transfer into ectopic sites show different patterns of posttranslational modification. For example, Epo secreted from muscle is demonstrably different from the endogenous Epo secreted from the kidney (Lasne *et al.* 2004).

It is possible to detect minute traces of gene transfer vectors using highly sensitive polymerase chain reaction (PCR)-based techniques. However, the window for detection of vector after administration is relatively small, particularly for nonviral vectors. A number of groups have developed quantitative methods for PCR for viral and nonviral transgenes, reporting improved detection with a number of protocol modifications (e.g. Baoutina *et al.* 2013). An alternative is the use of a primer-internal, intron-spanning PCR approach (Beiter *et al.* 2008, 2011), and a similar approach has been developed by another group (Baoutina *et al.* 2010). Small interfering RNA (siRNA) has been shown to decrease gene expression for a number of targets and could be used to decrease genes that limit muscle mass, such as myostatin (Takemasa *et al.* 2012). A liquid chromatography–high-resolution/high-accuracy mass spectrometry method has been developed to detect such siRNA (Thomas *et al.* 2013).

When regulated promoters are used, it may be possible to detect the activating molecule, such as tetracycline, rapamycin, or tamoxifen. However, each of these has another nondoping therapeutic action. Finally, it may be possible to detect evidence of prior administration of viral vectors by looking for evidence of an antibody response to the virus. However, this could be explained by inadvertent exposure to the natural infectious virus.

An alternative approach is to use indirect techniques to detect gene doping by looking for the consequence of the genetic manipulation, such as changes in patterns of target gene expression (transcriptomics), proteins (proteomics), or their metabolites (metobolomics). The transcriptomic approach has been reviewed (Rupert 2009), and the use of the proteomics approach for detecting androgenic steroid abuse in racehorses is another example (Barton *et al.* 2009). However, these methods require the establishment of normal standards, and some individuals are likely to fall outside of a normal range as a consequence of natural genetic variation. Indeed, the problem of ethnic and individual variation has been highlighted with assessment of the metabolism of testosterone (Strahm *et al.* 2009). A solution to this problem would be the use of an athlete's endocrinological passport based on the results of repeated tests over time (Sottas *et al.* 2008), as has been done for 'blood passports' for the detection of blood doping (Robinson *et al.* 2007). This would provide testers with a lifelong biological fingerprint of competitors to compare against drug-test samples.

12.7. Summary

The potential use of gene doping is critically dependent on our increasing understanding of the genetic modifiers of exercise physiology and the medical development of gene therapy systems that are highly efficient in humans. It is now well established that, in laboratory animals, genes can be added to increase levels of specific proteins or manipulated with a range of technologies to decrease production of specific proteins.

A substantial number of candidate genes have been identified as possible targets for gene doping, of which PPAR-δ is perhaps the biggest concern because its detection is likely to be a problem. At present, the technology is not sufficiently well developed that it is likely to be abused by athletes, but the rapid pace of change in antisense and gene therapy makes it increasingly likely that medical progress will make gene doping a reality sooner rather than later. However, in many cases, it is also likely that screening methods that have been developed experimentally will be able to detect many of the forms of gene doping.

12.8. References

Amthor, H., Macharia, R., Navarrete, R., *et al.* (2007). Lack of myostatin results in excessive muscle growth but impaired force generation. *Proc Natl Acad Sci U S A* 104(6):1835–1840.

Arany, Z., Lebrasseur, N., Morris, C., *et al.* (2007). The transcriptional coactivator PGC-1beta drives the formation of oxidative type IIX fibers in skeletal muscle. *Cell Metab* 5(1):35–46.

Arruda, V. R., Stedman, H. H., Nichols, T. C., *et al.* (2005). Regional intravascular delivery of AAV-2-F.IX to skeletal muscle achieves long-term correction of hemophilia B in a large animal model. *Blood* 105(9):3458–3464.

Barton, C., Beck, P., Kay, R., *et al.* (2009). Multiplexed LC-MS/MS analysis of horse plasma proteins to study doping in sport. *Proteomics* 9(11):3058–3065.

Barton-Davis, E. R., Shoturma, D. I., Musaro, A., *et al.* (1998). Viral mediated expression of insulin-like growth factor I blocks the aging-related loss of skeletal muscle function. *Proc Natl Acad Sci U S A* 95(26):15603–15607.

Baoutina, A., Coldham, T., Bains, G. S., and Emslie, K. R. (2010). Gene doping detection: Evaluation of approach for direct detection of gene transfer using erythropoietin as a model system. *Gene Ther* 17(8):1022–1032.

Baoutina, A., Coldham, T., Fuller, B., and Emslie, K. R. (2013). Improved detection of transgene and nonviral vectors in blood. *Hum Gene Ther Methods* 24(6):345–354.

Beiter, T., Zimmermann, M., Fragasso, A., *et al.* (2008). Establishing a novel single-copy primer-internal intron-spanning PCR (spiPCR) procedure for the direct detection of gene doping. *Exerc Immunol Rev* 14:73–85.

Beiter, T., Zimmermann, M., Fragasso, A., *et al.* (2011). Direct and long-term detection of gene doping in conventional blood samples. *Gene Ther* 18(3):225–231.

Boman, I. A., Klemetsdal, G., Blichfeldt, T., *et al.* (2009). A frameshift mutation in the coding region of the myostatin gene (MSTN) affects carcass conformation and fatness in Norwegian White Sheep (*Ovis aries*). *Anim Genet* 40(4):418–422.

Boutin, S., Monteilhet, V., Veron, P., *et al.* (2010). Prevalence of serum IgG and neutralizing factors against adeno-associated virus (AAV) types 1, 2, 5, 6, 8, and 9 in the healthy population: Implications for gene therapy using AAV vectors. *Hum Gene Ther* 21(6):704–712.

Calvo, J. A., Daniels, T. G., Wang, X., *et al.* (2008). Muscle-specific expression of PPARgamma coactivator-1alpha improves exercise performance and increases peak oxygen uptake. *J Appl Physiol* 104(5):1304–1312.

Chenuaud, P., Larcher, T., Rabinowitz, J. E., *et al.* (2004). Autoimmune anemia in macaques following erythropoietin gene therapy. *Blood* 103(9):3303–3304.

Chicoine, L. G., Montgomery, C. L., Bremer, W. G., *et al.* (2014). Plasmapheresis eliminates the negative impact of AAV antibodies on microdystrophin gene expression following vascular delivery. *Mol Ther* 22(2):338–347.

Coleman, M. E., DeMayo, F., Yin, K. C., *et al.* (1995). Myogenic vector expression of insulin-like growth factor I stimulates muscle cell differentiation and myofiber hypertrophy in transgenic mice. *J Biol Chem* 270(20):12109–12116.

de la Chapelle, A., Träskelin, A. L., and Juvonen, E. (1993). Truncated erythropoietin receptor causes dominantly inherited benign human erythrocytosis. *Proc Natl Acad Sci U S A* 90(10):4495–4499.

Denti, M. A., Rosa, A., D'Antona, G., *et al*. (2006). Body-wide gene therapy of Duchenne muscular dystrophy in the *mdx* mouse model. *Proc Natl Acad Sci U S A* 103(10):3758–3763.

Fattori, E., Cappelletti, M., Zampaglione, I., *et al*. (2005). Gene electro-transfer of an improved erythropoietin plasmid in mice and non-human primates. *J Gene Med* 7(2):228–236.

Fischetto, G., and Bermon, S. (2013). From gene engineering to gene modulation and manipulation: Can we prevent or detect gene doping in sports? *Sports Medicine* 43(10):977–990.

Friedmann, T., Rabin, O., and Frankel, M. S. (2010). Ethics. Gene doping and sport. *Science* 327 (5966):647–648.

Gao, G. P., Alvira, M. R., Wang, L., *et al*. (2002). Novel adeno-associated viruses from rhesus monkeys as vectors for human gene therapy. *Proc Natl Acad Sci U S A* 99(18):11854–11859.

Gao, G., Lebherz, C., Weiner, D. J., *et al*. (2004). Erythropoietin gene therapy leads to autoimmune anemia in macaques. *Blood* 103(9):3300–3302.

Gregorevic, P., Blankinship, M. J., Allen, J. M., *et al*. (2004). Systemic delivery of genes to striated muscles using adeno-associated viral vectors. *Nat Med* 10(8):828–834.

Grobet, L., Martin, L. J., Poncelet, D., *et al*. (1997). A deletion in the bovine myostatin gene causes the double-muscled phenotype in cattle. *Nat Genet* 17(1):71–74.

Hacein-Bey-Abina, S., Garrigue, A., Wang, G. P., *et al*. (2008). Insertional oncogenesis in 4 patients after retrovirus-mediated gene therapy of SCID-X1. *J Clin Invest* 118(9):3132–3142.

Hagstrom, J. E., Hegge, J., Zhang, G., *et al*. (2004). A facile nonviral method for delivering genes and siRNAs to skeletal muscle of mammalian limbs. *Mol Ther* 10(2):386–398.

Hakimi, P., Yang, J., Casadesus, G., *et al*. (2007). Overexpression of the cytosolic form of phosphoenolpyruvate carboxykinase (GTP) in skeletal muscle repatterns energy metabolism in the mouse. *J Biol Chem* 282(45):32844–32855.

Herweijer, H., and Wolff, J. A. (2007). Gene therapy progress and prospects: Hydrodynamic gene delivery. *Gene Ther* 14(2):99–107.

Hill, E. W., Gu, J., Eivers, S. S., *et al*. (2010). A sequence polymorphism in MSTN predicts sprinting ability and racing stamina in thoroughbred horses. *PLoS One* 5(1):e8645.

Houtman, C.J., Sterk, S.S., van de Heijning, M.P., *et al*. (2009) Detection of anabolic androgenic steroid abuse in doping control using mammalian reporter gene bioassays. *Anal Chim Acta* 637(1–2): 247–258.

Iezzi, S., Di Padova, M., Serra, C., *et al*. (2004). Deacetylase inhibitors increase muscle cell size by promoting myoblast recruitment and fusion through induction of follistatin. *Dev Cell* 6(5):673–684.

Journal of Gene Medicine. (2014). Gene therapy clinical trials worldwide. Available online at http://www.wiley.com/legacy/wileychi/genmed/clinical/ (accessed 16 July 2014).

Kastelein, J. J., Ross, C. J., and Hayden, M. R. (2013). From mutation identification to therapy: Discovery and origins of the first approved gene therapy in the Western world. *Hum Gene Ther* 24(5):472–478.

Kim, S., Peng, Z., and Kaneda, Y. (2008). Current status of gene therapy in Asia. *Mol Ther* 16(2):237–243.

Krämer, D. K., Ahlsén, M., Norrbom, J., *et al*. (2006). Human skeletal muscle fibre type variations correlate with PPAR alpha, PPAR delta and PGC-1 alpha mRNA. *Acta Physiol (Oxf)* 188(3–4):207–216.

Lasne, F., Martin, L., de Ceaurriz, J., *et al*. (2004). Genetic doping with erythropoietin cDNA in primate muscle is detectable. *Mol Ther* 10(3):409–410.

Lee, S., Barton, E. R., Sweeney, H. L., and Farrar, R. P. (2004). Viral expression of insulin-like growth factor-I enhances muscle hypertrophy in resistance-trained rats. *J Appl Physiol* 96(3):1097–1104.

Lin, J., Wu, H., Tarr, P. T., *et al*. (2002). Transcriptional co-activator PGC-1 alpha drives the formation of slow-twitch muscle fibres. *Nature* 418(6899):797–801.

Lunde, I. G., Ekmark, M., Rana, Z. A., *et al*. (2007). PPAR{delta} expression is influenced by muscle activity and induces slow muscle properties in adult rat muscles after somatic gene transfer. *J Physiol* 582(Pt 3):1277–1287.

McPherron, A. C., Lawler, A. M., and Lee, S. J. (1997). Regulation of skeletal muscle mass in mice by a new TGF-beta superfamily member. *Nature* 387(6628):83–90.

Midoux, P., Breuzard, G., Gomez, J. P., and Pichon, C. (2008). Polymer-based gene delivery: A current review on the uptake and intracellular trafficking of polyplexes. *Curr Gene Ther* 8(5):335–252.

Miura, S., Tomitsuka, E., Kamei, Y., *et al.* (2006). Overexpression of peroxisome proliferator-activated receptor gamma co-activator-1alpha leads to muscle atrophy with depletion of ATP. *Am J Pathol* 169(4):1129–1139.

Mosher, D. S., Quignon, P., Bustamante, C. D., *et al.* (2007). A mutation in the myostatin gene increases muscle mass and enhances racing performance in heterozygote dogs. *PLoS Genet* 3(5):e79.

Nakatani, M., Takehara, Y., Sugino, H., *et al.* (2008). Transgenic expression of a myostatin inhibitor derived from follistatin increases skeletal muscle mass and ameliorates dystrophic pathology in *mdx* mice. *FASEB J* 22(2):477–487.

Narkar, V. A., Downes, M., Yu, R. T., *et al.* (2008). AMPK and PPARdelta agonists are exercise mimetics. *Cell* 134(3):405–415.

Newman, C. M., and Bettinger, T. (2007). Gene therapy progress and prospects: Ultrasound for gene transfer. *Gene Ther* 14(6):465–475.

Nordstrom, J. L. (2003). The antiprogestin-dependent GeneSwitch system for regulated gene therapy *Steroids* 68(10–13):1085–1094.

O'Hara, A. J., Howell, J. M., Taplin, R. H., *et al.* (2001). The spread of transgene expression at the site of gene construct injection. *Muscle Nerve* 24(4):488–495.

Perry, J. K., Emerald, B. S., Mertani, H. C., and Lobie, P. E. (2006). The oncogenic potential of growth hormone. *Growth Horm IGF Res* 16(5–6):277–289.

Phelps, S. F., Hauser, M. A., Cole, N. M., *et al.* (1995). Expression of full-length and truncated dystrophin mini-genes in transgenic *mdx* mice. *Hum Mol Genet* 4(8):1251–1258.

Ponce, S., Orive, G., Hernández, R. M., *et al.* (2006). *In vivo* evaluation of EPO-secreting cells immobilized in different alginate-PLL microcapsules. *J Control Release* 116(1):28–34.

Qiao, C., Li, J., Jiang, J., *et al.* (2008). Myostatin propeptide gene delivery by adeno-associated virus serotype 8 vectors enhances muscle growth and ameliorates dystrophic phenotypes in *mdx* mice. *Hum Gene Ther* 19(3):241–254.

Qiao, C., Li, J., Zheng, H., *et al.* (2009). Hydrodynamic limb vein injection of AAV8 canine myostatin propeptide gene in normal dogs enhances muscle growth. *Hum Gene Ther* 20(1):1–10.

Raper, S. E., Chirmule, N., Lee, F. S., *et al.* (2003). Fatal systemic inflammatory response syndrome in a ornithine transcarbamylase deficient patient following adenoviral gene transfer. *Mol Genet Metab* 80(1–2):148–158.

Rivera, V. M., Gao, G. P., Grant, R. L., *et al.* (2005). Long-term pharmacologically regulated expression of erythropoietin in primates following AAV-mediated gene transfer. *Blood* 105(4):1424–1430.

Robinson, N., Sottas, P. E., Mangin, P., and Saugy, M. (2007). Bayesian detection of abnormal hematological values to introduce a no-start rule for heterogeneous populations of athletes *Haematologica* 92(8):1143–1144.

Rupert, J. L. (2009). Transcriptional profiling: A potential anti-doping strategy. *Scand J Med Sci Sports* 19(6):753–763.

Sartori, R., Schirwis, E., Blaauw, B., *et al.* (2003). BMP signaling controls muscle mass. *Nat Genet* 45(11):1309–1318.

Schertzer, J. D., and Lynch, G. S. (2006). Comparative evaluation of IGF-I gene transfer and IGF-I protein administration for enhancing skeletal muscle regeneration after injury. *Gene Ther* 13(23): 1657–1664.

Schuelke, M., Wagner, K. R., Stolz, L. E., *et al.* (2004). Myostatin mutation associated with gross muscle hypertrophy in a child. *N Engl J Med* 350(26):2682–2688.

Schuler, B., Rieger, G., Gubser, M., *et al.* (2014). Endogenous α-calcitonin-gene-related peptide promotes exercise-induced, physiological heart hypertrophy in mice *Acta Physiol (Oxf)* 211(1):107–121.

Sottas, P. E., Saudan, C., Schweizer, C., *et al.* (2008). From population- to subject-based limits of T/E ratio to detect testosterone abuse in elite sports. *Forensic Sci Int* 174(2–3):166–172.

Stieger, K., Belbellaa, B., Le Guiner, C., *et al.* (2009). *In vivo* gene regulation using tetracycline-regulatable systems. *Adv Drug Deliv Rev* 61(7–8):527–541.

Strahm, E., Sottas, P. E., Schweizer, C., *et al.* (2009). Steroid profiles of professional soccer players: An international comparative study. *Br J Sports Med* 43(14):1126–1130.

Takemasa, T., Yakushiji, N., Kikuchi, D. M., *et al.* (2012). Fundamental study of detection of muscle hypertrophy-oriented gene doping by myostatin knock down using RNA interference. *J Sports Sci Med* 11(2):294–303.

Thevis, M., Thomas, A., Kohler, M., *et al.* (2009). Emerging drugs: Mechanism of action, mass spectrometry and doping control analysis. *J Mass Spectrom* 44(4):442–460.

Thomas, A., Walpurgis, K., Delahaut, P., *et al.* (2013). Detection of small interfering RNA (siRNA) by mass spectrometry procedures in doping controls. *Drug Test Anal* 5(11–12):853–860.

Trollet, C., Scherman, D., and Bigey, P. (2008). Delivery of DNA into muscle for treating systemic diseases: Advantages and challenges. *Methods Mol Biol* 423:199–214.

Vandenberghe, L. H., Wilson, J. M., and Gao, G. (2009). Tailoring the AAV vector capsid for gene therapy. *Gene Ther* 16(3):311–319.

Vitiello, C., Faraso, S., Sorrentino, N. C., *et al.* (2009). Disease rescue and increased lifespan in a model of cardiomyopathy and muscular dystrophy by combined AAV treatments. *PLoS One* 4(3):e5051.

Wang, Y. X., Zhang, C. L., Yu, R. T., *et al.* (2004). Regulation of muscle fiber type and running endurance by PPARdelta. *PLoS Biol* 2(10):e294.

Welch, E. M., Barton, E. R., Zhuo, J., *et al.* (2007). PTC124 targets genetic disorders caused by nonsense mutations *Nature* 447(7140):87–91.

Wells, D. J., Wells, K. E., Asante, E. A., *et al.* (1995). Expression of human full-length and minidystrophin in transgenic *mdx* mice: Implications for gene therapy of Duchenne muscular dystrophy. *Hum Mol Genet* 4(8):1245–1250.

Wells, D. J. (2004). Gene therapy progress and prospects: electroporation and other physical methods *Gene Ther* 11(18):1363–1369.

Whittemore, L. A., Song, K., Li, X., *et al.* (2003). Inhibition of myostatin in adult mice increases skeletal muscle mass and strength. *Biochem Biophys Res Commun* 300(4):965–971.

World Anti-Doping Agency. (2014). The 2014 Prohibited List international standard. Available online at https://www.wada-ama.org/en/what-we-do/prohibited-list (accessed 9 September 2014).

Yue, Y., Ghosh, A., Long, C., *et al.* (2008). A single intravenous injection of adeno-associated virus serotype-9 leads to whole body skeletal muscle transduction in dogs. *Mol Ther* 16(12):1944–1952.

Zhu, T., Zhou, L., Mori, S., *et al.* (2005). Sustained whole-body functional rescue in congestive heart failure and muscular dystrophy hamsters by systemic gene transfer. *Circulation* 112(17):2650–2659.

Chapter 13

Stimulants

David R. Mottram

13.1. Introduction

The class of drugs referred to as stimulants encompasses a group of drugs with diverse pharmacological activities. There are limited applications for the use of these drugs as therapeutic agents, but many are used in a recreational context. Statistics recorded by World Anti-Doping Agency (WADA) laboratories (see Chapter 25, Table 25.2) reveal that the annual number of adverse analytical findings for stimulants is second only to anabolic agents. It is claimed that many of these adverse findings were a result of inadvertent use, not associated with attempted performance enhancement. This fact is reflected in the complex WADA regulations associated with this class of drugs.

13.2. Types of stimulants and their modes of action

Figure 13.1 shows the interrelationship between the various nervous systems of the body. Overall control of body function lies with the central nervous system (CNS). The CNS receives information about the body's environment, such as sight, sound, touch, and taste, through sensory nerves. The CNS then relays information through either the motor nervous system to the skeletal muscles or through the autonomic nervous system (ANS) to control the parts of the body that are not under conscious control, such as the heart, blood vessels, respiratory tract, gastrointestinal tract, and various glands. The ANS is divided into the parasympathetic nervous system, which controls function under times of rest, and the sympathetic nervous system (SNS), which controls function under times of stress. Under extreme stress conditions, the SNS is augmented by the hormone adrenaline (epinephrine).

There are numerous neurotransmitters within the CNS and ANS. The principal neurotransmitters through which stimulants exert their effects are adrenaline, noradrenaline, dopamine, and, to a lesser extent, 5-hydroxytryptamine. The effects produced by stimulants are due to increasing the levels of these neurotransmitters at their sites of action, either centrally or peripherally. This is achieved by increasing the release, preventing the re-uptake, reducing the metabolism, or mimicking the effect of these neurotransmitters (Jones 2008).

The classifications of stimulants used by the International Olympic Committee (IOC) in its original Prohibited List in 1967 were sympathomimetic amines, psychomotor stimulants, and CNS stimulants. These classifications distinguished stimulants on the basis of their mode of action.

Sympathomimetic amines mimic or potentiate the effects of the sympathetic nervous system. The principal neurotransmitter for the sympathetic nervous system is noradrenaline

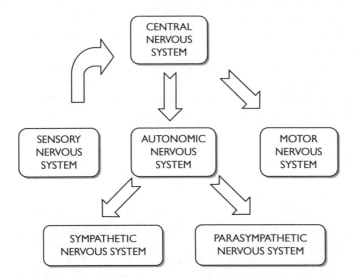

Figure 13.1 The organisation and interplay of the nervous system.

(norepinephrine). Sympathomimetics, such as ephedrine, pseudoephedrine, and phenylephrine, increase the release of noradrenaline or act on the same receptors as the noadrenaline to potentiate its effect.

CNS stimulants have relatively little effect on mental function but increase the activity of the respiratory and vasomotor centres of the CNS or increase reflex excitability. There are few CNS stimulants that are used in sport, although strychnine remains on the Prohibited List, having been used for over 100 years.

Psychomotor stimulants have a number of effects related to mental function and behaviour. They can induce excitement and euphoria, increase motor activity, or reduce fatigue. Psychomotor stimulants include amphetamines, cocaine, and methylxanthines, such as caffeine.

A large number of stimulants are listed on the WADA Prohibited List (see Table 13.2). A review of the pharmacology of these different types of stimulants was provided by Docherty (2008). Some of the stimulants that are more commonly used within sport are described in the following sections.

Ephedrines and cathine

The principal mode of action of ephedrines (ephedrine and pseudoephedrine) and cathine is as sympathomimetics, although they do exhibit some central stimulant properties. They are structurally related to amphetamine and exert their effect indirectly on neurones of the sympathetic and central nervous systems by displacing noradrenaline, and possibly other monoamine transmitters, from neuronal storage sites. They also exert direct effects on adrenergic α and β receptors and are weak inhibitors of monoamine uptake.

Ephedrine occurs naturally in the plant genus *Ephedra* and has been a component of ancient Chinese medicine for many centuries. Ephedrine and other herbal sources of stimulants were reviewed by Bucci (2000). Ephedrine is similar in structure and function to amphetamine but is reported to have a 25-fold lower biological potency (Robergs *et al*. 2003). The effects of ephedrines are produced within 40 minutes after administration and can last up to 3 hours.

Adverse effects of ephedrines are, most commonly, tachycardia, hypertension, headache, and dizziness. These drugs may cause anorexia, insomnia, irritability, and nervousness at low to medium doses. High doses are associated with mania and a psychosis similar to that occasionally seen with amphetamine.

Cathine is derived from the khat plant, which contains a number of active constituents. The most potent of its constituents is cathinone, which has amphetamine-like actions (Kalix 1992).

Amphetamines

Several structurally related drugs are known as amphetamines, including dextroamphetamine, methamphetamine, phenmetrazine, and methylphenidate. Amphetamine is a phenyl isopropylamine and was first synthesized in 1920. It was originally prescribed for the treatment of nasal congestion. In 1935, amphetamine was used to treat the neurological condition narcolepsy, and its use in the treatment of depression, anxiety, and hyperactivity in children followed from this. Amphetamine was used widely during the Second World War to reduce fatigue and increase alertness. The rapid development of tolerance to amphetamine and the occurrence of dependence have led to the drug's being withdrawn from clinical use.

The mode of action of amphetamine

There are four mechanisms by which amphetamine may produce its effects:

- Release of a neurotransmitter (dopamine, noradrenaline, or 5-hydroxytryptamine) from its respective nerve terminal
- Inhibition of monoamine oxidase activity
- Inhibition of neurotransmitter re-uptake
- Direct action on neurotransmitter receptors.

Of these four possibilities, neurotransmitter release appears to be the most important (Brookes 1985).

Amphetamine is a potent anorectic and elevates plasma free fatty acid levels. Body temperature is also elevated. The cardiovascular, gastrointestinal, and respiratory effects of amphetamine are sympathomimetic in nature.

Amphetamines are readily absorbed, mainly from the small intestine. The peak plasma concentration occurs 1–2 hours after administration. Absorption is usually complete in 2.5–4 hours and is accelerated by food intake.

The principal amphetamine metabolites are p-hydroxyephedrine and p-hydroxyamphetamine. Both of these metabolites have similar pharmacological effects to the parent amphetamine. Amphetamine is lost from the blood by renal filtration.

The effect of amphetamines on human mood and performance

The desire to enhance mood or performance (or both) is usually the main reason for taking amphetamines. In the short term, amphetamine increases the speed of learning of new tasks. The effects of amphetamine on judgement are uncertain, and several conflicting studies have been published (Brookes 1985). There is general agreement that amphetamines cause a mild distortion of time perception, which may lead to misjudgement in planning manoeuvres or in manipulations such as driving a car.

Although there is considerable interindividual variation in the effects of amphetamine on mood, the general effects are of positive mood enhancement. These positive effects include an increase in physical energy, mental aptitude, talkativeness, restlessness, vigour, excitement, and good humour. Subjects taking amphetamine also report that they feel confident, efficient, and ambitious, and that their food intake is reduced. Many athletes report that they feel most aggressive when taking amphetamines and are unlikely to report or complain of injuries (Laties and Weiss 1981). Methamphetamine is a powerful, positive reinforcing agent in humans (Hart *et al.* 2001).

Adverse effects of amphetamines

Amphetamines produce a number of side effects, including anxiety, indifference, slowness in reasoning, irresponsible behaviour, irritability, restlessness, dry mouth, tremors, and insomnia. These effects of amphetamine on mood are dose dependent. There is much evidence to show that amphetamines induce drug dependence and the amphetamine-dependent person may become psychotic, aggressive, and antisocial. Withdrawal of amphetamines is associated with mental and physical depression.

Tolerance to the positive effects of methamphetamine does occur over time, at least in new abusers, while the severity of the negative effects increases over time (Comer *et al.* 2001). Other major side effects of amphetamine administration (excluding those following withdrawal of the drug) include confusion, delirium, sweating, palpitations, dilation of the pupils, rapid breathing, hypertension, tachycardia, tremors, and muscle and joint pain. Although amphetamines may initially stimulate libido, chronic amphetamine use often leads to a reduction in sex drive. Chronic amphetamine administration is also associated with myocardial pathology and with growth retardation in adolescents. Usually, the personality changes induced by chronic low doses of amphetamine are gradually reversed after the drug is stopped. However, high chronic doses may lead to a variety of persistent personality changes.

Cocaine

Cocaine is derived from leaves of the coca plant (*Erythroxylum coca*). Cocaine first became available commercially in the 1880s. Sigmund Freud took the drug in an attempt to cure his own bouts of depression and suggested it as a 'cure-all' for others. The drug fell out of medical use by the 1920s, only to reappear in the 1960s as a major drug of abuse. 'Crack' cocaine is a highly purified form of freebase cocaine. The name derives from the cracking sound produced when the freebase of cocaine is heated.

Cocaine affects the brain in a complex way. The most obvious initial effects are a decrease in fatigue, an increase in motor activity, and an increase in talkativeness, coupled with a general feeling of euphoria and well-being. These mood changes soon subside and are replaced by dysphoria (mood lowering).

The mechanism by which cocaine produces these effects is not known fully. Animal studies show that cocaine is a powerful reinforcer and rewarding agent. It stimulates elements of the brain's pleasure and reward centres, which are distributed throughout the limbic system of the brain and include the dopamine-rich mesocortical and mesolimbic systems (Fibiger *et al.* 1992).

This acute effect of cocaine on dopamine has been demonstrated in many investigations (Chen and Reith 2000).

Cocaine may be administered by injection, orally, intranasally, or by inhalation. Oral administration produces peak effects at variable times, with behavioural changes lasting up to 1 hour. The most popular route is via nasal 'snorting,' which produces peak effects in 5–15 min, lasting for an hour. Inhalation of freebase cocaine produces peak effects in less than 1 minute but also a short-lived physiological effect measured in minutes. The route of cocaine administration influences the time course and onset of other actions of cocaine. Effects of the drug, such as increases in heart rate and blood pressure, are longer lasting via the oral compared to the intravenous route (Smith *et al*. 2001). Inhalation of cocaine results in the most intense cravings compared to other routes of administration (Wadler and Hainline 1989). The frequency of cocaine administration also influences the density of brain opioid and dopamine receptors (Unterwald *et al*. 2001). Cocaine is mainly metabolised by plasma and liver cholinesterases to benzoylecgonine and ecgonine methyl ester, which are excreted in the urine.

Adverse effects of cocaine

Cocaine is highly addictive – more so than amphetamine. The abuser may experience acute psychotic symptoms and undertake irrational actions, in addition to the well-known effects of euphoria. Chronic symptoms include a paranoid psychosis, similar to that induced by amphetamine, coupled with spells of delirium and confusion. Other CNS side effects include epileptogenesis (i.e. stimulation of epileptic seizures).

Cocaine abuse is strongly associated with cerebrovascular accidents arising either from the rupture or spasm of cerebral blood vessels. Some of these incidents may be due to preexisting vascular pathologies, but there are several cases where no predisposing cause has been found at autopsy (Wadler and Hainline 1989). Cocaine is also responsible for a number of cardiovascular side effects. Smith and Perry (1992) suggested that increases in the cardiovascular and cerebrovascular side effects of cocaine are due to the rise in abuse of crack cocaine, which is rapidly absorbed and produces a concentrated effect on cerebral arterioles.

13.3. Clinical uses of stimulants

The majority of drugs classified as stimulants are used as substances of abuse in a recreational context. There are a limited number of clinical uses for stimulants. The use of stimulants by athletes for the treatment of valid clinical conditions is subject to Therapeutic Use Exemption (TUE) regulations.

Attention-deficit/hyperactivity disorder

Attention-deficit/hyperactivity disorder (ADHD) is a common neuropsychiatric disorder with an estimated prevalence of 5–10 per cent among school-age children and adolescents (Kreher 2012). Stimulants such as methylphenidate and dexamfetamine are used for severe and persistent symptoms of ADHD in children and, if needed, may be continued into adolescence and adulthood. These drugs are not licenced for the initiation of treatment for ADHD in adulthood.

Centrally acting appetite suppression

Phentermine, fenfluramine, and sibutramine produce appetite suppression. However, they are not recommended for the treatment of obesity.

Sleep disorders

Excessive episodes of sleepiness associated with narcolepsy, sleep apnoea/hypopnoea syndrome, and shift-work sleep disorders may be treated with modafinil.

Anaphylaxis

Severe, life-threatening hypersensitivity reactions may be induced by poorly controlled asthma, insect bites, allergy to certain foods, or medicinal products. First-line treatment for such anaphylactic reactions includes the administration of adrenaline.

Dental anaesthesia

Adrenaline is widely used with dental anaesthetics, such as lidocaine, in order to restrict the area of anaesthesia through vasoconstriction at the site of injection.

Bronchodilation

Ephedrine will produce bronchodilation, but it is less suitable for conditions requiring this treatment than selective beta-2 agonists.

Nasal congestion

Sympathomimetics, such as ephedrine, methylephedrine, pseudoephedrine, and cathine, reduce nasal congestion through vasoconstriction in the nasal passages. The WADA regulations with respect to these drugs have undergone significant changes in recent years (see Section 13.4). The current regulations are shown in Table 13.1. Alternative drugs such as xylometazoline and ipratropium, which are not prohibited in sport, are safer alternative treatments for nasal congestion.

13.4. History of stimulant use in sport

Stimulants have a long history of use as potential performance-enhancing agents in sport. The potent but nonselective and highly toxic stimulant strychnine was used as long ago as the end of the nineteenth century. Amphetamines, first developed in the 1920s, have been a favourite of athletes in many sporting disciplines. Stimulants, along with narcotic analgesics, were therefore the first classes of drugs to be included on an IOC list of prohibited substances in 1967. At that time, stimulants were divided into three classes: sympathomimetic amines, psychomotor stimulants, and central nervous system stimulants. In 1988, the IOC grouped all these classes of drugs under the overall heading of stimulants.

It can be seen from the statistics released by WADA-accredited laboratories that, in recent years, the annual number of adverse analytical findings for stimulants have been second only to anabolic agents (see Chapter 25, Table 25.2). To what extent stimulants have been used in an attempt to enhance performance or used simply as recreational drugs is impossible to ascertain. The most frequently used stimulants, according to WADA statistics, are shown in Table

Table 13.1 Statistics from WADA-accredited laboratories for adverse analytical findings for substances classed as stimulants (2003–2012)

	2003	2004	2005	2006	2007	2008	2009	2010	2011	2012
Methylhexaneamine	–	–	–	–	–	1	31	123	283	320
Pseudoephedrine*	189	–	–	–	–	–	–	17	9	13
Amphetamine	43	112	194	199	430	166	27	112	133	58
Cocaine	48	75	85	85	101	77	60	65	40	59
Ephedrine	100	102	93	66	50	54	44	32	33	12
Methylphenidate	9	7	17	32	38	40	31	73	59	47
Cathine	2	9	14	22	33	15	15	4	5	6
Sibutramine	–	–	–	3	20	17	11	25	14	14
Phentermine	5	13	14	13	9	8	6	5	32	3
Methamphetamine	7	8	12	8	21	5	9	6	29	31
Others	113	56	80	62	91	89	91	112	81	134
Total	516	382	509	490	793	472	325	574	718	697

* Pseudoephedrine was removed from the WADA Prohibited List and placed on a monitoring list in 2004, returning to the Prohibited List in 2010.

13.1. Of particular interest is the dramatic increase in the number of adverse findings related to methylhexaneamine, which is discussed in Section 13.5.

Case studies related to stimulants

A number of landmark cases have been related to the use of stimulants by athletes, as discussed here.

Tommy Simpson (1967)

Tommy Simpson, the British cyclist, died of heat stroke and cardiac arrest whilst climbing the infamous Mont Ventoux during the thirteenth stage of the 1967 Tour de France. Simpson was trying to make up time lost in earlier stages, resulting from the fact that he had been suffering from a stomach bug. The postmortem examination found that Simpson had taken amphetamines and alcohol. The effect of these drugs was compounded by the facts that the temperatures on the mountain were extremely high on that day, the upper slopes of the mountain offer no shade from the sun, and, in those days, the Tour organisers limited the fluid intake of riders during each stage, as the effects of dehydration were poorly understood at that time.

Kelli White (2003)

Kelli White, an American sprinter, tested positive for modafinil at the World Athletics Championships in 2003. She claimed that her physician was prescribing modafinil for narcolepsy. Arising from the 2003 Bay Area Laboratory Cooperative investigation, the US Anti-Doping Agency also found evidence for the use of tetrahydrogestrinone and erythropoietin. White was banned for 2 years and stripped of her medals. The athlete had also claimed that modafinil was not on the Prohibited List. However, although not specifically cited on the list of examples of stimulants, modafinil was banned because it had the pharmacological properties of a stimulant and fell under the umbrella phrase of 'related substances,' a situation discussed by Kaufman (2005).

A situation that has consistently caused problems for athletes has involved drugs that are available to purchase over-the-counter (OTC), without a prescription. Athletes have therefore been able to purchase OTC medicines that have contained stimulants that appear on the Prohibited List. Despite the fact that the testing authorities used cut-off levels for these drugs, below which the athlete would not be sanctioned, it has been shown that these cut-off levels were unrealistic (Chester *et al.* 2004). This has led to a number of high-profile cases involving elite athletes.

Andreea Răducan (2000)

At the 2000 Olympic Games in Sydney, the Romanian gymnast Andreea Răducan tested positive for the drug pseudoephedrine, which was present in an OTC cough-and-cold product that the gymnast had taken (Dikic *et al.* 2013). Despite the fact that she had taken the drug on advice from her team doctor, strict liability rules prevailed and she was stripped of her gold medal. The Romanian physician was also sanctioned, being expelled from the Games and barred from Olympic Games for 4 years (Hilderbrand *et al.* 2003).

Alain Baxter (2002)

The Scottish skier Alain Baxter won a bronze medal in the men's slalom event at the Winter Olympic Games in Salt Lake City in February 2002. He then tested positive for methamphetamine and was stripped of his bronze medal. Baxter had used an American product (Vicks Vapor Inhaler) as a nasal decongestant to treat a cold. This product contains levmetamfetamine, the levo isomer of methamphetamine, a relatively inactive isomer compared with the dextro isomer. Baxter claimed that he was unaware that the product contained a banned substance because the medicine looked the same as a similar product that Baxter had used in the United Kingdom, which did not contain levmetamfetamine.

The International Ski Federation (ISF) accepted that Baxter had taken the drug inadvertently but imposed a ban of 3 months from all competitions. This ban was lifted by the Court of Arbitration in Sport, which accepted that Baxter 'did not intend to obtain a competitive advantage.' However, the IOC refused to overturn the medal disqualification. A subsequent study on the effects of inhaled levmetamfetamine on athlete performance showed that modest doses of the drug did not improve performance (Dufka *et al.* 2009).

These and other similar cases led WADA to remove most of the OTC stimulants from the Prohibited List in 2004. These drugs have been placed on a monitoring list, and their use by athletes is being recorded by WADA's accredited laboratories. It appears that athletes still do not fully understand the status and function of these OTC medicines, and many consider that they should be returned to the Prohibited List (Mottram *et al.* 2008). Indeed, pseudoephedrine was returned to the WADA Prohibited List in 2010.

A number of cases have involved the claim by athletes of the inadvertent use of cocaine.

Martina Hingis (2007)

The A and B urine samples taken from the Swiss tennis player Martina Hingis at the 2007 Wimbledon Tennis Championships both showed a positive result for cocaine. She was banned from competition for 2 years but announced her retirement from tennis in November 2007. Hingis claimed that she had never used cocaine and independently submitted a hair sample for testing, which was negative for drugs. Furthermore, she argued that the urine samples must have been handled improperly. However, she stated that she did not wish to contest the finding or the 2-year ban.

Richard Gasquet (2009)

On 28 March 2009, the French tennis player Richard Gasquet submitted a urine sample at a tournament in Florida. Both the A and B samples tested positive for cocaine. Gasquet was charged with a doping offence and was banned from competition. An independent anti-doping tribunal appointed by the International Tennis Federation (ITF) held a hearing on 29–30 June 2009, at which Gasquet claimed his positive result was a result of cocaine entering his body when he kissed a girl who had been using cocaine at a nightclub. The tribunal stated that because the amount of cocaine found in Gasquet's system was 'about the size of a grain of salt,' he was cleared to return to competition. On 6 August 2009, the ITF and WADA announced that they were appealing to the Court of Arbitration for Sport (CAS) against the tribunal's decision. However, in December 2009, the CAS dismissed the appeal and Gasquet returned to competitive tennis.

Frankie Dettori (2012)

The jockey Frankie Dettori, was given a 6-month ban from racing after testing positive for a banned substance in September 2012. It was later revealed that the substance was cocaine.

A dramatic rise in the number of adverse analytical findings relating to methylhexaneamine has been seen since 2009, when this drug was added to the WADA Prohibited List (see Table 13.1). This was exemplified by a case at the London 2012 Games.

Ghfran Almouhamad (2012)

The Syrian hurdler Ghfran Almouhamad provided an adverse analytical finding for methylhexaneamine at the London 2012 Olympic Games, from which she was disqualified. Methylhexaneamine, also known as Geranamine, is found in many supplements that are used by athletes (see Section 13.5).

Three further cases relating to the use of methylhexaneamine were recorded at the Sochi Winter Olympic games in February 2014.

Vitalijs Pavlovs, William Frullani, and Evi Sachenbacher-Stehle (2014)

The IOC announced that men's ice hockey player Vitalijs Pavlovs of Latvia, Italian bobsledder William Frullani, and biathlete Evi Sachenbacher-Stehle of Germany had been excluded from the XXII Olympic Winter Games in Sochi. All had tested positive for methylhexaneamine (dimethylpentylamine).

The potential for inadvertent ingestion of stimulants through supplement use was further illustrated in 2013.

Asafa Powell (2013)

In July 2013, it was revealed that the Jamaican sprinter Asafa Powell was alleged to have used the stimulant oxilofrine. He was given an 18 month suspension which was reduced to 6 months on appeal to the Court of Arbitration for Sport.

13.5. Action and use of stimulants in sport

The use of legal and illegal stimulating agents in sport is widespread, and they remain an important abused class of doping agents (Deventer *et al.* 2011). In addition to the ethical consideration of using stimulants as performance-enhancing agents in sport or their use in a social context, the health consequences of athletes using stimulants is a prime concern (Angell *et al.* 2013).

Ephedrine and other sympathomimetics in sport

Ephedrine and other sympathomimetics have been promoted for weight loss as well as enhancement of athletic performance. The first comprehensive study of the possible ergogenic effects of these drugs was carried out by Sidney and Lefcoe (1977). In this comprehensive experiment, ten variables were measured, including strength, endurance, reaction time, anaerobic capacity, and speed of recovery from effort. The results showed that exercise heart rate and resting pulse pressure increased, postexercise recovery rate slowed, and none of the physical performance measures improved. In Canada, Bell *et al.* (2001) measured the effects of 120 mg of ephedrine on power output, oxygen debt, and VO_2 max in sixteen healthy volunteers. They found that, compared to placebo, ephedrine significantly increased power output during the first 10 sec of cycle exercise but had no effect after this time. Ephedrine also had no effect on O_2 deficit or accumulated VO_2.

In 2003, Jacobs *et al.* carried out a controlled trial of ephedrine (0.8 mg/kg) alone or in combination with caffeine compared with placebo on males undertaking a weight-training circuit. The authors reported that acute ingestion of ephedrine or ephedrine plus caffeine increased muscular endurance during the first set of resistance-training exercises. However, they concluded that the performance enhancement was attributed primarily to the effects of ephedrine, with no additive effect of caffeine.

With respect to weight loss and enhanced performance due to ephedrine, Shekelle *et al.* (2003) undertook a meta-analysis of several trials. They showed that ephedrine can promote modest weight loss in the short term (approximately 0.9 kg/month more than placebo) for up to 6 months, but that the differences in the parameters used to measure performance within the various trials mean that conclusive evidence for performance enhancement could not be achieved. Indeed, Robergs *et al.* (2003) advised exercise physiologists and dieticians not to recommend the use of ephedrines as ergogenic aids or stimulants for increased weight loss because they expose the user to unacceptable health risks relative to the minimal weight loss or ergogenic potential of the supplements.

Pseudoephedrine was removed from the WADA Prohibited List in 2004 but reintroduced in 2010, in part due to evidence of performance-enhancing effects of the drug (Hodges *et al.* 2006; Betteridge *et al.* 2010; Pritchard-Peschek *et al.* 2010).

Ephedrine may be included in supplements that are used by athletes. The natural source of the ephedrine, such as ma huang (*Ephedra sinica*), is frequently mentioned on the label rather than the name of the active ingredients. Herbal supplements containing ma huang are frequently promoted for their performance-enhancing effects or their positive effects on weight reduction. In addition to ma huang, such herbal supplements may also contain additional ephedrine (Deventer *et al.* 2011). This may lead to inadvertent use of a banned substance by the athlete (Geyer *et al.* 2011).

Adverse effects of sympathomimetics in athletes

In the study by Jacobs *et al.* (2003), systolic blood pressure was increased significantly in subjects given ephedrine. The meta-analysis by Shekelle *et al.* (2003) showed that ephedrine was associated with a two- to threefold increase in adverse effects, including heart palpitations, and an increased risk of psychiatric and upper gastrointestinal symptoms. More serious side effects due to ephedrine within dietary supplements, such as seizures, stroke, and even death, have been reported by Haller *et al.* (2000).

Amphetamines in sport

In a review of CNS stimulants, Avois *et al.* (2009) concluded that amphetamines may have the following effects:

* Improve reaction time when fatigued
* Increase muscular endurance and strength
* Increase acceleration
* Raise lactic acid levels during maximal exercise
* Increase aerobic endurance capacity
* Stimulate metabolism by inducing a loss of body fat.

Many of the studies on the effects of amphetamine in athletic performance have been carried out on cyclists. Wyndham *et al.* (1971) carried out a wide-ranging placebo-controlled biochemical and physiological investigation on two champion cyclists exercising on a bicycle ergometer. There was no difference between amphetamine and placebo in terms of submaximal or maximal oxygen uptake, heart rate, or minute ventilation. However, there were significant increases in blood lactate levels. The authors concluded that amphetamines have no effect on the ability to do aerobic work, but they insignificantly increased the cyclists' ability to tolerate higher levels of anaerobic metabolism. The dangers inherent in these results are that an athlete taking amphetamine might be better able to ignore the usual internal signals of overexertion and heat stress, which may therefore explain the incidence of heat stroke and cardiac problems in cyclists who take amphetamines during long-distance cycling events.

Several reviewers, including Conlee (1991), have remarked on the considerable inconsistency of amphetamine effects in humans, particularly with regard to ergogenicity. A poorly explored feature of amphetamine action is its effect on fatigue. Most studies have concentrated on the central aspects of fatigue while neglecting peripheral contributions. The few studies of amphetamine effects on muscle glycogen stores before and during exercise have been contradictory (Conlee 1991).

Because no significant improvement in performance is associated with amphetamine use, why does it continue to be taken? The answer could be an effect on mental attitude in terms of improved mood, greater confidence and optimism, and increased alertness. Amphetamines could be abused for different reasons by different athletes. Baseball and football players may use them to increase alertness and concentration, whereas runners or swimmers may use them to increase energy and endurance (Smith and Perry 1992).

Several studies indicate that the effect of amphetamine on the psychological state of athletes might be self-induced and occur as a result of the athlete expecting to perform better and be more alert. A review of the confounding influences in psychostimulant results has been presented by Clarkson and Thompson (1997).

Another feature of most studies is the failure to control for trained or untrained subjects. This is very important if we are considering that amphetamine may have an effect on motivation, as trained athletes often exhibit higher motivational levels than the untrained, and the untrained therefore may not exercise fully to exhaustion (Clarkson and Thomson 1997).

Methylphenidate, a drug commonly used to treat ADHD, has been found to increase performance, but only in warm (30 °C) conditions (Kreher 2012).

Adverse side effects of amphetamines in athletes

Some important side effects of amphetamine have been revealed in individuals undertaking extremely arduous training or sporting schedules. One of the most widely publicised side effects of amphetamine, from which a number of fatalities have occurred, is heat stroke. This has been most prominent in cyclists owing to the intensity of their exercise, the endurance required, and the high ambient temperatures at which the exercise often occurs. Amphetamines cause a redistribution of blood flow away from the skin, thus limiting the cooling of the blood. As a result, two cyclists (Jenson and Simpson) who had both been taking amphetamine died of heat stroke and cardiac arrest, respectively, during gruelling road races. The former occurred in the intense summer heat of Rome, the latter whilst climbing the infamous Mont Ventoux during the 1967 Tour de France.

The side effects of amphetamine on behaviour are also important in sport. There were several accounts quoted by Golding (1981) in which the euphoriant effects of amphetamines rendered the takers unaware of the errors and misjudgements they were making on the field of play.

The prescription and administration of amphetamines are strictly controlled by law in most developed countries. They produce powerful stimulating effects on the CNS, which include euphoria, excitation, and increased aggression and alertness. These effects are achieved at the expense of judgement and self-criticism. Amphetamine administration may be followed by severe bouts of depression and dependence. Increases in athletic performance induced by amphetamines are very small, and several studies have failed to show that amphetamine use produces any physical advantage.

The adverse effects of amphetamine use in sport are largely focussed on CNS effects. However, significant cardiovascular events are associated with their use, with long-term atherosclerotic risk even with moderate usage (Angell *et al*. 2013).

The induction of dependence and the increased susceptibility to heat stroke and cardiac abnormalities seem to suggest that amphetamine is of little value as a performance-enhancing drug in the long term.

Effects of cocaine on athletes and exercise

Cocaine was used by native South Americans for centuries to increase efficiency, vigour, and physical endurance. In 1930, Theil and Essing reported that 0.1 g of cocaine administered to subjects before exercising on a cycle ergometer improved work efficiency, as determined by VO_2 measurements per unit work, and that exercise could be maintained for longer. The results were attributed to reduced CNS perception of fatigue. A second study using the same cocaine dose revealed no increase in work efficiency but a more rapid increase in recovery after exercise (Conlee 1991). In his review of pre-1983 studies of the effects of cocaine on exercise, Conlee (1991) concluded that they were all contradictory and were usually poorly controlled and carried out.

In 1991, Conlee *et al*. demonstrated, in rats exercising voluntarily, that cocaine increases glycogen metabolism and enhances the exercise-induced sympathetic responses. They suggested three possible mechanisms to explain cocaine's action, which could operate in parallel:

- Cocaine releases catecholamines, which increase glycogenolysis and lactate production, thus leading to early fatigue.
- Cocaine may induce skeletal muscle vasoconstriction, reducing oxygen delivery, oxidative metabolism, strength, and reaction time, as well as stimulating glycogen breakdown.
- Cocaine may have a direct effect on muscle glycogen breakdown.

Indirect evidence originally suggested that the second mechanism is less likely because cocaine-induced reduction of myocardial blood flow is not associated with increased myocardial glycogen breakdown. In 1994, Braiden *et al*. demonstrated a threefold increase in muscle lactate accumulation in the white vastus muscle of rats treated with cocaine under exercise conditions.

A study of the effects of the coca leaf has been described by Spielvogel *et al*. (1996). In this experiment, metabolic and hormonal changes in habitual coca chewers were compared to non-coca chewers during incremental exercise to exhaustion. During sustained exercise, oxygen uptake and work efficiency were similar in both groups. During incremental exercise, habitual chewers demonstrated lower arterial oxygen saturation, which was not due to reduced ventilatory response. Free fatty acid (FFA) levels were increased during incremental exercise in the coca chewers. This interesting study remains inconclusive because the possible benefits of raised FFA levels could not be determined. There were no simultaneous measurements of changes in carbohydrate metabolism or endurance. Therefore, it is unclear whether a carbohydrate-sparing mechanism was activated by coca chewing. Also, because catecholamine (i.e. noradrenaline and adrenaline) plasma levels remained unaltered, the mechanism for the elevation of plasma FFA levels was unknown.

A similar increase in FFA concentration following coca chewing was described by Favier *et al.* (1996), although they observed increased adrenaline and FFA levels during exercise, coupled with lower blood glucose concentrations. Their conclusion was that this might be evidence that cocaine could prolong work and postpone fatigue by increasing fat mobilisation and sparing glycogen utilisation, but it did not increase time to exhaustion.

Clarkson and Thompson (1997) questioned the validity of experiments using coca leaves rather than pure cocaine, even where the plasma cocaine concentration has been subsequently determined. The pharmacokinetics of cocaine may be altered by ingesting it via this route. Also, the coca leaf may contain other naturally occurring ingredients, which might influence cocaine metabolism and disposition, affect cocaine action at receptors or transporters, and/or have metabolic effects of their own. Habitual and naïve cocaine/coca users may exhibit different responses, and experiments in rats seem to support this (Conlee *et al.* 2000).

The effect of cocaine on catecholamine secretion could be the basis of the ergolytic effect of cocaine on exercise. Cocaine effects may not be caused by a vascular action of noradrenaline because the blockade of α_1-receptors does not block the action of cocaine on glycogenolysis or lactic acid production (Conlee *et al.* 2000). Because it is quite likely that athletes abusing cocaine will be chronic abusers, a comparison was made between cocaine responses in naïve and chronic cocaine-administered rats. It was found that responses to cocaine in terms of noradrenaline and adrenaline release were greater in rats that had previously received cocaine on a regular basis (Kelly *et al.* 1995).

Adverse effects of cocaine in athletes

There have been reports of athletes combining cocaine use with other drugs, such as alcohol and anabolic steroids. According to Welder and Melchert (1993), heavy alcohol consumption combined with cocaine abuse enhances cocaine's cardiotoxicity, possibly by the production of a unique metabolite called cocaethylene. The existence and structure of cocaethylene, as the ethyl ester of the cocaine metabolite benzoylecgonine, has been established by Farre *et al.* (1993), and its actions in animals and man have been reviewed and investigated by McCance-Katz *et al.* (1998). They have detailed the following facts:

- Cocaine and alcohol taken together have additive deleterious effects.
- Simultaneous consumption of alcohol and cocaine leads to the formation of cocaethylene.
- Athough cocaethylene is less potent than cocaine, it is eliminated more slowly and could thus accumulate during or following an alcohol/cocaine binge.

Further dangers arise from the possibility that the increased sense of well-being produced by the cocaine/alcohol mixture would lead to further abuse, leading to increased toxicity from the drugs plus the toxicity of cocaethylene. Is this relevant to sport? Most certainly it is. This may well have been the ultimate cause of death of the Canadian ice-hockey player John Kordic, who abused cocaine, alcohol, and anabolic steroids. His downfall has been chronicled in detail by Scher (1992) and included frequent fights on the pitch with opponents, teammates, and officials.

Methylhexaneamine

Methylhexaneamine is classed as a stimulant due to its effect of releasing the neurotransmitter noradrenaline from nerve endings. It is also known as 1,3-dimethylamine, or DMAA. It was originally patented as a nasal decongestant; however, it is marketed extensively under many names as a dietary supplement. Other common names for methylhexaneamine include dimethylpentylamine or DMP, 2-amino-4-methylhexane, forthane, geranamine, geranium oil or root extract, among others. A study by Lisi *et al.* (2011) suggests that geranium oils do not contain methylhexaneamine and that products labelled as containing geranium oil, but which contain methylhexaneamine, can only arise from the addition of synthetic material.

The supplements in which methylhexaneamine appears focus on fat loss or increases in energy, but supplements are marketed for a wide variety of reasons. Attempts have been made in some countries to remove supplements containing methylhexaneamine from the market.

The recent dramatic increase in adverse analytical findings for methylhexaneamine (see Table 13.1) probably reflects the widespread use of supplements by athletes and the complex array of names for this drug that are used by companies on the list of ingredients. Members of the United States Anti-Doping Agency (2013) have provided valuable advice to athletes regarding the inadvertent use of methylhexaneamine through taking dietary supplements.

13.6. Stimulants and the WADA Prohibited List

Stimulants have the potential for performance enhancement at the time of competing. They are therefore classified by WADA under Substances and Methods Prohibited In-Competition. Out-of-competition testing for stimulants is not considered necessary, thereby saving resources. This decision was supported through a study by Boghosian *et al.* (2011), who investigated data from eleven WADA-accredited laboratories to determine whether athletes were using stimulants during the training phase (out-of-competition). Results showed that there was no significant prevalence (0.36 per cent of positive findings), suggesting that this does not pose a challenge to the fight against doping.

The WADA regulations relating to stimulants are shown in Table 13.2. In 2009, WADA categorised stimulants as specified or nonspecified. The move was made to align the 2009 Prohibited List with the more flexible sanctions set forth in revised World Anti-Doping Code of 2009 (WADA 2009). The objective of more flexible sanctions was to allow enhanced sanctions for deliberate doping offenders and reduced sanctions for inadvertent cheaters or for athletes who can unequivocally establish that the substance involved was not intended to enhance performance.

In 2010, WADA returned pseudoephedrine to the Prohibited List as a result of evidence from their monitoring programme of a sustained increase in use at high concentrations and scientific evidence of its performance-enhancing effects at certain doses.

With respect to ephedrine, methylephedrine, and cathine, WADA specified urinary cut-off levels. A previous study (Chester *et al.* 2004), however, questioned the levels at which such cut-offs are set. Subsequent pharmacokinetic studies were taken into consideration when WADA reintroduced pseudoephedrine to the Prohibited List in 2010, increasing the urinary threshold to 150 µg/ml from the 25-µg/ml threshold in operation prior to 2004 (Deventer *et al.* 2011).

The list of nonspecified stimulants includes cocaine. Therefore, athletes need to avoid the possibility of passive inhalation of cocaine when smoked by others as the highly volatile crack cocaine. However, Yonamine *et al.* (2004) reviewed the literature on this issue and concluded that only individuals exposed to cocaine smoke under 'extremely harsh conditions' would eliminate cocaine metabolites in the urine.

Table 13.2 WADA 2014 regulations regarding stimulants

All stimulants, including all optical isomers (e.g., *d-* and *l-*) where relevant, are prohibited, except imidazole derivatives for topical use and those stimulants included in the 2014 Monitoring Program.* Stimulants include the following:

Nonspecified stimulants

Adrafinil, amfepramone, amfetamine, amfetaminil, amiphenazole, benfluorex, benzylpiperazine, bromantan, clobenzorex, cocaine, cropropamide, crotetamide, fencamine, fenetylline, fenfluramine, fenproporex, fonturacetam [4-phenylpiracetam (carphedon)], furfenorex, mefenorex, mephentermine, mesocarb, metamfetamine(*d*-), p-methylamphetamine, modafinil, norfenfluramine, phendimetrazine, phenmetrazine, phentermine, prenylamine, prolintane

A stimulant not expressly listed in this section is a Specified Substance.

Specified stimulants (examples)

Benzfetamine, cathine**, cathinone and its analogues (e.g. mephedrone, methedrone, α-pyrrolidinovalerophenone), dimethylamphetamine, ephedrine***, epinephrine**** (adrenaline), etamivan, etilamfetamine, etilefrine, famprofazone, fenbutrazate, fencamfamin, heptaminol, hydroxyamfetamine (parahydroamphetamine), isometheptene, levmetamfetamine, meclofenoxate, methylenedioxymethamphetamine, methylephedrine***, methylhexaneamine (dimethylpentylamine), methylphenidate, nikethamide, norfenefrine, octopamine, oxilofrine (methylsynephrine), pemoline, pentetrazol, phenpromethamine, propylhexedrine, pseudoephedrine*****, selegiline, sibutramine, strychnine, tenamfetamine (methylenedioxyamphetamine), trimetazidine, tuaminoheptane, and other substances with a similar chemical structure or similar biological effect(s).

* The following substances included in the 2014 Monitoring Program are not considered as prohibited substances: bupropion, caffeine, nicotine, phenylephrine, phenylpropanolamine, pipradol, synephrine.
** Cathine is prohibited when its concentration in urine is greater than 5 μg/ml.
*** Each of ephedrine and methylephedrine is prohibited when its concentration in urine is greater than 10 μg/ml.
**** Local administration (e.g. nasal, ophthalmologic) of epinephrine (adrenaline) or co-administration with local anaesthetic agents is not prohibited.
***** Pseudoephedrine is prohibited when its concentration in urine is greater than 150 μg/ml.
Source: World Anti-Doping Agency. (2013). The 2014 Prohibited List international standard. Available online at http://www.wada-ama.org/Documents/World_Anti-Doping_Program/WADP-Prohibited-list/2014/WADA-prohibited-list-2014-EN.pdf (accessed 18 July 2014).

Therapeutic use exemptions for stimulants

TUEs for stimulants have been approved by WADA for ADHD and narcolepsy (Fitch 2012). ADHD may have significant effects on competing athletes (Kreher 2012). Stringent conditions must be met to approve the use of stimulants, such as dexamfetamine or mephenidate, to manage ADHD in adults.

The approval to grant a TUE for modafinil or other stimulants for narcolepsy requires expert opinion from a consultant physician in sleep medicine plus a comprehensive investigation, including a positive multiple sleep latency test (Fitch 2012).

13.7. Summary

- Stimulants are a broad class of drugs with a number of clinical uses.
- Some stimulants, such as amphetamines and cocaine, are abused in a social context as recreational drugs. Other stimulants, such as methylhexaneamine, are found in supplements.

- The potential benefit of many stimulants as performance-enhancing agents is equivocal.
- Stimulants are one of the classes of drugs that appear most frequently on WADA's statistics on adverse analytical findings.
- There have been several high-profile cases involving athletes who have deliberately or inadvertently taken stimulants. Consequently, WADA regulations for stimulants, including Therapeutic Use Exemptions, are complex.

13.8. References

Angell, P. J., Chester, N., Sculthorpe, N. *et al.* (2013). Performance enhancing drug abuse and cardiovascular risk in athletes: Implications for the physician. *British Journal of Sports Medicine* 46(Suppl 1):i78–i84.

Avois, L., Robinson, N., Saudan, C., *et al.* (2009). Central nervous system stimulants and sport practice. *British Journal of Sports Medicine* 40(Suppl 1):i16–i20.

Bell, D. G., Jacobs, I., and Ellerington, K. (2001). Effect of caffeine and ephedrine ingestion on anaerobic exercise performance. *Medicine and Science in Sports Exercise* 33(8): 1399–1403.

Betteridge, S., Mündel, T., and Stannard, S. (2010). The effect of pseudoephedrine on self-paced endurance cycling performance. *European Journal of Sports Science* 10(1):53–58.

Boghosian, T., Mazzoni, I., Barroso, O., *et al.* (2011). Investigating the use of stimulants in out-of-competition sport samples. *Journal of Analytical Toxicology* 35(9):613–616.

Braiden, R. W., Fellingham, G. W., and Conlee, R. K. (1994). Effects of cocaine on glycogen metabolism and endurance during high intensity exercise. *Medicine and Science in Sports Exercise* 26(6): 695–700.

Brookes, L. G. (1985). Central nervous system stimulants. In S. D. Iverson (Ed.), *Psychopharmacology: Recent Advances and Future Prospects* (pp. 264–277). Oxford, UK: Oxford University Press.

Bucci, L. R. (2000). Selected herbals and human performance. *American Journal of Clinical Nutrition* 72(2):624S–636S.

Chen, N., and Reith, M. E. A. (2000). Structure and function of the dopamine transporter. *European Journal of Pharmacology* 405(4):329–339.

Chester, N., Mottram, D. R., Reilly, T., *et al.* (2004). Elimination of ephedrines in urine following multiple dosing: The consequences for athletes, in relation to doping control. *British Journal of Clinical Pharmacology* 57(1):62–67.

Clarkson, P. M., and Thompson, H. S. (1997). Drugs and sport: Research findings and limitations. *Sports Medicine* 24(6):366–384.

Comer, S. D., Hart, C. L., Ward, A. S., *et al.* (2001). Effects of repeated oral methamphetamine administration in humans. *Psychopharmacology* 155(4):397–401.

Conlee, R. K. (1991). Amphetamine, caffeine and cocaine. In D. R. Lamb and M. H. Williams (Eds.), *Perspectives in Exercise Science and Sports Medicine* (pp. 285–328). New York, NY: Brown and Benchmark.

Conlee, R. K., Han, D. H., Kelly, K. P. *et al.* (1991). Effects of cocaine on plasma catecholamine and muscle glycogen concentrations during exercise in the rat. *Journal of Applied Physiology* 70(3):1323–1327.

Conlee, R. K., Kelly, K. P., Ojuka, E. O. *et al.* (2000). Cocaine and exercise: Alpha-1 receptor blockade does not alter muscle glycogenolysis or blood lactacidosis. *Journal of Applied Physiology* 88(1):77–81.

Deventer, K., Roels, K., Delbeke, F. T., *et al.* (2011). Prevalence of legal and illegal stimulating agents in sport. *Annals of Bioanalytical Chemistry* 401(2):421–432.

Dikic, N., McNamee, M., Günter, H., *et al.* (2013). Sports physicians, ethics and antidoping governance: Between assistance and negligence. *British Journal of Sports Medicine* 47(11):701–704.

Docherty, J. R. (2008). Pharmacology of stimulants prohibited by the World Anti-Doping Agency (WADA). *British Journal of Pharmacology* 154(3):606–622.

Dufka, F., Galloway, G., Baggott, M., *et al.* (2009). The effects of inhaled L-methamphetamine on athlete performance while riding a stationary bike, a randomised placebo-controlled trial. *British Journal of Sports Medicine* 43(11):832–835.

Farre, M., De La Tour, R., Llorente, M., *et al.* (1993). Alcohol and cocaine interactions in humans. *Journal of Pharmacology and Experimental Therapeutics* 266(3):1364–1373.

Favier, R., Caceres, E., and Koubi, H. (1996). Effects of coca chewing on metabolic and hormonal changes during prolonged submaximal exercise. *Journal of Applied Physiology* 80(2):650–655.

Fibiger, H. C., Phillips, A. G., and Brown, E. E. (1992). The neurobiology of cocaine-induced reinforcement. In G. E. W. Wolstenholme (Ed.), *Cocaine: Scientific and Social Dimensions. Ciba Foundation Symposium 166* (pp. 96–124). Chichester, UK: John Wiley.

Fitch, K. (2012). Proscribed drugs at the Olympic Games: Permitted use and misuse (doping) by athletes. *Clinical Medicine* 12(3):257–260.

Geyer, H., Braun, H., Burke, L. M., *et al.* (2011). A–Z of nutritional supplements: Dietary supplements sports nutrition foods and ergogenic aids for health and performance – Part 22. *British Journal of Sports Medicine* 45(9):752–754.

Golding, L. A. (1981). Drugs and hormones. In W. P. Morgan (Ed.), *Ergogenic Aids and Muscular Performance* (pp. 368–397). New York, NY: Academic Press.

Haller, C. A.., and Benowitz, N. L. (2000). Adverse cardiovascular and central nervous system events associated with dietary supplements containing ephedra alkaloids. *New England Journal of Medicine* 343(25):1833–1838.

Hart, C. L., Ward, A. S., Haney, M., *et al.* (2001). Methamphetamine self-administration by humans. *Psychopharmacology* 157(1):75–81.

Hilderbrand, R. L., Wanninger, R., and Bowers, L. D. (2003). An update on regulatory issues in antidoping programs in sport. *Current Sports Medicine Reports* 2(4):226–232.

Hodges, K., Hancock, S., Currell, K., *et al.* (2006). Pseudoephedrine enhances performance in 1500-m runners. *Medicine and Science in Sports and Exercise* 38(2):329–333.

Jacobs, I., Pasternak, H., and Bell, D. G. (2003). Effects of ephedrine, caffeine and their combination on muscular endurance. *Medicine and Science in Sports and Exercise* 35(6):987–994.

Jones, G. (2008). Caffeine and other sympathomimetic stimulants: Modes of action and effects on sports performance. *Drugs and Ergogenic Aids to Improve Sport Performance* 44(1):109–123.

Kalix, P. (1992). Cathinone, a natural amphetamine. *Pharmacology and Toxicology* 70(2):77–86.

Kaufman, K. R. (2005). Modafinil in sports: Ethical considerations. *British Journal of Sports Medicine* 39(4):241–244.

Kelly, K. P., Han, D. H., Fellingham, G. W., *et al.* (1995). Cocaine and exercise: Physiological responses of cocaine-conditioned rats. *Medicine Science in Sports Exercise* 27(1):65–72.

Kreher, J. B. (2012). Attention deficit/hyperactivity disorder (ADHD) in athletes. *International Journal of Athletic Therapy and Training* 17(3):15–19.

Laties, V. G., and Weiss, B. (1981). The amphetamine margin in sports. *Federation Proceedings* 40 (12):2689–2692.

Lisi, A., Hasick, N., Kazlauskas, R., *et al.* (2011). Studies of methylhexaneamine in supplements and geranium oil. *Drug Testing Analysis* 3(11–12):873–876.

McCance-Katz, E. F., Kosten, T. R., and Jatlow, P. (1998). Concurrent use of cocaine and alcohol is more potent and potentially more toxic than use of either alone: A multi-dose study. *Biological Psychiatry* 44(4):250–259.

Mottram, D., Chester, N., Atkinson, G., *et al.* (2008). Athletes' knowledge and views on OTC medication. *International Journal of Sports Medicine* 29(10):851–855.

Pritchard-Peschek, K. R., Jenkins, D. G., Osborne, M. A., *et al.* (2010). Pseudoephedrine ingestion and cycling time-trial performance. *International Journal of Sports Nutrition and Exercise Metabolism* 20(2):132–138.

Robergs, R. A., Boone, T., and Lockner, D. (2003). Exercise physiologists should not recommend the use of ephedrine and related compounds as ergogenic aids or stimulants for increased weight loss. *Journal of Exercise Physiology* 6(4):42–52.

Scher, J. (1992). Death of a goon. *Sports Illustrated* 76(August 24th):112–116.

Shekelle, P. G., Hardy, M. L., Morton, S. C., *et al*. (2003). Efficacy and safety of ephedra and ephedrine for weight loss and athletic performance: A meta-analysis. *Journal of the American Medical Association* 289(12):1537–1545.

Sidney, K. H., and Lefcoe, W. M. (1977). The effects of ephedrine on the physiological and psychological responses to submaximal and maximal exercises in man. *Medicine and Science in Sports* 9(2): 95–99.

Smith B. J., Jones, H. E., and Griffiths, R. R. (2001). Physiological, subjective and reinforcing effects of oral and intravenous cocaine in humans. *Psychopharmacology* 156(4):435–444.

Smith, D. A., and Perry, P. J. (1992). The efficacy of ergogenic agents in athletic competition Part II: Other performance-enhancing agents. *Annals of Pharmacotherapy* 26(5):653–659.

Spielvogel, H., Caceres, E., Karbritt, B., *et al*. (1996). Effects of coca chewing on metabolic and hormonal changes during graded incremental exercise to maximum. *Journal of Applied Physiology* 80(2): 643–649.

Theil, D., and Essing, B. (1930). Cocaine und muskelarbeit I. Der einfluss auf leistung und gastoffwechsel. *Arbeitsphysiologie* 3:287–297.

United States Anti-Doping Agency. (2011). Available online at http://www.usada.org/athlete-advisory-methylhexaneamine-and-dietary-supplements (accessed 17 July 2014).

Unterwald, E. M., Kreek, M. J., and Cuntapay, M. (2001). The frequency of cocaine administration impacts cocaine-induced receptor alteration. *Brain Research* 900(1):103–109.

Wadler, G. A., and Hainline, B. (1989). *Drugs and the athlete*. Philadelphia, PA: F.A. Davis.

Welder, A. A., and Melchert, R. B. (1993). Cardiotoxic effects of cocaine and anabolic-androgenic steroids in the athlete. *Journal of Pharmacology and Toxicological Methodology* 29(1):61–68.

World Anti-Doping Agency. (2009). World Anti-Doping Code 2009. Available online at https://www.wada-ama.org/en/resources/the-code/2009-world-anti-doping-code#.VA-HP8stDX4 (accessed 9 September 2014).

Wyndham, G. H., Rogers, G. G., Benade, A. J. S., *et al*. (1971). Physiological effects of the amphetamines during exercise. *South African Medical Journal* 45(10):247–252.

Yonamine, M., Garcia, P. R., and de Moraes Moreau, R. L. (2004). Non-intentional doping in sports. *Sports Medicine* 34(1):697–704.

Chapter 14

Narcotics

David R. Mottram

14.1. Introduction

The use of certain drugs by athletes is prohibited because there is a potential for achieving enhanced levels of performance. With some drugs, the potential to induce serious harm to the user is an issue. In most countries, the use of certain drugs for nontherapeutic, recreational use is against the law. All three of these criteria apply to the class of drugs known as narcotics.

14.2. What are narcotics?

Narcotics are drugs that can induce narcosis, which can be defined as a state of insensibility. This class of drugs possesses significant analgesic activity, in which context they are frequently referred to as narcotic analgesics or opioid analgesics.

This group of drugs was originally derived from the opium poppy (*Papaver somniferum*). The active constituents of the poppy, of which morphine is the most potent, are extracted from the latex that exudes from incisions made in the unripe capsule of the flowering head. Opium has been used by humans for thousands of years. Morphine was first isolated in 1806 and was named after the Greek god of dreams, Morpheus.

The potency of morphine can be significantly enhanced by acetylation to diamorphine (heroin), which has the convenience of greater solubility. Codeine (3-methylmorphine) has only a fifth of the potency of morphine, but it is more reliably absorbed from the gastrointestinal system. Dihydrocodeine is similar in potency to codeine when given orally, although it is about twice codeine's potency when injected.

Morphine-like drugs are not just analgesics. It is clear from a variety of sources that they exhibit multiple activities, including respiratory depression, emesis, and smooth muscle relaxation. In addition, they have profound effects on perception. It can be argued that their analgesic effect has more to do with a change in concern about pain than in a physical reduction of pain. Euphoria is a common experience, too.

14.3. Clinical uses of narcotic analgesics

Narcotic analgesics have a number of clinical uses, the most significant of which is the alleviation of pain.

Analgesia

Nonopioid analgesics, such as aspirin, paracetamol, and nonsteroidal anti-inflammatory drugs such as ibuprofen and diclofenac, are suitable for pain in musculoskeletal conditions.

Opioid (narcotic) analgesics are more suitable for moderate to severe pain, particularly of visceral origin.

Pain

Pain is a subjective phenomenon, the scale of which is dependent on many factors apart from the severity of an injury. Pain is subjective and is notoriously difficult to measure.

Mechanism of action of narcotic analgesics

In the 1970s, it was independently discovered by Kosterlitz and Hughes (1977) and Simantov and Snyder (1976) that the body produces neuropeptides called endorphins, which stimulate neural receptors, resulting in a reduction of nociception and inducing a sense of well-being. Narcotic analgesics stimulate the same receptors, inducing similar or more profound levels of analgesia and euphoria. Opioid receptors in the central nervous system mediate the actions of endogenous peptides, such as enkephalins and dynorphins. There are three main types of opioid receptors in humans: μ (mu), κ (kappa), and δ (delta). The euphoria and physical dependence attributable to opioids are thought to be mediated through μ receptors in the brain.

Narcotic analgesics relieve most types of pain, including that associated with traumatic injuries. Their analgesic effect is achieved by a variety of concomitant activities. They inhibit the generation of nerve impulses in the peripheral pain fibres, inhibit transmission of impulses in the dorsal horn neuron, and stimulate the descending inhibitory pathway (which also suppresses the activity of the dorsal horn neuron).

Other clinical uses for narcotics

Acute diarrhoea

There are a number of types of medicines that can be used to manage cases of acute diarrhoea. The primary goal should be to counter the dehydrating effects of this condition using oral rehydration preparations. Gut motility can be controlled using antimotility drugs, including the opioids codeine and morphine. These medicines can be purchased over-the-counter, without a prescription. The reason that morphine can be obtained in this way is that it is administered, in small doses, in combination with an absorbent, such as kaolin.

Cough suppression

Cough may result from a number of causes, such as irritation to the respiratory epithelium due to an infection, exposure to environmental pollutants, or as a symptom of another underlying disorder. A cough may be productive, with mucus, or nonproductive. For most cases of cough, particularly a productive cough, the use of a cough suppressant is ill advised. However, for a dry, nonproductive cough, it may be appropriate to use a cough suppressant; mild opioids, such as codeine and pholcodine, are widely used.

Side effects of narcotic analgesics

Significant differences exist in the extent and severity of side effects between the mild and the more potent examples of this class of drugs. Narcotic analgesics are powerful drugs that produce a significant number of side effects, the most common of which include the following:

- Nausea, vomiting, and constipation
- Sweating
- Mental confusion and drowsiness
- Enhanced libido, but depressed sexual drive and performance

More serious side effects are experienced if opioids are taken in overdose. These may affect the cardiovascular, respiratory, and central nervous systems.

Narcotics have achieved notoriety due to their propensity toward tolerance and psychic and physical dependence, when used regularly. Tolerance is the need for an increased dose of the drug to produce the same pharmacological effect. Psychic dependence is characterised by the continued desire or craving for a substance. Physical dependence is observed when a substance is no longer administered and physical withdrawal symptoms are experienced.

Dependence is a compulsion to take a substance regularly, which may lead to impairment of physical, mental, and behavioural actions. The user is compelled to take the drug in order to feel good and to avoid withdrawal symptoms.

Opioid dependence is common, particularly if the drug is taken for long periods of time. Users become tolerant to the pleasurable effects, which leads to the use of increased doses in order to regain the pleasurable effects. Opioid withdrawal syndrome, sometimes referred to as going 'cold turkey,' results in serious adverse effects. Methadone is frequently prescribed to substitute for opioids during withdrawal.

It is for these reasons that the possession and use of the more potent narcotics are controlled by legislation in most countries.

14.4. The history of narcotics in sport

Classification of narcotics on prohibited lists

Narcotic analgesics were one of the four classes of drugs listed on the first International Olympic Committee (IOC) Prohibited List, published in 1967 (see Chapter 2). The mild narcotic analgesic, codeine, was removed from the IOC Prohibited List in 1993 following a number of cases in which athletes tested positive for this drug, having purportedly taken the drug inadvertently through over-the-counter medication.

The first Prohibited List drawn up by the World Anti-Doping Agency (WADA), in 2004, designated narcotics as prohibited only within competition.

Prevalence of narcotics use in sport

There have been relatively few cases of adverse analytical findings for narcotics reported by WADA-accredited laboratories. However, the numbers reported annually have been consistent (Table 14.1). The figures include cases where Therapeutic Use Exemption may have applied.

Cases involving narcotics

Some cases relate to serial use of narcotics by athletes within teams.

Table 14.1 WADA statistics for the number of adverse analytical findings for substances classified as narcotics (2004–2012)

	2004	2005	2006	2007	2008	2009	2010	2011	2012
Morphine	10	15	11	19	21	17	6	11	14
Methadone	2	1	3	1	2	1	2	6	1
Dextromoramide	1	–	–	–	–	–	–	–	–
Hydromorphone	1	1	1	1	2	1	2	1	–
Oxycodone	1	–	–	–	1	4	3	2	6
Pethidine	–	–	1	–	1	–	–	–	–
Heroin	–	–	–	–	1	–	–	–	–
Buprenorphine	–	–	–	–	–	1	2	–	–
Hydrocodone	–	–	–	–	–	–	1	–	–
Pentazocine	–	–	–	–	–	–	1	–	–
Oxymorphone	–	–	–	–	–	–	1	–	–
Diamorphine	–	–	–	–	–	–	1	–	–
Fentanyl	–	–	–	–	–	–	1	–	5
Total	15	17	16	21	28	24	20	20	26

Results on narcotics include adverse findings for which the athlete may have been granted a Therapeutic Use Exemption under WADA regulations.

Cycling has been a sport in which narcotic abuse cases have occurred in recent years. To be successful in long-distance cycling races, it is necessary for the cyclist to be able to overcome significant pain barriers. A mixture of drugs, including a narcotic analgesic, such as heroin, and stimulants, such as amphetamines and cocaine, was nicknamed the 'Belgian Mix' or *Pot Belge*. Its use has certainly not been limited to cyclists in Belgium, where cycling is a very popular sport, but this country may well have been its original source.

Festina Affair 1998

In the 1998 Tour de France, the Festina team was suspended when its physiotherapist, Willy Voet, was found to have a large number of drugs, including narcotics, in his possession.

Cahors Affair 2006

Perhaps the most significant case involving the use of narcotics in cycling was the infamous Cahors Affair. Emanating from cases in the year 2004, the trial opened in 2005 and culminated in 2006 with twenty-three convictions relating to the illicit use of performance-enhancing drugs, including *Pot Belge*. These convictions included some custodial sentences. Those testifying and those mentioned in testimonies included the top athletes in European cycling. The former French professional cyclist, Laurent Roux, intimated that some teams spent more on 'doctors' than on riders.

Other cases are attributable to use by individual athletes.

Christophe Brandt 2004

The Belgian cyclist Christophe Brandt tested positive for methadone in the 2004 Tour de France. Methadone is a drug that shares many of the properties of morphine; however, it is principally used as a heroin substitute for heroin addicts in some countries.

Endurance events, other than cycling, have also had cases involving narcotic usage.

Ambesse Tolossa 2007

The Ethiopian runner Ambesse Tolossa, who had already experienced success in other marathon events (San Diego and Tokyo), was the winner of the December 2007 Honolulu race. He was subsequently disqualified because of a positive test for morphine, and his prize money of $40,000 was withheld. Despite Tolossa's insistence that he had no idea how the drug came to be in his body, because of the strict liability policy associated with Olympic events, he also received a 2-year ban.

As a measure of the seriousness with which governing bodies take illegal drug abuse, one only has to consider the case of British runner Kate Reed.

Kate Reed 2008

Kate Reed, who was part of the 2008 Beijing Olympics team, had been suffering from an injury to her leg, and she had apparently joked with teammates about taking morphine for the pain. Shortly afterwards, her room was searched for drugs by British Olympic Association officials. None were found and she duly passed a doping test.

14.5. The action and use of narcotics in sport

Inflammation is a key response to sports injuries, a component of which is pain. Pain is an important, protective cue to the individual that all is not well. It is a stimulus that should promote rest – an important adjunct to recovery. It is also associated with a learning process that encourages the individual to avoid a repetition of the incident. Pain is also unpleasant and, at a moderate to severe level, frequently requires alleviation.

Because the pain associated with a sports injury will inevitably be associated with a traumatic inflammatory reaction, there is a strong case for using anti-inflammatory drugs, which will serve to reduce the overall scale of the body's reaction to trauma as well as reduce the level of pain. In some circumstances, however, the level of pain associated with a serious injury will require the use of more powerful analgesic drugs, such as narcotic analgesic drugs (possibly in association with anti-inflammatory drugs).

Given that one of the barriers to optimal performance is pain, there has been much speculation over many years as to whether powerful analgesic drugs could raise levels of performance. There is no convincing evidence that narcotics can provide such an enhancement, but they are nevertheless banned substances in competition. The therapeutic use of narcotic analgesics is permissible outside of competition periods.

Equestrian sport

The abuse of narcotics is not restricted to humans. Twenty British-owned or -trained racehorses tested positive for morphine. The most celebrated horse involved in this scandal was Be My Royal, winner of the 2002 Hennessy Cognac Gold Cup at Newbury. Despite appeals by the trainer, Willie Mullins, the horse was disqualified from the race. It was claimed that the horse was fed with contaminated feed.

14.6. Narcotics and the WADA prohibited list

The current WADA regulations regarding narcotics are shown in Table 14.2. With respect to morphine, WADA-accredited laboratories declare a test result as an adverse analytical finding if the urinary concentration of morphine exceeds 1 µg/ml (WADA 2013). This limit is used because morphine is one of the metabolites of codeine, a narcotic that is permitted in sport.

Monitoring programme

The World Anti-Doping Code states that a monitoring programme should be established regarding substances that are not on the Prohibited List but that WADA wishes to monitor to detect patterns of misuse in sport. The first monitoring programme, in January 2004, included a number of stimulants, principally available over-the-counter, which were removed from the Prohibited List. The programme also listed narcotics, particularly related to in-competition morphine/codeine ratios in order to monitor the use of these narcotics by athletes. In 2012, the narcotics hydrocodone and tramadol were added to the monitoring programme, with tapentadol being added in 2013 and mitragynine in 2014.

Therapeutic use exemptions

Narcotics are only prohibited in competition, not training. Detailed background information, including medical records, is required. These applications are considered by an independent panel of three medical experts.

Table 14.2 WADA 2014 regulations with respect to narcotics

The following are prohibited:

Buprenorphine, dextromoramide, diamorphine (heroin), fentanyl and its derivatives, hydromorphone, methadone, morphine, oxycodone, oxymorphone, pentazocine, and pethidine

Source: World Anti-Doping Agency. (2014). The 2014 Prohibited List international standard. Available online at https://elb.wada-ama.org/en/what-we-do/prohibited-list (accessed 5 September 2014).

Recreational use of narcotics

As previously discussed, narcotics are a class of drugs that are misused recreationally. Although drug abuse in society is increasing, it is drugs other than narcotics that are mainly implicated. However, athletes who indulge in recreational drug use risk an adverse analytical finding for narcotics, as well as for other prohibited drugs, such as amphetamines, cocaine, and cannabinoids.

14.7. Summary

- Narcotics are a group of drugs originally derived from the opium poppy, the main active constituent of which is morphine.
- Narcotics possess significant analgesic activity. For this reason, they are used both clinically and as a performance aid in sport.
- These drugs exhibit serious side effects, including the onset of dependence, which may lead to addiction.
- The annual number of adverse analytical findings for narcotics is low. However, narcotics remain a potent class of pharmacological agents with a potential for abuse in sport.

14.8. References

Kosterlitz, H. W., and Hughes, J. (1977). Peptides with morphine-like action in the brain. *British Journal of Psychiatry* 130(3):298–304.

Simantov, R., and Snyder, S. H. (1976) Morphine-like peptides in mammalian brain: Isolation, structure elucidation, and interactions with the opiate receptor. *Proceedings of the National Academy of Sciences USA* 73(7):2515–2519.

World Anti-Doping Agency. (2013). Decision limits for the confirmatory quantification of threshold substances. Available online at https://www.wada-ama.org/en/resources/science-medicine/td2013-dl-20#.VA-IUsstDX4 (accessed 9 September 2014).

Chapter 15

Cannabinoids

David R. Mottram

15.1. Introduction

Cannabinoids are derived from cannabis, which is commonly taken as a recreational drug. Although the pharmacological effects of cannabinoids are more likely to produce performance deterioration rather than enhancement, cannabinoids are one of the most frequently detected classes of drugs during doping control tests through World Anti-Doping Agency (WADA) laboratories. It has been suggested by some that cannabinoids should be removed from the WADA Prohibited List. These issues will be explored within this chapter.

15.2. What are cannabinoids?

Source of cannabinoids

Cannabinoids are defined, chemically, as aryl-substituted meroterpenes. They are derived principally from the plant *Cannabis sativa*. This plant contains more than 400 chemical constituents. Of these constituents, more than sixty are chemically classed as cannabinoids. The most potent of these cannabinoids, which produces psychoactive effects, is Δ^9-tetrahydrocannabinol (Δ^9-THC). Other plant cannabinoids include cannabinol and cannabidiol that, along with other cannabinoids, produce complex pharmacological actions and interactions when herbal cannabis is smoked (Ashton 2001).

The Δ^9-THC content varies to a great extent depending on the source of the plant and how the drug is taken (Ashton 2001). New varieties of cannabis plants have been bred in recent years, leading to more potent products than those that were available in the 1960s and 1970s (Ashton 1999).

The cannabis plant, when used for recreational purposes, is processed in various ways in order to derive the effects of the active constituents. The two most common are cannabis resin (hashish) and marijuana, which is normally associated with the dried and ground leaves, flower, and other parts of the plant prepared for smoking (Campos *et al.* 2003). When inhaled, in addition to the cannabinoids, the smoke from cannabis contains many of the constituents of tobacco smoke (Ashton 1999).

Tetrahydrocannabinol-like derivatives, such as dronabinol and nabilone, have been synthesised and are prescribed in some countries to treat weight loss, nausea, and vomiting associated with cancer therapy (Campos *et al.* 2003).

Mode of action of cannabinoids

Specific receptors for cannabinoids have been identified in humans. These are termed CB_1 receptors, which are located in the plasma membrane of nerve endings in the brain.

Stimulation of these receptors inhibits transmitter release, particularly acetylcholine, within the hippocampus (the area of the brain responsible for learning and memory) and noradrenaline in the cerebral cortex and cerebellum (responsible for alertness and motor coordination; Pertwee 1997). They are amongst the most numerous receptors in the brain. The second type of receptor, termed CB_2, is mainly found peripherally, associated with the immune system.

The discovery of cannabinoid receptors led to a search for endogenous mediators, of which a number have been identified. The two well-established endocannabinoids are anandamide and 2-arachidonoyl glycerol (Porter and Felder 2001). Anandamide has a high affinity for CB_1 receptors and has most of the actions of Δ^9-THC (Ashton 2001).

The effects of cannabinoids are perceived within minutes when cannabis is smoked. Oral cannabis results in absorption of approximately 25–30 per cent of the amount of cannabinoids obtained by smoking; the onset of effects is around 30 minutes to 2 hours, although the duration of action may be more prolonged by the oral route (Maykut 1985). Following absorption, cannabinoids are rapidly and widely distributed throughout the body. They tend to accumulate in fatty tissue, from where they are slowly released over extended periods of time. Complete elimination from the body may take as long as 30 days (Huestis *et al.* 1995), which may have consequences with respect to dope testing. Another reason for the extended period of elimination is that the metabolites are only partially excreted in the urine (approximately 25 per cent); most (65 per cent) is excreted into the gastrointestinal tract, from where they are reabsorbed into the body – a process that continues over a considerable period of time (Ashton 2001).

Effects and side effects of cannabinoids

It is difficult to distinguish between the effects and side effects of cannabinoids. The desired effect in one individual under one set of circumstances may be perceived as an undesired effect by another person under different conditions.

Cannabinoids produce both physical and psychological effects, the extent of which will vary depending on patterns of use. Therefore, isolated or infrequent use can lead to mild intoxication, drowsiness and sedation, slower reaction times, and memory deficiency. Regular consumption can lead to social detachment and psychological dependence (Saugy *et al.* 2006).

Cannabinoids can affect almost any system in the body and combine many of the properties of alcohol, tranquillisers, opiates, and hallucinogens. They are therefore anxiolytic, sedative, analgesic, and psychedelic in their action (Ashton 2001).

The main central effects of cannabinoids are impairment of short-term memory, learning tasks, and motor coordination along with catalepsy, hypothermia, analgesia, an increase in appetite, and an anti-emetic action. The main peripheral effects are tachycardia, bronchodilation, vasodilation, and a reduction of intraocular pressure (Rang *et al.* 2007). Users of cannabis develop a mild form of tolerance and dependence to the drug.

The incidence of serious, acute toxic side effects due to cannabinoids is low, and no deaths directly attributable to acute cannabis use have been reported (Ashton 1999). However, Ashton (1999, 2001) reviewed a number of significant adverse effects of cannabinoids on the cardiovascular and respiratory systems as well as on the central nervous system.

Cannabis use in society

There is no doubt that cannabis use as a recreational drug in society is widespread, with figures up to 16 per cent being quoted for use by young adults in Europe and the United States (Saugy *et al.* 2006). Even higher figures for prevalence have been reported in a review by Ashton (2001). It is not surprising, therefore, that a similar trend has happened in sport (Mottram 1999). Cannabinoids are amongst the most frequently detected substances, according to the annual statistics from WADA-accredited laboratories.

Apart from their recreational use, cannabinoids are increasingly being used therapeutically to treat pain, particularly for palliative care (Peat 2010), chemotherapy-induced nausea and vomiting (Delmás 2010), and spasticity in multiple sclerosis (Rog 2010).

15.3. History of cannabis in sport

Addition to the Prohibited List

The International Olympic Committee (IOC) first included cannabis on its list of prohibited substances in 1989. At that time, the decision was left to the governing international sports federation (ISF) as to whether cannabinoids were prohibited in their respective disciplines and whether anti-doping tests for cannabinoids should be conducted. This led to confusion within sport and in the minds of athletes, as exemplified in the case studies presented in the next section. A study by Venema et al. (1999) illustrated the inconsistency, which persisted for many years, in the attitude of ISFs with respect to whether they considered cannabis to be performance enhancing or not.

In 2004, WADA placed cannabinoids on their Prohibited List for all athletes in all sports, within competition. Whether that decision was rational remains open to debate.

Case studies relating to cannabinoids

A number of high-profile case studies have been reported in which cannabinoids have been involved.

Ross Ribagliati (1998)

Ross Ribagliati, a Canadian snowboarder, won the inaugural men's giant slalom event at the 1998 Winter Olympic Games in Nagano. Immediately after the event, he tested positive for cannabinoids and was stripped of his gold medal. He claimed that he had not taken marijuana himself but that he was a victim of passive smoking (Hilderbrand 2011). Regardless of the veracity of this claim, he had his medal reinstated 3 days later. Although the IOC had marijuana on its Prohibited List, Rebagliati's governing body, the International Ski Federation, did not prohibit the use of the drug at that time. This landmark case further highlighted the inconsistency in the application of rules between sporting organisations, which eventually led to harmonization through the establishment of the World Anti-Doping Agency.

Despite the introduction of a harmonised approach to the application of rules for doping violations, cases involving cannabinoids have been treated very differently.

Tomas Enge (2002)

In August 2002, the Czech motor racing driver Tomas Enge tested positive for cannabinoids after a Formula 3000 race in Hungary. He was conditionally suspended from racing for 12 months by his governing body, the International Automobile Federation (Campos et al. 2003).

> ### Michael Phelps (2009)
>
> A photograph of Michael Phelps, a holder of fourteen Olympic Gold Medals, smoking marijuana at a party in South Carolina was published by a British newspaper in January 2009. Although this incident was not the subject of a dope test violation, USA Swimming decided to suspend Michael Phelps for 3 months under its code of conduct.

A case involving cannabinoids was reported at the London 2012 Olympic Games.

> ### Nicholas Delpopolo (2012)
>
> At the London 2012 Olympic games, Nicholas Delpopolo, an American judoka, was disqualified by the IOC after metabolites of cannabis were identified in a urine sample. The athlete insisted that it was the result of eating food containing the banned substance; however, this was not deemed a sufficient defence. It should be noted that the period designated as 'in-competition' for the Olympic Games begins from the time when the Games Athlete Village opens and applies to anywhere that the athlete may be training.

15.4. Cannabinoids in sport

The use of cannabinoids within sport

Few studies have been undertaken relating to the use of cannabinoids in athletes. A study by Lorente *et al*. (2005), involving French university sports students, suggested that approximately 12 per cent of students had used cannabis in an attempt to enhance performance. The authors noted that using cannabis to enhance performance in a recreational manner can lead to its use in an attempt to enhance sporting performance. These authors also showed that cannabis use to enhance sport performance was positively related to the level of competition and to particular sports, such as 'sliding sports' (e.g. skiing, snowboarding, surfing, windsurfing, sailing). Another study on college student athletes reported that 28.4 per cent of US National Collegiate Athletic Association students used marijuana (Green *et al*. 2001).

Results from an analysis of elite athletes tested at the Italian Anti-Doping Laboratory between 2000 and 2009 showed that, among positive results, there was a high prevalence of stimulants and drugs of abuse, of which cannabis was the most frequently found (Rossi and Botrè 2011).

Are cannabinoids performance enhancing?

The balance of evidence suggests that cannabinoids, in most sports, are ergolytic rather than ergogenic (Eichner 1993). Recreationally, cannabis use produces a feeling of euphoria and reduces anxiety. These properties may be beneficial in alleviating the stress induced by competition, either pre- or post-event. However, cannabis smoking impairs cognition and psychomotor and exercise performance (Saugy *et al*. 2006). When compared with control subjects, marijuana was shown to reduce maximal exercise performance (Renaud and Cornier 1986).

Adverse effects of cannabinoids in sport

The adverse effects of cannabinoids on physical and psychological function mean that cannabis consumption can be dangerous in sports that rely on clear thinking, quick reactions, and split-second timing (Campos *et al.* 2003). Particular adverse effects include somnolence, dizziness, euphoria, and feelings of paranoia. Anxiety and tachycardia may also occur. All these effects are incompatible with most athletic endeavours (Campos *et al.* 2003).

Hilderbrand (2011) observed that, whilst impairment of response or inappropriate decision making as a result of cannabis use may be compensated by individuals, this does not apply to elite sport. In competitive sport, the athlete cannot afford compensating actions.

The consequences of cannabinoid use for other competitors

Does cannabinoid use pose a threat to fellow competitors? This probably depends on the sport. Menetrey *et al.* (2005) assessed driving capability under the influence of cannabinoids. The authors concluded that cannabinoids have a negative effect that would impair alertness and reflexes in motor sports, leading to danger for both users and their fellow competitors.

15.5. Cannabinoids and the WADA Prohibited List

WADA regulations with respect to cannabinoids

Cannabinoids are prohibited in all sports, but an adverse analytical finding is only reported if a positive urine sample is detected in competition. Furthermore, cannabinoids are classed as Specified Substances, which allows for more flexible sanctions to be applied in the case of an adverse finding. WADA laboratories undertake urine analysis, using gas chromatography/mass spectrometry, of 11-nor-delta 9-tetrahydrocannabinol-9-carboxylic acid (THC-COOH), the principal metabolite of Δ^9-THC, in either its free or conjugated form. If the sum of the concentration of free and conjugated THC-COOH is greater than 15 ng/ml, an adverse analytical finding is reported by the laboratory (WADA 2013).

In 2010, WADA first included synthetic cannabinoids on the Prohibited List. In 2011, marijuana-like substances (cannabimimetics) were included. A review of these cannabimimetics was provided by Hilderbrand (2011). Table 15.1 shows the current (2014) WADA regulations regarding cannabinoids.

Prevalence of adverse findings for cannabinoids

Statistics from WADA-accredited laboratories, between 2006 and 2012, show that cannabinoids constitute between 7.8 per cent and 12.8 per cent of all adverse analytical findings.

Table 15.1 WADA 2014 regulations with respect to cannabinoids

Natural (e.g. cannabis, hashish, marijuana) or synthetic delta 9-tetrahydrocannabinol (THC) and cannabimimetics (e.g. 'Spice,' JWH018, JWH073, HU-210) are prohibited.

Source: World Anti-Doping Agency. (2014). The 2014 Prohibited List international standard. Available online at https://elb.wada-ama.org/en/what-we-do/prohibited-list (accessed 5 September 2014).

These percentages place cannabinoids as the third most reported prohibited substance in each of these years, except 2008 and 2009 when they were the second most reported following anabolic agents. It is worth noting that cannabinoids are only tested in competition; therefore, any positive results found in urine samples taken out of competition are not reported by the laboratory. The extent of cannabis use by athletes could therefore be significantly higher than that indicated by the WADA statistics.

Passive ingestion of cannabinoids

The WADA Anti-Doping Code states that urinary levels of THC-COOH must exceed a threshold of 15 ng/ml in order to trigger an adverse analytical finding. This has been established in part to distinguish between active consumers of cannabinoids and those athletes who may have been exposed, passively, to cannabis smoke (Campos *et al.* 2003).

Several studies have been conducted to determine the likelihood of passive inhalation of cannabinoids sufficient to trigger an adverse analytical finding (Yonamine *et al.* 2004). The extent of passive inhalation depends on factors such as the size of the room and the effectiveness of the ventilation within the room, as well as the amount of marijuana being smoked and the concentration of Δ^9-THC within the marijuana. The conclusion reached was that an individual could produce urinary levels of THC-COOH sufficient to exceed the 15 ng/ml threshold only after 'extremely severe' conditions of passive exposure to marijuana smoke (Yonamine *et al.* 2004; Anderson 2011).

Hilderbrand (2011) suggests that the concept of 'strict liability' applies in sport, and one can safely say that the presence of THC-COOH in urine at any level approaching the 15-ng/ml confirmation threshold could not occur without the knowledge of the athlete.

The threshold limit also reduces the chance of an adverse test result after the consumption of food products that may contain traces of cannabinoids (Saugy *et al.* 2006). In this context, there has been an increase in the sale of hemp-containing products, such as cakes, cookies, and brownies, or of hemp seed oil products (Yonamine *et al.* 2004). However, research into the chances of exceeding urinary threshold levels when consuming such products reveals very variable and inconsistent results (Cone *et al.* 1988; Bosy and Cole 2000; Leson *et al.* 2000).

Should cannabinoids be on the WADA Prohibited List?

There are arguments for and against removing cannabinoids from the WADA Prohibited List. Arguments for removing cannabinoids from the Prohibited List include the fact that, in most countries, the possession and consumption of cannabis products are illegal. Is it therefore appropriate for WADA to impose a further level of legislation? Of course, this argument is flawed because the laws relating to cannabis use are not universally in place or rigorously applied.

Other arguments for removing cannabinoids relate to the possibility of passive consumption, although this is countered by the presence of a threshold level for THC-COOH and the classification of cannabinoids as specified substances, which allows athletes to prove that they had not intended to use cannabinoids for performance-enhancing purposes. It should be noted, however, that the elimination of THC-COOH from the body is a slow and individually variable process, making it difficult to prove intent or otherwise (Saugy *et al.* 2006).

Huestis *et al.* (2011) reviewed the rationale for retaining cannabinoids on the WADA Prohibited List by relating the pharmacological and sociological implications of cannabinoid use to the three criteria specified in Section 4 of the World Anti-Doping Code to determine whether substances should be placed on the Prohibited List. The code specifies that only two of the three criteria need to be fulfilled. The authors argue that cannabinoids have the potential for health risks, not only for the athlete but also for their fellow competitors as a result of impaired decision making and the probability of accidents. Regarding the second criterion, cannabinoids can be performance enhancing, albeit only for some athletes in certain sport disciplines. Thirdly, considering the ethical and societal aspects of using a recreational drug, cannabinoids contravene the spirit of sport. Consequently, Huestis *et al.* concluded that the WADA decision to retain cannabinoids on the Prohibited List is correct, a view supported by Bergamaschi and Crippa (2013).

The international anti-doping community generally considers athletes to be portrayed as role models in society, which is intrinsically incompatible with the use of cannabinoids. It can therefore be argued that cannabinoids should be banned by WADA both within competition, as at present, but also out of competition.

15.6. Summary

- Cannabinoids produce a wide range of effects in the body, most of which would not be classified as performance enhancing.
- Despite this, cannabinoids are one of the most frequently detected prohibited classes of substances in athletes, according to WADA laboratory statistics.
- This high frequency of detection in athletes probably reflects their use as recreational drugs.
- Although it has been argued that cannabinoids should be removed from the WADA Prohibited List, balance of opinion is that they should remain.

15.7. References

Anderson, J. M. (2011). Evaluating the athlete's claim of an unintentional positive drug test. *Current Sports Medicine Reports* 10(4):191–196.

Ashton, C. H. (1999). Adverse effects of cannabis and cannabinoids. *British Journal of Anaesthesia* 83(4):637–649.

Ashton, C. H. (2001). Pharmacology and effects of cannabis: A brief review. *British Journal of Psychiatry* 178: 101–106.

Bergamaschi, M. M., and Crippa, J. A. S. (2013). Why should cannabis be considered doping in sports? *Frontiers in Psychiatry* 4:1–2.

Bosy, T. Z., and Cole, K. A. (2000). Consumption and quantititation of Δ^9-tetrahydrocannabinol in commercially available hemp seed oil products. *Journal of Analytical Toxicology* 24(7):562–566.

Campos, D. R., Yonamine, M., and de Moraes Moreau, R. L. (2003). Marijuana as doping in sports. *Sports Medicine* 33(6):395–399.

Cone, E. J., Johnson, R. E., Paul, B. D., *et al.* (1988). Marijuana-laced brownies: Behavioural effects, physiologic effects and urinalysis in humans following ingestion. *Journal of Analytical Toxicology* 12(4):169–175.

Delmás, M. D. (2010). Preliminary efficacy and safety of an oromucosal standardized cannabis extract in chemotherapy-induced nausea and vomiting. *British Journal of Clinical Pharmacology* 70(5): 656–663.

Eichner, E. R. (1993). Ergolytic drugs in medicine and sport. *American Journal of Medicine* 94(2):205–211.

Green, G. A., Uryasz, F. D., Petr, T. A., *et al.* (2001). NCAA study of substance use and abuse habits of college student-athletes. *Clinical Journal of Sports Medicine* 11(1):51–56.

Hilderbrand, R. L. (2011). High performance sport, marijuana and cannabimimetics. *Journal of Analytical Toxicology* 35(9):624–637.

Huestis, M. A., Mazzoni, I., and Rabin, O. (2011). Cannabis in sport. Anti-doping perspective. *Sports Medicine* 41(11):949–966.

Huestis, M. A., Mitchell, J. M., and Cone, E. J. (1995). Detection times of marijuana metabolites in urine by immunoassay and GC-MS. *Journal of Analytical Toxicology* 19(6):443–449.

Leson, G., Pless, P., Grotenhermen, F., *et al.* (2000). Evaluating the impact of hemp food consumption on workplace drug tests. *Journal of Analytical Toxicology* 25(8):691–698.

Lorente, F. O., Peretti-Watel, P., and Grelot, L. (2005). Cannabis use to enhance sportive and non-sportive performances among French sport students. *Addictive Behaviours* 30(7):1382–1391.

Maykut, M. O. (1985). Health consequences of acute and chronic marijuana use. *Progress in Neuropsychopharmacology and Biological Psychiatry* 9(3):209–238.

Menetrey, A., Augsburger, M., Favrat, B., *et al.* (2005). Assessment of driving capability through the use of clinical and psychomotor tests in relation to blood cannabinoids levels following oral administration of 20mg dronabinol or of a cannabis decoction made with 20 or 60mg delta 9-THC. *Journal of Analytical Toxicology* 29(5):327–338.

Mottram, D. R. (1999). Banned drugs in sport: Does the International Olympic Committee (IOC) list need updating? *Sports Medicine* 27(1):1–10.

Peat, S. (2010). Using cannabinoids in pain and palliative care. *International Journal of Palliative Nursing* 16(10):481–485.

Pertwee, R. G. (1997). Pharmacology of cannabinoid CB1 and CB2 receptors. *Pharmacological Therapeutics* 74(2):129 180.

Porter, A. C., and Felder, C. C. (2001). The endocannabinoid nervous system: Unique opportunities for therapeutic intervention. *Pharmacological Therapeutics* 90(1):45–60.

Rang, H. P., Dale, M. M., Ritter, J. M., *et al.* (2007). Cannabinoids. In H. P. Rang, J. M. Ritter, R. J. Fowler, and G. Henderson (Eds.), *Rang and Dale's Pharmacology* (6th ed., pp. 248–255). London, UK: Churchill Livingstone.

Renaud, A. M., and Cornier, Y. (1986). Acute effects of marijuana smoking on maximal exercise performance. *Medicine and Science in Sports and Exercise* 18(6):685–689.

Rog, D. J. (2010). Cannabis-based medicines in multiple sclerosis: A review of clinical studies. *Immunobiology* 215(8):658–672.

Rossi, S. S., and Botrè, F. (2011). Prevalence of illicit drug use among the Italian athlete population with special attention on drugs of abuse: A 10-year review. *Journal of Sports Sciences* 29(5):471–476.

Saugy, M., Avois, L., Saudan, C., *et al.* (2006). Cannabis and sport. *British Journal of Sports Medicine* 40(Suppl 1):i13–i15.

Venema, H., de Boer, D., Horta, L., *et al.* (1999). Different anti-doping policies of International Sport Federations towards the ban of the use of cannabis. In *Fifth World Congress of Sports Sciences: Book of Abstracts* (p. 218). Canberra, Australia: Sports Medicine Australia.

World Anti-Doping Agency. (2013). International standard for laboratories. Available online at https://www.wada-ama.org/en/resources/international-standards/international-standard-for-laboratories-isl#.VA-J9cstDX4 (accessed 9 September 2014).

Yonamine, M., Garcia, P. R., and de Moraes Moreau, R. L. (2004). Non-intentional doping in sports. *Sports Medicine* 34(11):697–704.

Chapter 16

Glucocorticosteroids

Nick Wojek

16.1. Introduction

Glucocorticosteroids, or glucocorticoids as they are often known, are adrenal steroid hormones with diverse physiological effects that can be anti-inflammatory, immunosuppressive, and metabolic in nature. They also affect central nervous system function and the activity of other endogenous hormones. Glucocorticoids are regulated by a negative feedback loop involving the hypothalamic-pituitary-adrenal (HPA) axis (Figure 16.1). Cortisol is the main hormone secreted from the adrenal cortex following the activation of the HPA axis; it is released during stressful situations, such as when encountering emotional stress, infection, trauma, and exercise. In addition to responding to stress stimuli, endogenous cortisol is released in an hourly pulsatile manner; it exhibits a circadian rhythm with peak concentrations occurring at the onset of the daily activity period (Young *et al.* 2004; Son *et al.* 2011).

Glucocorticoids exert their multiple actions through genomic and nongenomic mechanisms. In genomic-mediated mechanisms, glucocorticoids bind primarily to intracellular glucocorticoid receptors (GR), which translocate into the cell nucleus as a result of a conformational change in the GR. In the nucleus, this GR-glucocorticoid complex regulates gene transcription and consequently protein synthesis by either binding to glucocorticoid response elements in the promoter region of genes or by inhibiting the activity of other transcription factors, such as activator protein-1 and nuclear factor-κB (Czock *et al.* 2005; Stahn *et al.* 2007). In nongenomic mediated mechanisms, glucocorticoids exert rapid actions that cannot be explained by genomic mechanisms. Nongenomic modes of action may involve the binding of glucocorticoids with cell membrane-bound GRs, binding with intracellular GRs, or physiochemical interactions with cell membranes (Czock *et al.* 2005; Stahn *et al.* 2007).

The two isoforms of the intracellular GR, GR-alpha (α) and GR-beta (β), are widely expressed in almost all tissues, explaining why glucocorticoids have such diverse physiological effects. However, glucocorticoids only bind with GR-α, which is expressed at much higher levels than GR-β in most tissues (Oakley *et al.* 1997; Pujols *et al.* 2002). Instead, GR-β is thought to affect GR-α gene transcription by acting as a dominant negative inhibitor of GR-α signalling (Oakley *et al.* 1996; Charmandari *et al.* 2005) or by independently regulating genes not controlled by GR-α (Lewis-Truffin *et al.* 2007; Kino *et al.* 2009).

16.2. Clinical uses and adverse effects of glucocorticosteroids

Synthetic glucocorticoids are administered by systemic (i.e. oral, rectal, intravenous, intramuscular) or local routes (e.g. inhalation, intranasal, intraarticular, peritendinous, topical).

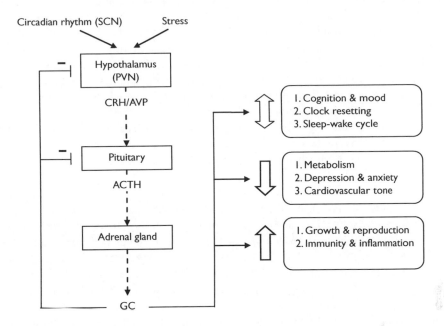

Figure 16.1 Simplified scheme of the synthesis, secretion, and actions of glucocorticoids (adapted from Son *et al.*, 2011).

ACTH, adrenocorticotropic hormone; AVP, arginine vasopressin; CRH, corticotropin-releasing hormone; GC, glucocorticoid; PVN, paraventricular nucleus; SCN, suprachiasmatic nucleus.

They are often used in a multitude of clinical applications, despite not having a reparative function to resolve injury or illness.

Systemic glucocorticoids are used for their potent anti-inflammatory and immunosuppressive effects in the treatment of allergies (e.g. urticaria), gastrointestinal disorders (e.g. inflammatory bowel disease), autoimmune diseases (e.g. systemic lupus erythematosus), respiratory diseases (e.g. exacerbation of asthma), rheumatologic diseases (e.g. arthritis), and musculoskeletal injuries (e.g. hamstring injuries) and in emergency medicine (e.g. anaphylactic reactions; Czock *et al.* 2005; Nichols 2005; Dvorak *et al.* 2006). They also possess analgesic properties that alleviate postoperative pain (Romundstad *et al.* 2004; De Oliveira *et al.* 2011). Prednisolone is the most commonly prescribed systemic glucocorticoid in the United Kingdom; other types include dexamethasone, budesonide, methylprednisolone, hydrocortisone, and triamcinolone.

In contrast, local glucocorticoids target specific sites of inflammation in an attempt to reduce the side effects that are often associated with systemic administration. Inhaled forms are considered to be the mainstay of asthma treatment; topically applied forms are routinely used to treat skin conditions such as eczema; and intranasal forms help to reduce nasal inflammation and symptoms associated with allergic rhinitis.

Local glucocorticoids are also frequently administered by intraarticular and peritendinous injections to treat athletic musculoskeletal injuries, such as tendinopathies, soft-tissue injuries, and overuse injuries. It is thought that by reducing inflammation and alleviating pain associated with the injury, glucocorticoid use in turn improves motion and function around the site of injury to hasten an athlete's return to competition. Although there is a rationale for their use in sport, there is little published evidence supporting the benefit of local glucocorticoid use in this way over the risk of complications to health (Harmon and Hawley 2003; Nichols 2005; Dvorak *et al*. 2006). Long-term complications may include tendon rupture, loss of tensile strength in ligaments, and cartilage degeneration (Brukner and Nicol 2004; Nichols 2005).

Systemic glucocorticoids have many other side effects that limit their clinical use, especially when used for long durations. In particular, long-term use may adversely affect bone (osteoporosis, increased bone fracture risk), muscle (wasting, weakness), the skin (thinning, delayed wound healing), the eyes (glaucoma, cataract), the immune system (increased risk of infection), metabolism and the endocrine system (insulin resistance, redistribution of fat), and the central nervous system (disturbances in mood, behaviour, memory, and cognition; Schäcke *et al*. 2002; Buttgereit *et al*. 2005).

The withdrawal of glucocorticoids can also lead to abnormalities in HPA axis function, characterised by a reduction in adrenal cortisol release. Suppression of the HPA axis seems to be temporary because adrenal function returns to normal in most individuals within 14 days after short-term (≤ 7 days) glucocorticoid treatment has ended (Streck and Lockwood 1979; Henzen *et al*. 2000; Jollin *et al*. 2010). However, suppression can occur for much longer if treatment continues for longer than 7 days (Henzen *et al*. 2000). The risk of adrenal insufficiency has also been found to be apparent following one-off intraarticular and epidural injections in elite cyclists (Duclos 2007; Guinot *et al*. 2007).

Abnormalities in HPA axis function arise because glucocorticoids provide negative feedback to the hypothalamus and pituitary glands, attenuating the release of corticotropin-releasing hormone and adrenocorticotropic hormone (ACTH), respectively (Figure 16.1). The reduction in ACTH levels ultimately leads to atrophy of the adrenal cortex and the appearance of secondary adrenal insufficiency when the withdrawal of the glucocorticoid occurs. This effect is evident at rest (Petrides *et al*. 1997; Marquet *et al*. 1999) and occurs during exercise where the normal increase in pituitary release of ACTH and dehydroepiandrosterone is blunted (Arlettaz *et al*. 2006; Collomp *et al*. 2008; Le Panse *et al*. 2009). The effect of adrenal insufficiency on athletic performance is unknown, but atypical forms of adrenal crisis (e.g. hypoglycaemia, sudden exhaustion, feelings of faintness) could possibly explain some of the unusual decreases in performance observed in athletes following glucocorticoid treatment (Duclos 2007).

Mode of action: Anti-inflammatory

The anti-inflammatory effects associated with glucocorticoids are mediated mainly via genomic modes of action, as outlined in the introduction to this chapter. There are two genomic modes of action: transrepression and transactivation.

Glucocorticoids primarily inhibit the synthesis of inflammatory proteins through the suppression of the genes that encode them (transrepression). In the cell nucleus, the interaction of GR-glucocorticoid complexes with transcription factors, such as activator protein-1 and nuclear factor-κB, leads to the inhibition of their transcriptional activity. This inhibition prevents the expression of proinflammatory proteins, such as cytokines (extracellular signalling proteins that induce cellular responses), chemokines (attract inflammatory cells to the site of inflammation), adhesion molecules (bind inflammatory cells to the site of inflammation), and inflammatory enzymes (mediators of the inflammatory response), which are known to be involved in the inflammatory process (Czock *et al*. 2005; Barnes 2006).

Glucocorticoids also switch on genes with anti-inflammatory effects through the binding of GR-glucocorticoid complexes with glucocorticoid response elements (transactivation). This interaction leads to an increase in the transcription of genes coding for anti-inflammatory proteins, such as lipocortin-1 (inhibits the inflammatory enzyme phospholipase A2), interleukin-10 (inhibits the activity of various pro-inflammatory cytokines), and interleukin-1 receptor antagonist (blocks the action of the pro-inflammatory chemokine interleukin-1; Schäcke *et al*. 2002; Czock *et al*. 2005; Barnes 2006). In addition, glucocorticoids increase the transcription of the mitogen-activated kinase phosphatise-1 gene, which inhibits signal transduction of the mitogen-activated protein kinase pathways (Barnes 2006). These pathways would normally activate pro-inflammatory transcription factors, leading to inflammation.

16.3. Uses of glucocorticosteroids in sport

The physiological effects of glucocorticoids suggest that they could enhance performance and therefore appeal to athletes for nontherapeutic reasons. This section outlines why glucocorticoids have the potential to be misused in sport, focussing on their effects on metabolism and the central nervous system. Speculative modes of action are also described.

Central nervous system effects

One-off and short-term ($\leq$14 days) glucocorticoid intake moderately increases vigour and reduces feelings of fatigue at rest in patients (Swinburn *et al*. 1988) and healthy individuals (Plihal *et al*. 1996; Tops *et al*. 2006). There is no research that exists to confirm whether glucocorticoids exert similar ergogenic effects during exercise. However, such an effect seems likely at low to moderate exercise intensities because high serum cortisol levels, induced by a single ACTH injection, delay the onset of fatigue during submaximal but not maximal exercise (Soetens *et al*. 1995; Baume *et al*. 2008), and has a positive influence on mood by increasing vigour following successive days of exercise (Soetens *et al*. 1995).

It is difficult to determine the significance of how these central effects translate into performance gains based on the limited research. Nevertheless, experiencing an increase in vigour and a reduction in the feelings of fatigue, even only at submaximal exercise intensities, may convince athletes of the in-competition benefits of glucocorticoids. These central effects may especially appeal to athletes in sports involving prolonged exertion where exercise is not maximal throughout or in sports where repetition of performance over several successive days is required.

Mode of action: Central nervous system

These central effects are likely to occur through glucocorticoid-induced activation of the mesolimbic dopaminergic transmission pathway – the area of the brain that is associated with reward and desire. It is evident that both acute and short-term glucocorticoid administration stimulates an increase in extracellular dopamine (the neural substrate for reward) in the nucleus accumbens of rats and leads to an increase in wheel-running activity (Piazza *et al*. 1996b; Duclos *et al*. 2009). Glucocorticoid treatment also restores dopamine levels in the nucleus accumbens of adrenalectomised rats, which further demonstrates its stimulatory effect on the mesolimbic dopaminergic pathway (Piazza *et al*. 1996a).

The precise mechanism by which glucocorticoids stimulate increases in extracellular dopamine is unknown. Nevertheless, glucocorticoids are likely to exert their central effects through the inhibition of dopamine reuptake at presynaptic dopaminergic neurons and through inhibiting monoamine oxidase activity to reduce dopamine degradation (Piazza *et al.* 1996b). GRs are likely to be involved in this mechanism because they are largely expressed on dopaminergic neurons that project to the mesolimbic areas of the brain (Härfstrand *et al.* 1986).

Dopamine also inhibits the secretion of prolactin from the anterior pituitary gland. Prolactin is considered to reflect alterations in 5-hydroxytryptamine (serotonin) and dopaminergic activity in the brain and is used as a marker of central fatigue (Davis 1995). Prolactin remains suppressed during submaximal exercise following a short-term course, which may be a contributing factor to delaying the perceived onset of fatigue in time to exhaustion protocols (Arlettaz *et al.* 2007; Le Panse *et al.* 2009).

Metabolic effects

Glucocorticoids play a key role in accelerating carbohydrate, lipid, and protein metabolism (McMahon *et al.* 1988; Del Corral *et al.* 1998). These metabolic effects are apparent during exercise as both glucocorticoid and ACTH administration increase plasma glucose (Soetens *et al.* 1995; Arlettaz *et al.* 2007; Collomp *et al.* 2008), free fatty acid (FFA; Gorostiaga *et al.* 1988; Soetens *et al.* 1995), and amino acid levels (Thomasson *et al.* 2011), increasing the availability of these substrates for energy ahead of glycogen stores. Following endurance exercise, hypercortisolemia may also assist metabolic recuperation as glucocorticoid intake enhances muscle and liver glycogen store content in insulin-resistant rats (Gorostiaga *et al.* 1988; Ruzzin and Jensen 2005); this recovery effect has yet to be studied in humans.

In addition, acute and short-term ($\leq$7 days) glucocorticoid intake seems to increase energy expenditure and shift substrate utilisation from carbohydrates towards lipids at rest (Brillon *et al.* 1995; Qi *et al.* 2004) and during submaximal exercise (Arlettaz *et al.* 2008a). These effects, coupled with the catabolic energy-mobilising effects of high circulating glucocorticoid levels, suggest that glucocorticoid intake may induce weight loss in individuals undertaking high-volume, low-intensity endurance training on calorie-maintained diets. This proposed alteration in body composition may be specific to fat loss because low-intensity exercise training seems to also negate the catabolic effects of glucocorticoids on muscle glycogen and protein in rat and human skeletal muscle (Horber *et al.* 1985; Barel *et al.* 2010).

Mode of action: Substrate utilisation

Glucocorticoids increase the transcription of enzymes involved in gluconeogenesis, lipolysis, and proteolysis through binding to GRs located in the liver, adipose tissue, and muscle. Glucocorticoids exert their metabolic effects through the following actions (Sarpolsky *et al.* 2000; Vegiopoulos and Herzig 2007):

*   They stimulate hepatic gluconeogenesis by increasing the expression of phosphoenol-pyruvate carboxykinase (PEPCK) and glucose-6-phosphatase (G6Pase) enzymes, which are normally rate-limiting steps in the gluconeogenic pathway. This leads to an increase in glucose production from nonhexose substrates, such as amino acids and glycerol.
*   They stimulate lipolysis in peripheral adipose tissue by increasing the expression of hormone-sensitive lipase and decreasing the expression of lipoprotein lipase (a key enzyme in the formation of triglycerides) and PEPCK (a key enzyme in glyceroneogenesis). This leads to the release of FFAs (substrate for β-oxidation) and glycerol (substrate for gluconeogenesis).

- They stimulate proteolysis by inhibiting the protein kinase b (Akt)/mammalian target of rapamycin signalling pathway in muscle. This pathway normally promotes protein synthesis and decreases protein degradation. Glucocorticoids inhibit the transcription of phosphoinositide 3-kinase or AKt, which removes the inhibition of the adenosine triphosphate (ATP)-dependent ubiquitin-proteasome proteolysis pathway, allowing an increase in protein degradation to occur. This increase in proteolysis leads to the mobilisation of amino acids (substrate for gluconeogenesis).

Mode of action: Body composition

An athlete's power-to-weight ratio is an important factor that contributes to success in weight-bearing endurance sports. Anecdotal reports suggest that weight loss in the region of 4–5 kg over a 3–4 week period may occur when combining low-intensity exercise with a short-term (~7 days) course of glucocorticoids administered by intramuscular injection or orally.

Such a dramatic weight loss could be the result of glucocorticoid-induced increases in circulating plasma FFA levels, which are then preferentially used as the predominant fuel source if an athlete trains at a relatively low intensity for long durations. Studies on mitochondrial functioning show that high rates of FFA uptake by skeletal and cardiac muscle activates the nuclear transcription factor peroxisome proliferator-activated receptor alpha (PPAR-α). PPAR-α activation not only increases the expression of fatty acid oxidation enzymes but also upregulates the expression of uncoupling protein-3, peroxisome proliferator-activated receptor γ co-activator 1α, and mitochondria thioesterase-1 (Stavinoha et al. 2004; Murray et al. 2005; Turner et al. 2007; Cole et al. 2011), which are indicators of mitochondrial uncoupling. This combination of increased fatty acid oxidation and mitochondrial uncoupling raises the metabolic rate by decreasing metabolic efficiency (a higher consumption of oxygen to produce the same amount of ATP) in mitochondrial, leading to the observed reduction in adipose tissue. Glucocorticoid administration over 5 days has been shown to decrease the efficiency of oxidative phosphorylation in rat liver mitochondria, supporting the theory of metabolic inefficiency (Roussel et al. 2004).

Summary of studies measuring performance

No consensus exists regarding whether the ergogenic effects of glucocorticoids on metabolism, central nervous system, and body composition outlined in this chapter translate into performance gains. Short-term glucocorticoid use (5–7 days) increases time to exhaustion during cycling at ≤ 75 per cent VO_{2max} (Arlettaz et al. 2008a; Collomp et al. 2008; Le Panse et al. 2009), but not at exercise intensities of >75 per cent VO_{2max} (Marquet et al. 1999). In contrast, acute glucocorticoid use does not improve submaximal cycling or high-intensity intermittent running (Petrides et al. 1997; Arlettaz et al. 2006, 2008b), although acute supratherapeutic doses have yet to be explored at exercise intensities of ≤ 75 per cent VO_{2max}. Acute ACTH administration also fails to improve maximal exercise (Soetens et al. 1995) or time-trial performance (Baume et al. 2008).

These inconsistent findings may be attributable to the dose, duration, or type of glucocorticoid used, as well as the duration, intensity, and type of exercise protocols selected. Performance indicators such as VO_{2max}, maximal heart rate, ventilatory threshold, and maximal blood lactate may be inappropriate to confirm the ergogenic effects of glucocorticoids in comparison to other central and metabolic variables that may indirectly enhance performance. Furthermore, the ergogenic effects of glucocorticoids on prolonged exercise tests lasting 3–4 hours, sport-specific intermittent exercise tests, or one-off sprint tests following a fatiguing protocol are unknown (Duclos 2010). It seems that an ergogenic effect at least occurs at submaximal exercise intensities following a short course of a glucocorticoid.

16.4. Glucocorticosteroids and the WADA Prohibited List

All glucocorticoids are prohibited in-competition when administered by oral, intravenous, intramuscular, or rectal routes, but they are not prohibited out-of-competition (World Anti-Doping Agency [WADA] 2014). This means that athletes should not have a synthetic glucocorticoid or its metabolites present in their urine following an in-competition drug test, even when the administration of a systemic dose has occurred out-of-competition. The only exception to the presence in the urine following an in-competition test is when an athlete has obtained a Therapeutic Use Exemption (TUE) to authorise such use.

All glucocorticoids administered by local injection routes (e.g. epidural, intraarticular, intradermal, periarticular, peritendinous) or by inhalation are permitted at all times, regardless if administered in- or out-of-competition. Topical preparations, when used for auricular, buccal, dermatological, gingival, nasal, ophthalmic, and perianal disorders, are also not prohibited in- or out-of-competition.

The interpretation of analysed urine samples showing the presence of glucocorticoids is complicated by this mix of regulations. As a result, WADA-accredited laboratories are directed by WADA to only report urinary concentrations if detected in-competition above the minimum required performance limit of 30 ng/mL (WADA 2013). This strategy seems to be based on the assumption that a low concentration is more likely to be due to the legitimate therapeutic use of a glucocorticoid by permitted routes rather than the systemic use close to a competition for nontherapeutic reasons.

WADA laboratory data reporting on the adverse analytical findings (AAFs) for 2009, 2010, 2011, and 2012 showed 265, 234, 274, and 365 in-competition instances of the presence of a glucocorticoid, respectively. Of all AAFs reported in these years, glucocorticoid detection represents 5.2 per cent (sixth), 4.2 per cent (fifth), 4.9 per cent (fifth), and 8.1 per cent (fourth), respectively, of the proportion of prohibited substances detected per WADA drug category; this indicates an increase in the proportion of samples that contain a glucocorticoid in comparison to other prohibited drug categories. However, these statistics are likely to include many samples from athletes who have been granted TUEs, so they are not necessarily an accurate reflection of the number of athletes to have received an anti-doping rule violation as a result of glucocorticoid misuse. Indeed, UK TUE data revealed that 60–64 per cent of all TUE approvals in 2010, 2011, and 2012 were for the use of systemic glucocorticoids (UK Anti-Doping, unpublished data).

16.5. Summary

- Glucocorticoids are adrenal steroid hormones with diverse physiological effects that are regulated by a negative feedback loop involving the hypothalamic-pituitary-adrenal axis.
- They are widely used in medicine for their potent anti-inflammatory and immunosuppressive effects.
- The ergogenic effects of glucocorticoids on metabolism and on the central nervous system have been observed during exercise intensities of ≤ 75 per cent VO_{2max} but no higher.

Performance is likely to be indirectly enhanced through glucocorticoid-induced weight loss in sports where power-to-weight ratio is a limiting performance factor.

- Glucocorticoids have deleterious effects that can cause several side effects, thus limiting their clinical use, especially when used for long durations.
- Glucocorticoids exert their multiple actions primarily through genomic mechanisms, in which they bind to intracellular glucocorticoid receptors that regulate the transcription of key proteins that are involved in inflammation, metabolism, and the activation of the central nervous system.
- They are currently only prohibited by WADA in-competition when administered by systemic routes.
- There is an argument that the systemic use of glucocorticoids should be prohibited in- and out-of-competition, especially because short-term systemic use induces weight loss with low-intensity exercise training. Weight loss indirectly enhances performance in weight-bearing endurance sports and weight classification sports where 'making weight' is critical and maintaining power following weight loss is advantageous.

16.6. References

Arlettaz, A., Collomp, K., Portier, H., Lecoq, A.-M., Pelle, A., and De Ceaurriz, J. (2006). Effects of acute prednisolone intake during intense submaximal exercise. *Int J Sports Med* 27(9):673 679.

Arlettaz, A., Collomp, K., Portier, H., Lecoq, A-M., Rieth, N, Le Panse, B., and De Ceaurriz, J. (2008b). Effects of acute prednisolone administration on exercise endurance and metabolism. *Br J Sports Med* 42(4):250–254.

Arlettaz, A., Portier, H., Lecoq, A.-M., Labsy, Z., De Ceaurriz, J., and Collomp, K. (2008a). Effects of acute prednisolone intake on substrate utilization during submaximal exercise. *Int J Sports Med* 29 (1):21–26.

Arlettaz, A., Portier, H., Lecoq, A.-M., Rieth, N., De Ceaurriz, J., and Collomp, K. (2007). Effects of short-term prednisolone intake during submaximal exercise. *Med Sci Sports Exerc* 39 9):1672–1678.

Barel, M., Perez, O. A., Giozzet, V. A., Rafacho, A., Bosqueiro, J. R., and do Amaral, S. L. (2010). Exercise training prevents hyperinsulinemia, muscular glycogen loss and muscle atrophy induced by dexamethasone treatment. *Eur J Appl Physiol* 108(5):999–1007.

Barnes, P. J. (2006). Corticosteroid effects on cell signalling. *Eur Respir J* 27(2):413–426.

Baume, N., Steel, G., Edwards, T., Thorstensen, E., and Miller, B. F. (2008). No variation of physical performance and perceived exertion after adrenal gland stimulation by synthetic ACTH (Synacthen®) in cyclists. *Eur J Appl Physiol* 104(4):589–600.

Brillon, D. J., Zheng, B., Campbell, R. G., and Matthews, D. E. (1995). Effect of cortisol on energy expenditure and amino acid metabolism in humans. *Am J Physiol* 268(3 Pt 1):E501–E513.

Brukner, P., and Nicol, A. (2004). Use of oral corticosteroids in sports medicine. *Curr Sports Med Rep* 3(4):181–183.

Buttgereit, F., Burmester, G.-R., and Lipworth, B. J. (2005). Optimised glucocorticoid therapy: The sharpening of an old spear. *Lancet* 365(9461):801–803.

Charmandari, E., Chrousos, G. P., Ichijo, T., Bhattacharyya, N., Vottero, A., Souvatzoglou, E., and Kino, T. (2005). The human glucocorticoid receptor (hGR) β isoforms suppresses the transcriptional activity of hGRα by interfering with formation of active coactivator complexes. *Mol Endocrinol* 19(1):52–64.

Cole, M. A., Murray, A. J., Cochlin, L. E., Heather, L. C., McAleese, S., *et al.* (2011). A high fat diet increases mitochondrial fatty acid oxidation and uncoupling to decrease efficiency in rat heart. *Basic Res Cardiol* 106(3):447–457.

Collomp, K., Arlettaz, A., Portier, H., Lecoq, A.-M., Le Panse, B., Rieth, N., and De Ceaurriz, J. (2008). Short-term glucocorticoid intake combined with intense training on performance and hormonal responses. *Br J Sports Med* 42(12):983–988.

Czock, D., Keller, F., Rasche, F. M., and Häussler, U. (2005). Pharmacokinetics and pharmacodynamics of systemically administered glucocorticoids. *Clin Pharmacokinet* 44(1):61–98.

Davis, J. M. (1995). Central and peripheral factors in fatigue. *J Sports Sci* 13:S49–S53.

De Oliveira, G. S., Almeida, M. D., Benzon, H. T., and McCarthy, R. J. (2011). Perioperative single dose systemic dexamethasone for postoperative pain. *Anesthesiology* 115(3):575–588.

Del Corral, P., Howley, E. T., Hartsell, M., Ashraf, M., and Younger, M. S. (1998). Metabolic effects of low cortisol during exercise in humans. *J Appl Physiol* 84(3):939–947.

Duclos, M. (2010). Glucocorticoids: A doping agent? *Endocrinol Metab Clin N Am* 39(1):107–126.

Duclos, M., Gatti, C, Bessiere, B., and Mormède, P. (2009). Tonic and phasic effects of corticosterone on food restriction-induced hyperactivity in rats. *Psychoneuroendocrinology* 34(3):436–445.

Duclos, M., Guinot, M., Colsy, M., Merle, F., Baudot, C., Corcuff, J. B., and Lebouc, Y. (2007). High risk of adrenal insufficiency after a single articular steroid injection in athletes. *Med Sci Sports Exerc* 39(7):1036–1043.

Dvorak, J., Feddermann, N., and Grimm, K. (2006). Glucocorticosteroids in football: Use and misuse. *Br J Sports Med* 40(suppl 1):i48–i54.

Gorostiaga, E. M., Czerwinski, S. M., and Hickson, R. C. (1988). Acute glucocorticoid effects on glycogen utilization, O_2 uptake, and endurance. *J Appl Physiol* 64(3):1098–1106.

Guinot, M., Duclos, M., Idres, N., Souberbielle, J. C., Megret, A., and Le Bouc, Y. (2007). Value of basal serum cortisol to detect corticosteroid-induced adrenal insufficiency in elite cyclists. *Eur J Appl Physiol* 99(3):205–216.

Härfstrand, A., Fuxe, K., Cintra, A., Agnati, L.F., Zini, I., Wikström, A. C., *et al*. (1986). Glucocorticoid receptor immunoreactivity in monoaminergic neurons of rat brain. *Proc Natl Acad Sci USA* 83 (24):9779–9783.

Harmon, K. G., and Hawley, C. (2003). Physician prescribing patterns of oral corticosteroids for musculoskeletal injuries. *J Am Board Fam Pract* 16(3):209–212.

Henzen, C., Suter, A., Lerch, E., Urbinelli, R., Schorno, X. H., and Briner, V. A. (2000). Suppression and recovery of adrenal response after short-term, high-dose glucocorticoid treatment. *Lancet* 355 (9203):542–545.

Horber, F. F., Scheidegger, J. R., Grünig, B. E., and Frey, F. J. (1985). Evidence that prednisone-induced myopathy is reversed by physical training. *J Clin Endocrinol Metab* 61(1):83–88.

Jollin, L., Thomasson, R., Le Panse, B., Baillot, A., Vibarel-Rebot, N., Lecoq, A. M., *et al*. (2010). Saliva DHEA and cortisol responses following short-term corticosteroid intake. *Eur J Clin Invest* 40(2):183–186.

Kino, T., Manoli, I., Kelkar, S., Wang, Y., Su, Y. A., and Chrousos, G. P. (2009). Glucocorticoid receptor (GR) β has intrinsic, GRα-independent transcriptional activity. *Biochem Biophys Res Comm* 381 (4):671–675.

Le Panse, B., Thomasson, R., Jollin, L., Lecoq, A.-M., Amiot, V., Rieth, N., *et al*. (2009). Short-term glucocorticoid intake improves exercise endurance in healthy recreationally trained women. *Eur J Appl Physiol* 107(4):437–443.

Lewis-Truffin, L. J., Jewell, C. M., Bienstock, R. J., Collins, J. B., and Cidlowski, J. A. (2007). Human glucocorticoid receptor β binds RU-486 and is transcriptionally active. *Mol Cell Biol* 27(6):2266–2282.

Marquet, P., Lac, G., Chassain, A. P., Habrioux, G., and Galen F. X. (1999). Dexamethasone in resting and exercising men. I. Effects on bioenergetics, minerals, and related hormones. *J Appl Physiol* 87(1):175–182.

McMahon, M., Gerich, J., and Rizza, R. (1988). Effects of glucocorticoids on carbohydrate metabolism. *Diabetes Metab Rev* 4(1):17–30.

Murray, A. J., Panagia, M., Hauton, D., Gibbons, G. F., and Clarke, K. (2005). Plasma free fatty acids and peroxisome proliferator-activated receptor α in the control of myocardial uncoupling protein levels. *Diabetes* 54(12):3496–3502.

Nichols, A. W. (2005). Complications associated with the use of corticosteroids in the treatment of athletic injuries. *Clin J Sports Med* 15(5):370–375.

Oakley, R. H., Sar, M., and Cidlowski, J. A. (1996). The human glucocorticoid receptor beta isoforms. Expression, biochemical properties, and putative function. *J Biol Chem* 271(16):9550–9559.

Oakley, R. H., Webster, J. C., Sar, M., Parker, R., and Cidlowski, J. A. (1997). Expression and subcellular distribution of the β-isoform of the human glucocorticoid receptor. *Endocrinology* 138(11):5028–5038.

Petrides, J. S., Gold, P. W., Mueller, G. P., Singh, A., Stratakis, C., *et al.* (1997). Marked differences in functioning of the hypothalamic-pituitary-adrenal axis between groups of men. *J Appl Physiol* 82(6):1979–1988.

Piazza, P. V., Barrot, M., Rougé-Pont, F., Marinelli, M., Maccari, S., Abrous, D. N., *et al.* (1996a). Suppression of glucocorticoid secretion and antipsychotic drugs have similar effects on the mesolimbic dopaminergic transmission. *Proc Natl Acad Sci USA* 93(26):15445–15450.

Piazza, P. V., Rougé-Pont, F., Deroche, V., Maccari, S., Simon, H., and Le Moal, M. (1996b). Glucocorticoids have state-dependent stimulant effects on the mesencephalic dopaminergic transmission. *Proc Natl Acad Sci USA* 93(16):8716–8720.

Plihal, W., Krug, R., Pietrowsky, R., Fehm, H. L., and Born, J. (1996). Corticosteroid receptor mediated effects on mood in humans. *Psychoneuroendocrinology* 21(6):515–523.

Pujols, L., Mullol, J., Roca-Ferrer, J., Torrego, A., Xaubet, A., Cidlowski, J. A., and Picado, C. (2002). Expression of glucocorticoid receptor α- and β-isoforms in human cells and tissues. *Am J Physiol Cell Physiol* 283(4):C1324–C1331.

Qi, D., Pulinilkunnil, T., An, D., Ghosh, S., Abrahani, A., Pospisilik, J. A., *et al.* (2004). Single-dose dexamethasone induces whole-body insulin resistance and alters both cardiac fatty acid and carbohydrate metabolism. *Diabetes* 53(7):1790–1797.

Romundstad, L., Breivik, H., Niemi, G., Helle, A., and Stubhaug, A. (2004). Methylprednisolone intravenously 1 day after surgery has sustained analgesic and opioid-sparing effects. *Acta Anaesthesiologica Scandinavica* 48(10):1223–1231.

Roussel, D., Dumas, J.-F., Simard, G., Malthiery, Y., and Ritz, P. (2004). Kinetics and control of oxidative phosphorylation in rat liver mitochondria after dexamethasone treatment. *Biochem J* 382(Pt 2):491–499.

Ruzzin, J., and Jensen, J. (2005). Contraction activates glucose uptake and glycogen synthase normally in muscles from dexamethasone-treated rats. *Am J Physiol Endocrinol Metab* 289(2):E241–E250.

Sarpolsky, R. M., Romero, M., and Munck, A. U. (2000). How do glucocorticoids influence stress responses? Integrating permissive, suppressive, stimulatory, and preparative actions. *Endocr Rev* 21(1):55–89.

Schäcke, H., Döcke, W.-D., and Asadullah, K. (2002). Mechanisms involved in the side effects of glucocorticoids. *Pharmacol Ther* 96(1):23–43.

Soetens, E., De Meirleir, K., and Hueting, J. E. (1995). No influence of ACTH on maximal performance. *Psychopharmacology* 118(3):260–266.

Son, G. H., Chung, S., and Kim, K. (2011). The adrenal peripheral clock: Glucocorticoid and the circadian timing system. *Front Neuroendocrinol* 32(4):451–465.

Stahn, C., Löwenberg, M., Hommes, D. W., and Buttgereit, F. (2007). Molecular mechanisms of glucocorticoid action and selective glucocorticoid receptor agonists. *Mol Cell Endocrinol* 275(1–2):71–78.

Stavinoha, M. A., RaySpellicy, J. W., Essop, M. F., Graveleau, C., Abel, E. D., Hart-Sailors, M. L., *et al.* (2004). Evidence for mitochondrial thioesterase 1 as a peroxisome proliferator-activated receptor-α-regulated gene in cardiac and skeletal muscle. *Am J Physiol Endocrinol Metab* 287(5): E888–E895.

Streck, W. F., and Lockwood, D. H. (1979). Pituitary adrenal recovery following short-term suppression with corticosteroids. *Am J Med* 66(6):910–914.

Swinburn, C. R., Wakefield, J. M., Newman, S. P., and Jones, P. W. (1988). Evidence of prednisolone induced mood change ('steroid euphoria') in patients with chronic obstructive airways disease. *Br J Clin Pharmac* 26(6):709–713.

Thomasson, R., Rieth, N., Jollin, L., Amiot, V., Lasne, F., and Collomp, K. (2011). Short-term glucocorticoid intake and metabolic responses during long-lasting exercise. *Horm Metab Res* 43(3): 216–222.

Tops, M., Van Peer, J. M., Wijers, A. A., and Korf, J. (2006). Acute cortisol administration reduces subjective fatigue in healthy women. *Psychophysiology* 43(6):653–656.

Turner, N., Bruce, C. R., Beale, S. M., Hoehn, K. L., So, T., Rolph, M. S., and Cooney, G. J. (2007). Excess lipid availability increases mitochondrial fatty acid oxidative capacity in muscle. *Diabetes* 56(8):2085–2092.

Vegiopoulos, A., and Herzig, S. (2007). Glucocorticoids, metabolism and metabolic diseases. *Mol Cell Endocrinol* 275(1–2):43–61.

World Anti-Doping Agency. (2012). 2012 anti-doping testing figures report. Available online at https://wada-main-prod.s3.amazonaws.com/resources/files/WADA-2012-Anti-Doping-Testing-Figures-Report-EN.pdf (accessed 9 September 2014).

World Anti-Doping Agency. (2013). Minimum required performance levels for detection and identification of non-threshold substances. Available online at https://www.wada-ama.org/en/resources/science-medicine/td2013-mrpl#.VA-Lc8stDX4 (accessed 9 September 2014).

World Anti-Doping Agency. (2014). The 2014 list of prohibited substances and methods. Available online at https://www.wada-ama.org/en/what-we-do/prohibited-list (accessed 9 September 2014).

Young, E. A., Abelson, J., and Lightman, L. (2004). Cortisol pulsatility and its role in stress regulation and health. *Front Neuroendocrinol* 25(2):69–76.

Chapter 17

Alcohol

David R. Mottram

17.1. Introduction

Fermented beverages have been used since ancient times, and alcohol continues to feature prominently in contemporary life. With respect to sport, alcohol is closely associated with sponsorship and branding, as well as with consumption by players and spectators (Palmer 2011). Alcohol consumption is part of the social aspects of many sporting events and is claimed to be the most widely used drug among sport participants and athletes (El-Sayed *et al.* 2005).

17.2. Mode of action of alcohol

Metabolism of alcohol

The alcohols are a group of chemicals, most of which are toxic. The most common is ethanol or ethyl alcohol, which is obtained by the fermentation of sugar. It is nontoxic, except in large and chronic doses, and has been enjoyed as a beverage for many centuries.

Ethyl alcohol is both a drug and a food. Its energy value per unit weight is 7 kcal/g compared with a value of 9 kcal/g for fat, but it is higher than the value of 4 kcal/g for both carbohydrate and protein. The value of alcohol as a foodstuff is limited because it is metabolized mainly in the liver and at a fixed rate of about 100 mg/kg of body weight per hour. For a 70-kg individual, this amounts to 7 g of alcohol hourly. The energy is not available to active skeletal muscle, and consequently it is not possible to exercise oneself to sobriety. The diuretic effect of drinking beer makes it less than the ideal agent of rehydration after hard physical training.

Alcohol is a polar substance that is freely miscible in water. It easily penetrates biological membranes and can be absorbed unaltered from the stomach and more quickly from the small intestine. Absorption is quickest if alcohol is drunk on an empty stomach, if gas molecules are present in the drink, and if the alcohol content is high. Intense mental concentration, lowered body temperature, and physical exercise tend to slow the rate of absorption.

From the gastrointestinal tract, the alcohol is transported to the liver in the hepatic circulation. The activity of the enzyme alcohol dehydrogenase, present chiefly in the liver, governs the disappearance of alcohol from the body. In the liver, alcohol dehydrogenase converts the alcohol to acetaldehyde; it is then converted to acetic acid or acetate by aldehyde dehydrogenase. About 75 per cent of the alcohol taken up by the blood is released as acetate into the circulation. The acetate is then oxidized to carbon dioxide and water within the Krebs (or citric acid) cycle. An alternative metabolic route for acetate is its activation to acetyl coenzyme A and further reactions to form fatty acids, ketone bodies, amino acids, and steroids.

Ethyl alcohol is distributed throughout the body by means of the circulatory system; it enters all the body water pools and tissues, including the central nervous system. Initially, alcohol moves rapidly from blood into the tissues.

The metabolism of alcohol in the liver is unaffected by its concentration in the blood. Some alcohol is eliminated in the breath, but this is usually less than 5 per cent of the total amount metabolized. This route is used in assessing safe levels for driving, forming the basis of the breathalyser tests. Small amounts of alcohol are excreted in urine and also in sweat if exercise is performed whilst drunk. Higher excretion rates through the lungs, urine, and sweat are produced at high environmental temperatures and at high blood alcohol levels.

With a single drink, the blood alcohol level usually peaks about 45 minutes after ingestion. This is the point where any influence on performance will be most evident.

Action of alcohol on the nervous system

Alcohol has differential effects on the central neurotransmitters, acetylcholine, serotonin, noradrenaline, and dopamine. Alcohol decreases serotonin turnover in the central nervous system. Activity in the neurones of serotonergic pathways is important for the experience of anxiety; output of corticosteroid hormones from the adrenal cortex increases the activity in these neurones. Alcohol has an opposing action, so it may reduce the tension that is felt by the individual in a stressful situation.

An effect of alcohol is to increase activity in central noradrenergic pathways. This is transient and is followed, some hours later, by a decrease in activity. Catecholaminergic pathways are implicated in the control of mood states, with activation of these pathways promoting happy and merry states. The fall in noradrenaline turnover as the blood alcohol concentration drops ties in with the reversal of mood that follows the initial drunken euphoric state. This is exacerbated by large doses of alcohol, as these tend to give rise to depression.

Alcohol stimulates the brain to release dopamine. Dopamine is regarded as a pleasure-related hormone, and its release is triggered in the limbic system. Stimulation of sweat glands also affects the limbic system, whilst cerebral cortical activity is depressed. Pain sensors are numbed and later the cerebellum is affected, causing difficulty with balance.

Alcohol also affects cerebral energy metabolism by increasing glucose utilisation in the brain. Because glucose is the main substrate furnishing energy for nerve cells, the result is that the lowered glucose level may induce mental fatigue. This will be reflected in failing cognitive functions, as well as declines in mental concentration and in information processing.

The disruption of acetylcholine synthesis and release means that alcohol acts as a depressant, exerting its effect on the reticular activating system, whose activity represents the level of physiological arousal. It also has a depressant effect on the cortex. Alcohol first affects the reasoning centres in the frontal lobes and sedates inhibitory nerves; at higher levels of blood alcohol, the centres for speech, vision, and motor control are affected and eventually awareness is lost. In smaller doses, alcohol inhibits cerebral control mechanisms, freeing the brain from its normal inhibition. This release of inhibition has been blamed for aggressive and violent conduct of individuals behaving out of character when under the influence of alcohol.

Progressive effects of alcohol at different blood alcohol concentrations are summarized in Table 17.1. An important effect of alcohol, not listed, is that it diminishes the ability to process appreciable amounts of information arriving simultaneously from two different sources.

It is thought that moderate drinking provides a degree of protection against coronary heart disease. In a prospective cohort study over 20 years in Denmark, Pedersen *et al.* (2008)

Table 17.1 Demonstrable effects of alcohol at different blood alcohol concentrations

Concentration level (mg/100 ml blood)	Effects
30 (0.03%)	Enhanced sense of well-being
	Delayed simple reaction time
	Impaired hand-eye coordination
60 (0.06%)	Mild loss of social inhibition
	Impaired judgement
90 (0.09%)	Marked loss of social inhibition
	Coordination reduced
	Noticeably 'under the influence'
120 (0.12%)	Apparent clumsiness
	Loss of physical control
	Tendency towards extreme responses
	Definite drunkenness is noted
150 (0.15%)	Erratic behaviour
	Slurred speech
	Staggering gait
180 (0.18%)	Loss of control of voluntary activity
	Impaired vision

showed that engaging in physical activity was linked to a 25–30 per cent decrease in risk of death from heart disease; moderate alcohol intake was also linked to a smaller reduction, with the risk of death from heart disease reduced by 17 per cent in men and 24 per cent in women.

17.3. Adverse effects of alcohol

The effects of alcohol on health are usually viewed in terms of chronic alcoholism. Persistent drinking leads to a dependence on alcohol so that it becomes addictive. Most physicians emphasize that alcoholism is a disease or a behavioural disorder rather than a vice and devise therapy accordingly.

The result of excessive drinking is ultimately manifested in liver disease: cirrhosis, a serious hardening and degeneration of liver tissue, is fatal for many heavy drinkers. Cancer is also more likely to develop in a cirrhotic liver. Cancers of the bowel, pharynx, larynx, and oesophagus have also been linked to alcohol consumption.

Cardiomyopathy or damage to the heart muscle can result from years of heavy drinking. Other pathological conditions associated with alcohol abuse include generalized skeletal myopathy and pancreatitis. Impairment of brain function also occurs, with alcoholic psychoses being a common cause of hospitalization in psychiatric wards. There are also potentially fatal consequences of binge drinking, where excessive amounts of alcohol are drunk in one session.

Alcohol use modulates the immune system and impairs host defence mechanisms. Van der Horst Graat *et al.* (2007) reported an association between alcohol intake and frequency of respiratory infections in apparently healthy elderly people. Alcohol taken with a meal increases postprandial lipaemia, an effect that is the opposite of response to exercise. The suppression of fat oxidation would increase the propensity for weight gain and increased abdominal adiposity (Suter and Schutz 2008). Alcohol may impair absorption of minerals and vitamins. Vitamin D was deficient in 90 per cent of the men and 76 per cent of the women with alcoholism studied by Malik *et al.* (2009). The link between alcohol consumption and osteoporosis was more evident in the men, with raised levels of oestradiol providing a degree of protection for the women. Alcohol decreases resting levels of testosterone and cortisol; it also blunts the cortisol and growth hormone responses to submaximal exercise – factors that could impair performance.

17.4. Alcohol use in sport

Alcohol as an antianxiety drug

Amongst athletes, participation in sports brings its own unique form of stress, not only before important contests but also due to frequent competitive events. Although a certain amount of precompetition anxiety is inevitable, the anxiety response varies enormously between individuals, with some people coping extremely poorly. Many find their own solutions to attenuate anxiety levels, without exogenous aids. Anxiety may adversely affect performance, especially in activities highly demanding of mental concentration and steadiness of limbs. This likely impairment has prompted the use of antianxiety drugs.

The psychological reaction to impending sports competition is variously referred to as anxiety, arousal, stress, or activation. Anxiety suggests worry or emotional tension, arousal denotes a continuum from sleep to high excitement, stress implies an agent that induces strain in the organism, and activation refers to the metabolic state in the 'flight-or-fight' reaction. A moderate level of 'anxiety' about the forthcoming activity is desirable to induce the right levels of harnessed motivation for action. The simpler the task, the higher is the level of anxiety that can be tolerated before performance efficiency begins to fall.

Overanxiety has a detrimental effect on the physical and psychomotor elements that comprise sports performance. In such instances, anxiety-reducing strategies will have an ergogenic effect. The athlete or mentor may have to choose between mental relaxation techniques or drugs to alleviate anxiety. When alcohol is used to reduce stress in overanxious individuals, the benefits must be balanced against any adverse effects on physical and neuromotor performance that might be introduced.

Anxiety level depends very much on the nature of the sport as well as on the individual concerned. High anxiety is mostly associated with brief and high-risk activities. Anxiety responses before the start of competition, as reflected in emotional tachycardia, show motor racing, ski jumping, and downhill skiing to be top of the list (Reilly 1997). In aiming sports, such as archery, a steady limb is needed to provide a firm platform for launching the missile at its target or to keep the weapon still.

Residual effects of alcohol may carry over to the following day, affecting training or subsequent competitive performance. There are also possibilities of tolerance to the drug with chronic use or of drug dependence developing.

Alcohol use in a social sporting context

Heavy drinking is not compatible with serious participation in sport. For the athlete, drinking is usually done only in moderation – an infrequent respite for the ascetic regimens of physical training, although the occasional end-of-season binge may be customary. Nevertheless, drinking is a social convention in many sports, in which there may be peer-group pressure to take alcohol following training or competition or at club social functions. Even individuals who can tolerate competitive stress still need to relax following competition or at times of a series of important competitions. The same applies to athletes in team sports gathered together in training camps for a sustained period. In these cases, drinking alcohol is a frequent method of facilitating relaxation among athletes. The practice is sometimes condoned by the team's management as a means of 'bonding' among the players. Indeed, victories are celebrated and defeats accepted by postevent drinking in many sports.

In a study with elite Australian athletes, Dunn *et al*. (2011) found that alcohol was nominated as a drug of concern only by a small proportion of athletes. The sensible athlete drinks moderately and occasionally, avoiding alcohol for at least 24 hours before competing. Hangovers may persist for a day and disturb concentration in sports involving complex skills.

For a healthy athlete in a good state of training, occasional drinking of alcohol in moderation will have little adverse effect. It is important to emphasize that any such occasional bouts of drinking should be restrained and should follow rather than precede training sessions.

Adverse effects of alcohol in sport and exercise

The deleterious effects of alcohol on the nervous system will have consequences for performance in sports that require fast reactions, complex decision making, and highly skilled actions. It will also have an impact on hand–eye coordination, tracking tasks (e.g. driving), and vigilance tasks (e.g. long-distance sailing). An effect on tracking tasks is that control movements lose their normal smoothness and precision, becoming more abrupt or jerky. At high doses of alcohol, meaningful sport becomes impractical or even dangerous.

Alcohol ingestion lowers muscle glycogen at rest compared with control conditions. As prestart glycogen levels are important for sustained exercise at an intensity of approximately 70 80 per cent VO_2max, such as marathon running, taking alcohol in the 24 hours before such endurance activities is ill advised. The impairment in glucose production by the liver would lead to an increased likelihood of hypoglycaemia developing during prolonged exercise.

Alcohol intoxication may adversely affect a sportsperson's dietary choices by displacing carbohydrate from the diet at a time when restoration of glycogen stores should be a priority (Maughan 2006).

Impairment in carbohydrate synthesis postexercise would delay the restoration of muscle glycogen stores and adversely affect endurance performance. Burke *et al*. (2003) showed that alcohol delayed glycogen resynthesis the day after strenuous exercise, but not when carbohydrate intake was high.

Alcohol decreases peripheral vascular resistance. This response is because of the vasodilatory effect of alcohol on the peripheral blood vessels, which would increase heat loss from the surface of the skin and cause a drop in body temperature. This consequence would be dangerous if alcohol is taken in conjunction with exercise in cold conditions. Sampling whisky on the ski slopes may bring an immediate feeling of warmth, but its disturbance of normal thermoregulation may put the recreational skier at risk of hypothermia. Frostbitten mountaineers especially should avoid drinking alcohol because the peripheral vasodilation it induces would cause the body temperature to fall further. In hot conditions, alcohol is also inadvisable because it acts as a diuretic and would exacerbate problems of dehydration.

Alcohol and sports accidents

Peak effects on motor performance following administration of alcohol are typically observed 45–60 min later, but impairment is evident for up to 3 hours after dosing (Kelly *et al*., 1993).

This could render the drinker susceptible to accidents if alcohol is imbibed after sports competitions before driving home. Even at blood alcohol concentrations within the legal limit (about 0.03 per cent), accident risk is increased when driving after sleep restricted to 4 hours the previous night (Vakulin *et al.* 2007) or after a prolonged period (18–21 hours) of being awake (Howard *et al.* 2007).

Alcohol can compound the hangover effects of some sleeping tablets and is likely to disturb complex skills more than simpler motor tasks performed on the morning of the next day (Kunsman *et al.* 1992). Attention and reaction time tasks were impaired by concentrations of temazepam and ethanol in combinations that alone did not cause decrements in performance. Subjects tend to be unaware of their reduced performance capabilities when taking these drugs in combination, a factor likely to increase injury risk. Of 402 victims of ski accidents, 20 per cent were positive for alcohol, 8.5 per cent had taken benzodiazepines, and 2.5 per cent were positive for both drugs. There is also a diurnal variation in the effects of alcohol. Drinking at lunchtime has a more detrimental effect on psychomotor performance than alcohol taken in the evening (Horne and Gibbons, 1991). Consequently recreational skiers place themselves at increased risk of injury by drinking at lunchtime rather than solely *après ski*.

A review by El-Sayed *et al.* (2005) concluded that alcohol is the most frequently used drug among athletes and that it is directly linked to the rate of injury sustained in sport events. In addition, alcohol appears to evoke detrimental effects on exercise performance capacity.

Alcohol in sport: The wider picture

Apart from the specific issue of alcohol use by athletes, there is a much wider association between alcohol and sport. Palmer (2011) provided a detailed review of these wider issues, which include the commercial aspects of sponsorship and advertising in sport by manufacturers of alcoholic drinks. The social practices of spectators with associated issues of crime, violence, and health are also addressed.

A study was conducted in New Zealand in which sportspeople from various sporting codes were asked whether they personally, their team, or their club received free and/or discounted alcohol or funding from an alcohol industry body (O'Brien and Kypri 2008). Results showed that 47.8 per cent of respondents reported receiving alcohol industry sponsorship. The authors concluded that sports administration bodies should consider the health and ethical risks of accepting such sponsorship.

It is interesting to note that the Fédération Internationale de Football Association requested Brazil to suspend a national ban on the sale of alcoholic beverages in soccer stadiums during the 2014 World Cup (Caetano *et al.* 2012); although the ban was subsequently lifted.

17.5. Alcohol and the WADA Prohibited List

Alcohol was first included on the International Olympic Committee (IOC) Prohibited List in 1988 as part of a group of drugs referred to as Classes of Drugs Subject to Certain Restrictions. In 2003, following the establishment of the World Anti-Doping Agency (WADA), the joint IOC/WADA Prohibited List redefined the group of drugs that included alcohol as Classes of Prohibited Substances in Certain Sports. This Prohibited List stated that, where the rules of the governing body so provide, tests will be conducted for ethanol. This rather loose protocol was strengthened the following year when the first WADA Prohibited List came into force on 1 January 2004. Alcohol was then classified under Substances Prohibited in Particular

Table 17.2 Particular sports in which alcohol was prohibited in 2004

Aeronautics	Football	Roller sports
Archery	Gymnastics	Skiing
Automobile	Karate	Triathlon
Billiards	Modern pentathlon	Wrestling
Boules	Motorcycling	

Sports, with the international federations that had requested alcohol to be prohibited being clearly identified. This classification has continued to the current 2014 Prohibited List.

In which sports is alcohol prohibited?

In 2004, there were fourteen sports in which alcohol was prohibited (Table 17.2). There were variable threshold levels (between 0.02 g/l and 0.50 g/l) of alcohol being specified by some sport federations, whereas others instituted a complete ban.

By 2009, the number of sports in which alcohol was prohibited had reduced to nine and a standard threshold level of 0.10 g/l established. As a result of the continued annual review by international federations, by 2014 the WADA Prohibited List included just six sports in which alcohol was prohibited (Table 17.3).

The 2014 list of sports in which alcohol was prohibited included those sports in which participation under the influence of alcohol could have serious consequences, not just for the athlete but also for fellow competitors and spectators.

Prevalence of adverse analytical findings for alcohol

Although alcohol is undoubtedly used by many athletes in a social context, WADA prohibits its use in particular sports only within competition. Consequently, there have been few cases of adverse analytical findings involving alcohol from WADA-accredited laboratories (Table 17.4).

Table 17.3 Particular sports in which alcohol was prohibited in 2014

Air sports	Motorcycling
Archery	Power boating
Automobile	Triathlon
Karate	

Table 17.4 WADA statistics for the annual number of adverse analytical findings for alcohol

Year	Number of cases
2003–2008	0
2009	5
2010	9
2011	5
2012	5

17.6. Summary

- Alcohol is the most abused drug in society at large, and athletes are not immune to the social conventions of using alcohol to relax and reduce stress.
- Alcohol may be used as an ergogenic aid in a limited number of sports; consequently, in 2014, WADA prohibited the use of alcohol in just six sports.
- The use of alcohol in social contexts, including sport, is pervasive. Therefore, the acute and chronic effects of alcohol have potentially serious implications for the health of athletes who drink it.

17.7. References

Burke, L. M., Collier, G. R., Broad, E. M., *et al.* (2003). Effect of alcohol intake on muscle glycogen storage after prolonged exercise. *Journal of Applied Physiology* 95(3): 983–990.

Caetano, R., Pinsky, I., and Laranjeira, R. (2012). Should soccer and alcohol mix? Alcohol sales during the 2014 World Soccer Cup games in Brazil. *Addiction* 107(10):1722–1723.

Dunn, M., Thomas, J. O., Swift, W., *et al.* (2011). Recreational substance use among elite Australian athletes. *Drug and Alcohol Review* 30(1):63–68.

El-Sayed, M. S., Ali, N., and Ali, Z. E. (2005). Interaction between alcohol and exercise. *Sports Medicine*, 35(3):257–269.

Horne, J. A. and Gibbons, H. (1991). Effects on vigilance performance and sleepiness of alcohol given in the early afternoon (post lunch) vs. early evening. *Ergonomics* 34(1):67–77.

Howard, M. E., Jackson, M. L., Kennedy, G. A., *et al.* (2007). The interaction effects of extended wakefulness and low-dose alcohol on simulated driving and vigilance. *Sleep* 30(10):1334–1340.

Kelly, T. H., Fultin, R. W., Emurian, C. S., *et al.* (1993). Performance based testing for drugs of abuse: dose and time profiles of marijuana, amphetamine, alcohol and diazepam. *Journal of Analytical Toxicology* 17(5):264–272.

Kunsman, G. W., Manno, J. B., Przekop, M. A., *et al.* (1992). The effects of temazepam and ethanol on human psychomotor performance. *European Journal of Clinical Pharmacology* 43(6):603–611.

Malik, P., Gasser, R. W., Kemmler, G., *et al.* (2009). Low bone mineral density and impaired bone metabolism in young adolescent patients without cirrhosis: A cross-sectional study. *Alcoholism, Clinical and Experimental Research* 33(2):375–381.

Maughan, R. J. (2006). Alcohol and football. *Journal of Sports Science* 24(7):741–748.

O'Brien, K.S., and Kypri, K. (2008). Alcohol industry sponsorship and hazardous drinking among sportspeople. *Addiction* 103(12):1961–1966.

Palmer, C. (2011). Key themes and research agendas in the sport-alcohol nexus. *Journal of Sport and Social Issues* 35(2):168–185.

Pedersen, J. O., Heitmann, B. L., Schnoir, P., *et al.* (2008). The combined influence of leisure-time physical activity and weekly alcohol intake on fatal ischaemic heart disease and all-cause mortality. *European Heart Journal* 29(2):204–212.

Reilly, T. (1997). Alcohol: its influence in sport and exercise. In T. Reilly and M. Orme (Eds.), *The Clinical Pharmacology of Sport and Exercise* (pp. 281–290). Amsterdam, the Netherlands: Elsevier.

Suter, P. M., and Schutz, P. (2008). The effect of exercise, alcohol or both combined on health and physical performance. *International Journal of Obesity (London)* 32(Suppl. 6):548–552.

Vakulin, A., Baulk, S. D., Catcheside, P. G., *et al.* (2007). Effect of moderate sleep deprivation and low-dose alcohol on driving simulator performance and perception in young men. *Sleep* 30(10):1327–1333.

Van der Horst Graat, J. M., Terpstra, J. S., Kok, F. J., *et al.* (2007). Alcohol, smoking and physical activity related to respiratory infections in elderly people. *Journal of Nutrition Health and Aging* 11(1):80–85.

Chapter 18

Beta blockers

David R. Mottram

18.1. Introduction

Beta blockers are drugs that are used to treat a wide variety of clinical conditions, primarily associated with the cardiovascular system. Some of the more peripheral pharmacological properties of beta blockers, such as reducing anxiety and hand tremor, are used by some athletes to enhance performance. These potential enhancing effects only apply to a small number of sports.

18.2. What are beta blockers?

Beta blockers were first synthesised by the pharmaceutical industry in 1958. They have become one of the most frequently prescribed classes of drugs, providing therapeutic support for a wide range of clinical conditions, principally associated with the cardiovascular system.

Mode of action of beta blockers

Beta blockers antagonise beta receptors, one of the subclasses of receptors that noradrenaline (norepinephrine) and adrenaline (epinephrine) act upon. Noradrenaline and adrenaline are found in both the central nervous system (CNS), where they act as neurotransmitters, and in the periphery, where noradrenaline is a neurotransmitter in the sympathetic nervous system and adrenaline is a hormone, released from the adrenal medulla during conditions of stress.

Both noradrenaline and adrenaline act through receptor sites known as adrenoceptors. These are subclassified into two major classes: alpha (α) and beta (β). The β-adrenoceptors are further subclassified into at least three types of receptors: β_1, β_2, and β_3. These receptors are found in a variety of tissues and organs of the body. The main ones are shown in Table 18.1, which also shows the principal effects that occur when beta blockers affect these receptors. It can be seen, therefore, that the effects of beta blockers are wide ranging.

Over the years, the pharmaceutical industry has developed beta blockers that act selectively on particular subclasses of β-adrenoceptors, in an attempt to target their therapeutic action more precisely and to reduce unwanted side effects. Table 18.2 lists some of the more common beta blockers, indicating their respective selectivity for beta receptor subclasses.

In addition to receptor selectivity, there are a number of other characteristics that distinguish one beta blocker from another. Some beta blockers, such as oxprenolol, pindolol,

Table 18.1 The main tissues and organs of the body (other than the brain) that contain β-adrenoceptors and the pharmacological effects of beta blockers

Organ	Receptor type	Principal effects of beta blockers
Heart	β_1	Decrease rate and force of beating
Blood vessels		
Arteries	β_2	Constriction
Veins	β_2	Constriction
Respiratory tract	β_2	Bronchoconstriction
Gastrointestinal tract	β_2	Increase motility
Bladder	β_2	Contraction of the bladder wall
Kidney	β_1	Inhibition of renin secretion
Skeletal muscle	β_2	Reduction in tremor, reduction of glycogenolysis
Liver	β_2	Reduction of glycogenolysis
Fat tissue	β_3	Reduction of lipolysis

acebutolol, and celiprolol, possess intrinsic sympathomimetic activity (ISA) or partial agonist activity, which represents the capacity of these beta blockers to stimulate as well as block adrenergic receptors. They tend to produce less slowing of the heart (bradycardia) than other beta blockers and may also reduce coldness of extremities, a common side effect of beta blockers (Head 1999).

Beta blockers have variable degrees of solubility between the lipid and water phases. Atenolol, celiprolol, nadolol, and sotalol are the most water soluble. They are less likely to enter the brain, crossing the blood–brain barrier, and therefore they are less likely to cause centrally mediated side effects (Turner 1983).

Table 18.2 Some of the more common beta blockers and their receptor specificities

Nonselective beta blockers
  Alprenolol
  Carteolol
  Levobunolol
  Metipranolol
  Nadolol
  Oxprenolol
  Pindolol
  Propranolol
  Sotalol
  Timolol

Selective beta blockers (cardioselective for β_1-adrenoceptors)
  Acebutolol
  Atenolol
  Betaxolol
  Bisoprolol
  Celiprolol
  Esmolol
  Metoprolol
  Nevibolol

Beta blocker and alpha blocker combinations
  Carvedilol
  Labetalol

18.3. Clinical uses of beta blockers

Effects of beta blockers

The main clinical uses for beta blockers are shown in Table 18.3. Many of these uses relate to the effects of beta blockers on the cardiovascular system blocking the β_1-adrenoceptors in the heart, thereby reducing cardiac rate and force of beating. It was this pharmacological effect that prompted the search for effective drugs to treat patients with angina pectoris. This condition is characterised by severe chest pain due to insufficient oxygen reaching cardiac muscle during exertion in patients with compromised cardiac arteries. Beta blockers do not treat the symptoms of angina; however, by reducing heart rate, they act prophylactically to prevent the onset of an anginal attack by improving exercise tolerance.

Blockade of β_1-adrenoceptors in the heart is important in the management of some types of cardiac dysrhythmias, particularly supraventricular tachycardia and heart failure. Bisoprolol and carvedilol are particularly useful in stable heart failure.

Blockade of β_1-adrenoceptors in the heart is also used to therapeutic advantage by reducing blood pressure in hypertensive patients. Other pharmacological actions of beta blockers that contribute to their antihypertensive action include alteration of baroreceptor reflex sensitivity, depression of renin secretion, and possibly CNS effects, particularly with those beta blockers that can easily cross the blood–brain barrier.

Beta blockers have been shown to be effective in preventing secondary heart attacks in patients who have experienced a myocardial infarction, although for some patients with comorbidities such as uncontrolled heart failure, bradyarrhythmia, or obstructive airways disease, beta blockers are contraindicated.

Phaeochromocytoma is a benign cancer of the adrenal medulla, leading to increased release of the hormone adrenaline. Beta blockers, as well as alpha blockers, are used to block the systemic effects of this overproduction of adrenaline.

Migraine is a condition that is treated by beta blockers through effects on blood vessels. Not all migraine sufferers respond to beta blockers, and more effective treatment regimes are available.

Glaucoma, a condition characterised by increased intraocular pressure in the eye, is treated by beta blockers. Although their mode of action is not fully understood, beta blockers are one of the first-line classes of drugs for this condition.

Table 18.3 The main clinical conditions for which beta blockers are used

Cardiovascular
  Hypertension
  Angina pectoris
  Cardiac dysrhythmias
  Heart failure
  Prevention of secondary myocardial infarction

Other uses
  Phaeochromocytoma (benign cancer of the adrenal medulla)
  Migraine
  Glaucoma
  Anxiety
  Essential tremor

A more unusual clinical use for beta blockers is in the management of anxiety. The most widely used class of drugs to treat anxiety, the benzodiazepines, treat the psychological symptoms of anxiety, such as worry, tension, and fear, mediated through the CNS. Beta blockers, on the other hand, treat the symptoms of anxiety mediated through the peripheral autonomic nervous system. They decrease heart rate by blocking β_1-adrenoceptors, thereby reducing palpitations, and reduce hand tremor mediated through β_2-adrenoceptors in skeletal muscle (Bowman and Anden 1981).

Essential tremor is a condition characterised by an involuntary rhythmic shaking of a part of the body, most commonly the arms, hands, and head. Beta blockers, by blocking the β_2-adrenoceptors in skeletal muscle, can reduce the severity of tremor, particularly in the hands.

Side effects of beta blockers

Common side effects associated with beta blockers are fatigue due to reduced cardiac output and reduced muscle perfusion in exercise, coldness in the extremities (hands and feet) due to peripheral vasoconstriction, and sleep disturbances (Cruickshank 1981). Those beta blockers with associated ISA are less likely to produce cold extremities, whilst those which are water soluble are less likely to produce sleep disturbances such as nightmares, insomnia, and occasionally depression.

Beta blockers are contraindicated in certain patients because of their wide range of pharmacological effects. They are especially contraindicated in patients with asthma because they block the β_2-adrenoceptors in the respiratory tract, leading to bronchoconstriction with associated airway resistance. This effect is less pronounced in those beta blockers that have selectivity for β_1-adrenoceptors (see Table 18.2). However, it should be noted that, at higher doses, these beta blockers lose their cardioselectivity.

Hypoglycaemia is associated with beta blocker use. Glucose release in response to adrenaline is important to patients with diabetes and other patients prone to hypoglycaemic attacks. Hypoglycaemia triggers symptoms to warn patients of the urgent need for carbohydrate. Beta blockers reduce these symptoms; therefore, beta blockers are contraindicated in patients with poorly controlled diabetes.

18.4. History of beta blockers in sport

Beta blockers are of potential benefit in sports where hand tremor and high anxiety play a role. Beta blockers were, for many years, first-line drugs for the treatment of a number of cardiovascular diseases such as angina and hypertension. Under this pretext, a number of high-ranking professional snooker players tested positive for beta blockers at the 1987 World Professional Snooker Championships, as had occurred a few years earlier by competitors in shooting events at the 1984 Olympic Games in Los Angeles (Reilly 2005). The argument that beta blockers were indispensable drugs for these conditions was, however, unsustainable because other equally effective first-line drugs were available to treat the cardiovascular conditions in question.

At the 1984 Olympic Games, the International Olympic Committee (IOC) Medical Commission, aware that some athletes were taking beta blockers to improve performance in shooting events, demanded a medical certificate to justify their use. These 'medical certificates' were submitted by eighteen athletes (Fitch 2012).

Beta blockers were added to the IOC Prohibited List in 1985 as one of the major classes of prohibited substances. It was clear that the pharmacological effects of beta blockers would have an adverse, rather than enhancing, effect on performance in most sports. This led the

IOC Medical Commission to test for beta blockers only in high-risk sports where beta blockers may be used for their antianxiety effect or in sports where hand steadiness was important. This policy was adopted at the Summer and Winter Olympic Games from 1988 to 1993 (Reilly 2005). Thereafter, the IOC reclassified beta blockers from Section I, Doping Classes, to Section II, Class of Drugs Subject to Certain Restrictions, where they were only prohibited in specified sports. This policy continued when the World Anti-Doping Agency (WADA) took over responsibility for the Prohibited List in 2004, and beta blockers were classed as Classes of Prohibited Substances in Certain Sports.

Case studies related to beta blockers

There have been relatively few cases involving beta blockers.

Kim Jong-Su (2008)

During the 2008 Beijing Olympic Games, the North Korean shooter Kim Jong-Su was expelled from the games when he tested positive for the beta blocker propranolol (Wendt 2009).

18.5. The action and use of beta blockers in sport

Use of beta blockers in sport

Stress and anxiety are common responses to competitive sport. Therapeutically, benzodiazepines are widely used as tranquillizers and antianxiety drugs. They exert their effect in the CNS through inhibition of the release of a number of neurotransmitters, most notably scrotonin (Reilly 2005). However, beta blockers are usually preferred as antianxiety agents in sport because they exert their effects peripherally rather than centrally and do not possess the addictive properties of benzodiazepines. Their peripheral antianxiety effects are principally associated with blockade of β_1-adrenoceptors in the heart, where they reduce stress-induced tachycardia and the reduction of limb tremor by blockade of β_2-adrenoceptors in skeletal muscle. With respect to the reduction in tremor, a study on the effect of oxprenolol on pistol shooting found a significant improvement in shooting scores but only in slow-firing events (Antal and Good 1980).

In 1986, Kruse *et al.* showed that there was a clear (13.4 per cent) improvement in the shooting performance of pistol shooters with metoprolol compared with placebo control. The most skilled marksmen showed the greatest improvement. No correlation was found between shooting improvement and cardiovascular variables, such as heart rate and blood pressure, leading the authors to conclude that the improvement was caused by an effect of metoprolol on hand tremor.

One particular sport has been associated with high levels of anxiety, even leading to a specific term to describe the phenomenon – the 'yips' in golf (Smith *et al.* 2003). It has been defined as a motor phenomenon of involuntary movements affecting golfers and is associated with high stress levels and performance anxiety. The physical symptoms of the yips are tremor, jerks, or freezing of the hands and forearms, particularly associated with putting strokes. For this reason, some golfers have used alcohol and/or beta blockers to alleviate the symptoms. It was only in 2009 that WADA added golf to the list of sports in which beta blockers are prohibited within competition, at the request of the International Golf Federation. In 2009,

Doug Barron became the first golfer to test positive for beta blockers, although he argued that he took beta blockers and testosterone for legitimate medical needs (Chamblee 2012).

Beta blockers are also prohibited in sports requiring vehicle control. In a review by Shrivastav *et al.* (2010), the authors described the various analytical methods available for the detection of beta blockers in plasma and urine.

Adverse effects of beta blockers in sport

Beta blockers produce metabolic effects, including a decrease in the rate of glycogenolysis in skeletal muscle. This may have implications for performance at submaximal levels. Similarly, in sustained exercise, the inhibition of glycogenolysis in liver will affect performance by reducing blood glucose levels (Reilly 2005). These effects on glycogenolysis are mediated through blockade of β_2-adrenoceptors and are more evident with nonselective beta blockers, such as propranolol. Prolonged exercise may be adversely affected by the inhibition of lipolysis that is produced by beta blockers. The availability of free fatty acids is reduced, thereby causing an earlier onset of fatigue. A thorough description of the metabolic effects of beta blockers in exercise can be found in a review paper by Head (1999).

A study by Rusko *et al.* (1980) examined the effect of beta blockers on short-term, high-intensity exercise. A series of anaerobic tasks were performed by subjects comparing the beta blocker oxprenolol with placebo control. Oxprenolol reduced power output on a cycle ergometer with a concomitant reduction in heart rate and peak blood lactate. The drug had no effect on isometric strength of leg extension, stair running, or vertical jumping. In a study of alpine skiers, it was reported that short-term maximal muscle power, recorded during a 30-second submaximal cycling test, was reduced by beta blockers (Karlsson *et al.* 1983). Beta blockers have been shown to reduce maximal oxygen uptake (VO_{2max}; Head 1999).

In prescribing medication for hypertensive patients who participate in sport, Derman (2008) recommended caution in the use of beta blockers because they are not the most efficacious class of antihypertensives, and their effects on exercise are detrimental to competition.

18.6. Beta blockers and the WADA Prohibited List

WADA regulations with respect to beta blockers

The 2014 WADA Prohibited List classifies beta blockers as substances prohibited in particular sports. The 2014 WADA regulations for beta blockers are shown in Table 18.4.

Table 18.4 2014 WADA regulations for beta blockers

Unless otherwise specified, beta blockers are prohibited in competition only in the following sports:

Archery (also prohibited out-of-competition)
Automobile
Billiards (all disciplines)
Darts
Golf
Shooting (also prohibited out-of-competition)
Skiing/snowboarding: ski jumping, freestyle aerials/halfpipe, and snowboard halfpipe/big air

Source: World Anti-Doping Agency. (2014). The 2014 Prohibited List international standard. Available online at https://elb.wada-ama.org/en/what-we-do/prohibited-list (accessed 5 September 2014).

Table 18.5 WADA statistics for the number of positive results for substances classified as beta blockers (2004–2012)

	2004	2005	2006	2007	2008	2009	2010	2011	2012
Beta blockers									
Atenolol	8	6	9	3	6	8	4	4	2
Bisoprolol	5	10	2	6	5	7	6	5	1
Metoprolol	5	5	6	6	4	10	4	4	5
Acebutolol	–	1	–	–	2	–	2	–	1
Propranolol	6	16	6	8	9	11	10	4	1
Carteolol	–	–	–	1	–	1	–	–	–
Sotalol	1	–	–	–	–	–	1	–	1
Carvedilol	–	4	3	2	1	1	1	–	–
Timolol	–	–	2	1	–	–	–	1	–
Betaxolol	–	–	–	–	3	–	–	–	–
Labetalol	–	–	–	–	1	–	–	–	2
Nadolol	–	–	–	–	–	–	2	2	–
Celiprolol	–	–	–	–	–	–	–	1	–
Total	25	42	28	27	31	38	30	21	13

For most of these sports, beta blockers are prohibited in-competition only. However, in the sports of archery and shooting, beta blockers are also prohibited out-of-competition.

Prevalence of adverse findings for beta blockers

Annual statistics from WADA-accredited laboratories show that there are few adverse analytical findings for beta blockers. The annual statistics ranged from 13 to 42 over the period from 2003 to 2012, with a steady reduction each year since 2009. Table 18.5 shows the annual occurrence for individual drugs within the class.

Results are unremarkable and probably reflect the international prescribing patterns of the respective drugs. It is interesting to note that cardioselective and noncardioselective beta blockers are used equally.

It should be noted that beta blockers are first-line drugs in the treatment of the eye condition glaucoma. Ophthalmologists need to be aware of the need for a Therapeutic Use Exemption certificate for athletes receiving eyedrops containing beta blockers, particularly within competition, as reported by Nicholson et al. (2012) at the time of the London 2012 Olympic and Paralympic Games.

18.7. Summary

- Beta blockers are used widely to treat medical conditions, particularly associated with the cardiovascular system.
- There have been few cases of misuse of beta blockers in sport.
- For most sports, the adverse effects of beta blockers far outweigh any potential performance-enhancing effect.
- WADA regulations restrict the use of beta blockers in particular sports in which the reduction of hand tremor and high levels of anxiety may be beneficial.

18.8. References

Antal, L. C., and Good, C. S. (1980). Effects of oxprenolol on pistol shooting under stress. *Practitioner* 224(1345): 755–760.

Bowman, W., and Anden, N. (1981). Effects of adrenergic activators and inhibitors on the skeletal muscles. In L. Szekeres (Ed.), *Adrenergic Activators and Inhibitors* (pp. 47–128). Berlin, Germany: Springer-Verlag.

Chamblee, B. (2012). Keeping it clean. *Golf Magazine* 54(11):120.

Cruickshank, J. M. (1981). β-blockers, bradycardia, and adverse effects. *Acta Therapeutica* 7:309–321.

Derman, W. (2008). Antihypertensive medications and exercise. *International SportsMed Journal* 9(1):32–38.

Fitch, K. (2012). Proscribed drugs at the Olympic Games: permitted use and misuse (doping) by athletes. *Clinical Medicine* 12(3):257–260.

Head, A. (1999). Exercise metabolism and β-blocker therapy. *Sports Medicine* 27(2):81–96.

Karlsson, J., Kjessel, T., and Kaiser, P. (1983). Alpine skiing and acute beta-blockade. *International Journal of Sports Medicine* 4(3):190–193.

Kruse, P., Ladefoged, J., Nielsen, U., *et al.* (1986). Beta-blockade used in precision sports: Effect on pistol shooting performance. *Journal of Applied Physiology* 61(2):417–420.

Nicholson, R. G. H., Thomas, G. P. L., Potter, M. J., *et al.* (2012). London 2012: Prescribing for athletes in ophthalmology. *Eye* 26(8):1036–1038.

Reilly, T. R. (2005). Alcohol, antianxiety drugs and sport. In D. R. Mottram (Ed.), *Drugs in Sport* (4th ed., pp. 258–287). London, UK: Routledge.

Rusko, H., Kantola, H., Luhtanen, R., *et al.* (1980). Effect of beta-blockade on performances requiring force, velocity, coordination and/or anaerobic metabolism. *Journal of Sports Medicine and Physical Fitness* 20(2):139–144.

Shrivastav, P. S., Buha, S. M., Shailesh, M., *et al.* (2010). Detection and quantitation of beta blockers in plasma and urine. *Bioanalysis* 2(2):263–276.

Smith, A. M., Adler, C. H. Crews, D., *et al.* (2003). The 'yips' in golf. A continuum between a focal dystonia and choking. *Sports Medicine* 33(1):13–31.

Turner, P. (1983). β-blockade and the human central nervous system. *Drugs* 25 (Suppl 2):262–273.

Wendt, J. T. (2009). Reflections on Beijing. *Entertainments and Sports Lawyer* 26(4):10–18.

Substances and methods permitted in sport

Chapter 19

Nonsteroidal anti-inflammatory drugs

Nick Wojek

19.1. Introduction

Musculoskeletal and joint injuries are frequently encountered in sport and lead to time lost from training and competition. In most instances, these types of injuries are considered to be minor, but they can account for numerous days of inactivity and ultimately lead to losses in performance. The challenge faced in sports medicine is to find interventions that hasten an athlete's return to activity without compromising tissue repair.

One common intervention used in the management of acute or chronic musculoskeletal injuries is the use of nonsteroidal anti-inflammatory drugs (NSAIDs). They are used to control pain and to limit the amount and duration of inflammation. Although the use of NSAIDs has become a widely accepted treatment of minor musculoskeletal injuries in sport, there is a growing view that NSAIDs have only modest results in the management of such injuries (Almekinders 1999; Paoloni *et al*. 2009). This chapter describes how NSAIDs work, explores their effectiveness, and investigates how prevalent use is amongst athletes.

19.2. What are NSAIDs?

NSAIDs possess analgesic, anti-inflammatory, antipyretic, and antithrombotic properties (Joint Formulary Committee 2014b). They exert their effects by inhibiting cyclo-oxygenase (COX) enzyme activity, which is involved in the synthesis of prostaglandins from arachidonic acid (Figure 19.1). NSAID inhibition of COX enzyme activity causes a decrease in the formation of prostaglandins, which in turn diminishes the inflammatory response. Prostaglandins are mediators of the inflammatory process as they initiate vasodilation, increase capillary permeability, and attract inflammatory cells to areas of cell damage, leading to pain and inflammation (Smith *et al*. 1991; Mitchell *et al*. 1995). They also have important cardiovascular, renal, and gastrointestinal (GI) regulatory functions (Warden 2009).

NSAIDs are categorised by their selectivity for inhibiting the activity of the two isoforms of COX: COX-1 and COX-2. COX-1 is the constitutive form, which is expressed in a variety of cells including endothelial, gastric mucosal, blood platelet, and kidney cells. COX-2 is inducible and becomes overexpressed in cases of inflammation, such as when rheumatoid arthritis occurs or following skeletal muscle damage. Nonselective NSAIDs inhibit both COX-1 and COX-2 activity to some degree, whereas selective COX-2 inhibitors predominately inhibit COX-2 enzyme activity (Figure 19.1).

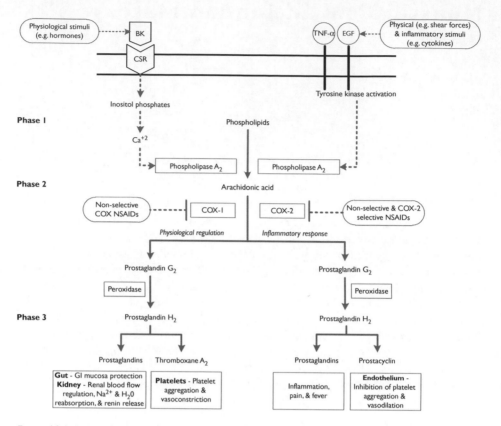

Figure 19.1 Biosynthesis of prostaglandins and the mode of action of NSAIDs.

There are three phases of prostaglandin production. **Phase 1**: mobilisation of arachidonic acid from cellular phospholipids which is caused by physiological, physical, and inflammatory stimuli; **Phase 2**: conversion of arachidonic acid to prostaglandin G_2 and then prostaglandin H_2; **Phase 3**: prostaglandin H_2 is converted to various derivatives including prostacyclin, prostaglandins, and thromboxane A_2 which have a number of physiological functions depending on in which cells they are produced and the types of stimuli that have activated their production.

BK, bradykinin; Ca^{2+}, calcium; CSR, cell surface receptor; COX, cyclo-oxygenase; EGF, endothelial growth factor; GI, gastrointestinal; H_2O, water; Na^{2+}, sodium; NSAIDs, non-steroidal anti-inflammatory drugs; TNF-α, tumour nuclear factor-alpha.

19.3. Clinical uses and efficacy of NSAIDs

NSAIDs are administered by oral, topical, intramuscular, and less commonly by intravenous routes. They are routinely used to relieve pain following operative procedures and when associated with fever, headaches, migraines, and dysmenorrhea (Day and Graham 2013). Low-dose aspirin, unlike other NSAIDs, is prescribed to individuals at high risk of having a heart attack or stroke because it has specific antiplatelet effects that reduce the likelihood of these cardiovascular events from occurring (Joint Formulary Committee 2014a). NSAIDs are also useful as adjunctive medication in the treatment of rheumatic conditions, such as rheumatoid arthritis, osteoarthritis, gout, and lupus. There are approximately twenty NSAIDs available for clinical use in the UK, some of which are available for general purchase (Table 19.1).

Table 19.1 Examples of selective and nonselective COX inhibitors available in the United Kingdom

Type	Nonproprietary name	Proprietary name
Nonselective NSAIDs (only available as POM)	Aceclofenac	Preservex
	Acemetacin	Emflex
	Dexibuprofen	Seractil
	Dexketoprofen	Keral
	Etodolac	Eccoxolac, Etopan, Lodine
	Indomethacin	Indocid, Indolar
	Ketorolac	Acular, Toradol
	Ketoprofen	Axorid, Ketocid, Orudis, Oruvail, Powergel
	Mefenamic acid	Ponstan
	Nabumetone	Reflex
	Piroxicam	Brexidol, Feldene
	Tenoxicam	Mobiflex
	Tiaprofenic acid	Surgam
	Tolfenamic acid	Clotam
Nonselective NSAIDs (available as GSL, P, or POM)	Aspirin (GSL, P, POM)	Anadin, Asasantin, Beechams, Codis, Disprin
	Diclofenac (P, POM)	Arthrotec, Diclomax, Dyloject, Econac, Fenactol, Motifene, Rheumatac, Rhumalgan, Solaraze, Volsaid, Voltarol
	Flurbiprofen (P, POM)	Froben, Ocufen, Strefen
	Ibuprofen (GSL, P, POM)	Anadin, Brufen, Calprofen, Cuprofen, Feminax, Fenbid, Fenpaed, Hedex, Ibuderm, Ibugel, Ibuleve, Ibumousse, Ibuspray, Lemsip, Nurofen, Nuromol, Pedea, Phorpain, Soleve, Solpadeine, Sudafed
	Naproxen (P, POM)	Feminax, Napratec, Naprosyn
Selective COX-2 inhibitors (only available as POM)	Celecoxib	Celebrex
	Etoricoxib	Arcoxia
	Parecoxib	Dynastat

COX, cyclo-oxygenase; GSL, general sales list; NSAID, nonsteroidal anti-inflammatory drug; P, pharmacy; POM, prescription-only medicine.

In sport, NSAIDs are used to treat a wide range of acute musculoskeletal injuries, such as ligament sprains, ligament and muscle tendon strains, muscle contusions, and muscle soreness (Almekinders 1999; Paoloni *et al.* 2009). They are also used in painful chronic musculoskeletal conditions, such as osteoarthritis, tenosynovitis, inflammatory bursitis, and soft-tissue injuries involving nerve impingement (Almekinders 1999; Paoloni *et al.* 2009). These acute and chronic injuries provoke an inflammatory response that results in pain, stiffness, swelling, and consequently a loss of function. Athletes require analgesic drugs to inhibit the pain component of the injury. However, because these injuries are also normally associated with an inflammatory element, the logical choice is to use an NSAID instead of an analgesic to counter both components together. The inflammatory process at times can also be excessive and cause oedema, resulting in anoxia and further cell death (Paoloni *et al.* 2009). In these instances, NSAIDs may be beneficial by acting to restrict the amount of inflammation and oedema that appears.

Inflammation is an important step in the healing process of injury because it facilitates the removal of cellular debris and damaged tissue, which allows healing to begin. There is increasing evidence, albeit mainly from animal studies, that NSAIDs have a deleterious effect on long-term tissue regeneration as a result of preventing inflammation. Indeed, long-term tendon (Marsolais *et al.* 2003; Cohen *et al.* 2006), ligament (Elder *et al.* 2001; Warden *et al.* 2006), and muscle (Thorsson *et al.* 1998; Shen *et al.* 2005) healing has been found to be impaired in animal models with acute injury. Regular use may also impair bone healing following fracture due to the inhibition of COX-2 (Simon and O'Connor 2007; Geusens *et al.* 2013).

Knowledge of the effect of NSAID use on tissue healing in humans is largely unknown. Whilst animal data may have limited translation to the clinical setting, the clinical implications of animal models infers that in humans prolonged use will likely enhance injury susceptibility, impair mechanical strength, and delay injury repair. There is also a potential concern that prolonged use of NSAIDs may impair the adaptive response to exercise by impairing protein metabolism (Trappe *et al.* 2002) and satellite cell activity (Mackey *et al.* 2007). Many athletes are thought to take NSAIDs prophylactically, which may be contraindicative to the aim of resistance training, although this has yet to be proven (Warden 2009). In contrast, short-term use of NSAIDs does not seem to have a detrimental effect on postexercise protein synthesis in humans, despite a detrimental effect in animal models (Schoenfield 2012).

NSAID use is controversial in the treatment of injuries where inflammation is not the primary feature (Magra and Maffulli 2006; Paoloni *et al.* 2009). In chronic tendinopathies, NSAIDs are used with the primary goal to relieve pain, which may lead to further damage if individuals ignore the early symptoms of the injury due to pain masking (Magra and Maffulli 2006). In such scenarios, the use of an NSAID over paracetamol is questionable because inflammation is not present and paracetamol has an analgesic action comparable to NSAIDs, but with fewer potential side effects (Woo *et al.* 2005; Dalton and Schweinie 2006). Furthermore, evidence-based working groups on pain management recommend using paracetamol as first-line treatment in chronic musculoskeletal pain management (Schnitzer 2006; Paoloni *et al.* 2009).

19.4. Adverse effects of NSAIDs

NSAIDs are not without their adverse effects, especially when administered at high doses or for a prolonged period. The use of nonselective NSAIDs can lead to GI side effects, including dyspepsia, haemorrhage, intestinal bleeding, peptic ulceration, and perforation (Wolfe *et al.* 1999; Michels *et al.* 2012). These side effects occur due to the direct toxic effects of NSAIDs on the gastroduodenal mucosa and their indirect effects, whereby they decrease the synthesis of prostaglandins that normally protect the gastroduodenal mucosa from hydrochloric acid damage (Schoen and Vender 1989; Wolfe *et al.* 1999).

Selective COX-2 inhibitors have been introduced to clinical practice, with the aim of inhibiting the formation of inflammatory prostaglandins without inhibiting COX-1 activity. A lower incidence of adverse GI effects has been observed with the use of selective COX-2 inhibitors compared to traditional nonselective NSAIDs (Deeks *et al.* 2002; Takemoto *et al.* 2008). However, COX-2 inhibitors have also been associated with cardiovascular events because they disturb the prostacyclin-thromboxane balance, thereby increasing the risk of the development of prothrombotic states (Burnier 2005; Warden 2005). The adverse cardiovascular effect profile of rofecoxib has even led this particular COX-2 inhibitor to be withdrawn from the market (Burnier 2005; Day and Graham 2013). It is unknown whether this is an isolated drug effect or a class-specific problem.

NSAIDs are known to have adverse effects on kidney function. The occurrence of renal dysfunction in the form of hyponatremia has been observed during endurance (Walker *et al.* 1994; Baker *et al.* 2005) and ultraendurance exercise (Wharam *et al.* 2006; Page *et al.* 2007) in athletes taking either selective or nonselective NSAIDs. Acute renal changes during exercise are thought to be regulated predominantly via COX-2 inhibition because selective COX-2 inhibitors and nonselective NSAIDs both induce significant inhibition of free water clearance (Baker *et al.* 2005). Changes in renal function as a result of prolonged use of NSAIDs can also lead to renal failure and consequently result in the need for a kidney transplant. In 2007, Croatian footballer Ivan Klasnic suffered kidney failure, which he associated with the prolonged use of NSAIDs to recover from injury (McGrath 2012).

Topical NSAIDs in the form of creams, gels, sprays, and patches may limit some of these adverse effects. Topical preparations are appealing to use because plasma levels remain low, reducing the likelihood of adverse effects, and these preparations show good penetration of the drug through the skin to the underlying tissues (Singh and Roberts 1994). Clinical trials generally demonstrate that topical NSAIDs are slightly more effective than topical placebo preparations when used to relieve musculoskeletal pain when used to treat acute musculoskeletal conditions and are without the associated side effects of systemic NSAIDs (Massey *et al.* 2010).

19.5. Prevalence of use of NSAIDs in sport

Reports identifying the frequent use of NSAIDs by athletes are well documented. Approximately one in four athletes drug tested at the Sydney 2000 Olympic Games declared the use of an NSAID, with use occurring within 3 days of doping control (Corrigan and Kazlauskas 2003). The estimated frequency of NSAID use decreased at the Athens 2004 Olympic Games to one in ten athletes drug tested, although NSAIDs were still the most declared type of medication (Tsitsimpikou *et al.* 2009). In addition to multisport events, just over half of all football players at some point during each of the three Fédération Internationale de Football Association World Cups from 2002 to 2010) have been prescribed with an NSAID (Tscholl and Dvorak 2012).

Although these reports indicate that NSAIDs are the most commonly used class of medication by athletes, prevalence of use seems to differ depending on the type of sport. Elite Finnish athletes competing in speed and power sports were found to be more frequent users of NSAIDs than athletes in endurance or motor skill-based sports (Alaranta *et al.* 2006). Similarly, international-level athletes competing in power and sprint disciplines in track-and-field athletics declared using more NSAIDs than middle- and long-distance runners (Tscholl *et al.* 2010). Team sports (e.g. football, handball, volleyball) and sports involving the extensive use of upper and lower limbs (e.g. baseball, fencing, gymnastics, rowing, softball, tennis) appear to have the highest incidence of NSAID use, even above power- and speed-based sports, according to data gathered from the 1996 and 2000 Canadian Olympic teams (Huang *et al.* 2006) and medication declarations monitored over a 4-year period from doping control forms analysed by the Ghent World Anti-Doping Agency (WADA)-accredited laboratory (van Thuyne and Delbeke, 2008).

The above reports do not explore the reasons why NSAIDs are the most frequently used type of medication amongst athletes. In a comparison study, it was estimated that athletes use approximately fourfold more NSAIDs than age-matched controls from the general population (Alaranta *et al.* 2006). Such higher usage rates are likely to be primarily reflective of the greater occurrence of musculoskeletal injuries as a result of the physical demands of sport over normal daily activities and common disorders encountered such as fever, headaches, and migraines. The specific injury profile (i.e. the rate of acute or chronic injuries) and the physical demands of a sport are also likely to account for some of the observed differences between the types of sports in which higher rates of use are observed.

There is also the potential for the overuse of NSAIDs within the athlete population. Athletes have relatively unrestricted access to these drugs because many can be purchased over the counter or via the internet, and the class of drug itself is not regulated by WADA (2014). It has become apparent that some athletes use at least two different preparations concurrently (Corrigan and Kazlauskas 2003; Tscholl *et al.* 2008; Tsitsimpikou *et al.* 2009), which increases the risk of experiencing side effects. In other cases, use has been found to occur on a prophylactic basis in an attempt to prevent the onset of pain associated with muscle contusions and the delayed onset of muscle soreness (Warner *et al.* 2002; Tscholl *et al.* 2008). Use may even form part of an athlete's precompetition routine or superstition rather than being due to an actual therapeutic need (Warden 2009).

19.6. Summary

- NSAIDs possess analgesic, anti-inflammatory, antipyretic, and antithrombotic properties as they inhibit COX activity, which prevents the production of prostaglandins.
- COX-1 and COX-2 are responsible for the production of different prostaglandins. Nonselective NSAIDs inhibit both COX-1 and COX-2 activity to some degree, whereas selective COX-2 inhibitors predominately inhibit COX-2 enzyme activity.
- NSAIDs are widely used in sports medicine to treat acute and chronic musculoskeletal injuries to reduce pain and inflammation and allow the early return of an athlete to activity.
- The potential beneficial effect of NSAIDs in the early phase of injury when inflammatory signs and symptoms are present is not maintained in the long term, and may even delay the repair process if use becomes prolonged.
- The use of NSAIDs in the treatment of fractures, muscle strains, and chronic tendinopathies is controversial. In these scenarios, paracetamol appears to be a more suitable first-line treatment option because it has a similar analgesic efficacy to NSAIDs and has a lower side-effect profile.
- NSAID-induced inhibition of prostaglandin formation can lead to adverse GI, renal, and cardiovascular effects if NSAIDs are used for prolonged periods of time, at high doses, or concurrently with multiple NSAIDs.
- NSAIDs are not prohibited in sport and are readily available over the counter.
- It would appear that NSAIDs are overused by athletes.

19.7. References

Alaranta, A., Alaranta, H., Heliövaara, M., Airaksinen, M., and Helenius, I. (2006). Ample use of physician-prescribed medications in Finnish elite athletes. *Int J Sports Med* 27(11): 919–925.

Almekinders, L. C. (1999). Anti-inflammatory treatment of muscular injuries in sport: An update of recent studies. *Sports Med* 28(6):383–388.

Baker, J., Cotter, J. D., Gerrard, D. F., *et al.* (2005). Effects of indomethacin and celecoxib on renal function in athletes. *Med Sci Sports Exerc* 37(5):712–717.

Burnier, M. (2005). The safety of rofecoxib. *Expert Opin Drug Saf* 4(3):491–499.

Cohen, D. B., Kawamura, S., Ehteshami, J. R., and Rodeo, S. A. (2006). Indomethacin and celecoxib impair rotator cuff tendon-to-bone healing. *Am J Sports Med* 34(3):362–369.

Corrigan, B., and Kazlauskas, R. (2003). Medication use in athletes selected for doping control at the Sydney Olympics. *Clin J Sports Med* 13(1):33–40.

Dalton, J. D., and Schweinie, J. E. (2006). Randomized controlled noninferiority trial to compare extended release acetaminophen and ibuprofen for the treatment of ankle sprains. *Ann Emerg Med* 48(5):615–623.

Day, R. O., and Graham, G. G. (2013). Republished research: Non-steroidal anti-inflammatory drugs (NSAIDs). *Br J Sports Med* 47(17):1127.

Deeks, J. J., Smith, L. A., and Bradley, M. D. (2002). Efficacy, tolerability, and upper gastrointestinal safety of celecoxib for treatment of osteoarthritis and rheumatoid arthritis: Systematic review of randomised controlled trials. *BMJ* 325(7365):619.

Elder, C. L., Dahners, L. E., and Weinhold, P. S. (2001). A cyclooxygenase-2 inhibitor impairs ligament healing in the rat. *Am J Sports Med* 29(6):801–805.

Geusens, P., Emans, P. J., de Jong, J. J., and van den Bergh, J. (2013). NSAIDs and fracture healing. *Curr Opin Rheumatol* 25(4):524–531.

Huang, S.-H., Johnson, K., and Pipe, A. L. (2006). The use of dietary supplements and medications by Canadian Athletes at the Atlanta and Sydney Olympic Games. *Clin J Sport Med* 16(1):27–33.

Joint Formulary Committee. (2014a). Cardiovascular system. London, UK: BMJ Group and Pharmaceutical Press. Available online at http://www.medicinescomplete.com/mc/bnf/current/PHP1519-antiplatelet-drugs.htm (accessed 26 February 2014).

Joint Formulary Committee. (2014b). Musculoskeletal and joint diseases. London, UK: BMJ Group and Pharmaceutical Press. Available online at http://www.medicinescomplete.com/mc/bnf/current/PHP6379-non-steroidal-anti-inflammatory-drugs.htm (accessed 26 February 2014).

Mackey, A. L., Kjaer, M., Dandanell, S., Mikkelsen, K. H., Holm, L., Døssing, S., et al. (2007). The influence of anti-inflammatory medication on exercise-induced myogenic precursor cell responses in humans. *J Appl Physiol* 103(2):425–431.

Magra, M., and Maffulli, N. (2006). Nonsteroidal antiinflammatory drugs in tendinopathy: Friend or foe. *Clin J Sport Med* 16(1):1–3.

Marsolais, D., Côté, C. H., and Frenetta, J. (2003). Nonsteroidal anti-inflammatory drug reduces neutrophil and macrophage accumulation but does not improve tendon regeneration. *Lab Invest* 83(7):991–999.

Massey, T., Derry, S., Moore, R. A., and McQuay, H. J. (2010). Topical NSAIDs for acute pain in adults. *Cochrane Database Syst. Rev* 6:1–99.

McGrath, M. (2012). FIFA alarmed at widespread 'abuse' of painkillers. Available online at http://www.bbc.co.uk/news/science-environment-18064904 (accessed 24 February 2014).

Michels, S. L., Collins, J., Reynolds, M. W., Abramsky, S., Paredes-Diaz, A., and McCarberg, B. (2012). Over-the-counter ibuprofen and risk of gastrointestinal bleeding complications: A systematic literature review. *Curr Med Res Opin* 28(1):89–99.

Mitchell, J. A., Larkin, S., and Williams, T. J. (1995). Cyclooxygenase-2: Regulation and relevance in inflammation. *Biochem Pharmacol* 50(10):1535–1542.

Page, A. J., Reid, S. A., Speedy, D. B., Mulligan, G. P., and Thompson, J. (2007). Exercise-associated hyponatremia, renal function, and nonsteroidal antiinflammatory drug use in an ultraendurance mountain run. *Clin J Sport Med* 17(1):43–48.

Paoloni, J. A., Milne, C., Orchard, J., and Hamilton, B. (2009). Non-steroidal anti-inflammatory drugs in sports medicine: Guidelines for practical but sensible use. *Br J Sports Med* 43(11):863–865.

Schnitzer, T. J. (2006). Update on guidelines for the treatment of chronic musculoskeletal pain. *Clin Rheumatol* 25(Suppl 1):S22–S29.

Schoen, R. T., and Vender, R. J. (1989). Mechanisms of nonsteroidal anti-inflammatory drug-induced gastric damage. *Am J Med* 86(4):449–458.

Schoenfeld, B. J. (2012). The use of nonsteroidal anti-inflammatory drugs for exercise-induced muscle damage: Implications for skeletal muscle development. *Sports Med* 42(12):1017–1028.

Shen, W., Li, Y., Tang, Y., Cummins, J., and Huard, J. (2005). NS-398, a cyclooxygenase-2-specific inhibitor, delays skeletal muscle healing by decreasing regeneration and promoting fibrosis. *Am J Pathol* 167(4):1105–1117.

Simon, A. M., and O'Connor, J. P. (2007). Dose and time-dependent effects of cyclooxygenase-2 inhibition on fracture-healing. *J Bone Joint Surg Am* 89(3):500–511.

Singh, P., and Roberts, M. S. (1994). Skin permeability and local tissue concentrations of nonsteroidal anti-inflammatory drugs after topical application. *J Pharmacol Exp Ther* 268(1):144–151.

Smith, W. L., Marnett, L. J., and DeWitt, D. L. (1991). Prostaglandin and thromboxane biosynthesis. *Pharmacol Ther* 49(3):153–179.

Takemoto, J. K., Reynolds, J. K., Remsberg, C. M., Vega-Villa, K. R., and Davies, N. M. (2008). Clinical pharmacokinetic and pharmacodynamic profile of etoricoxib. *Clin Pharmacokinet* 47(11):703–720.

Thorsson, O., Rantanen, J., Hurme, T., and Kalimo, H. (1998). Effects of nonsteroidal antiinflammatory medication on satellite cell proliferation during muscle regeneration. *Am J Sports Med* 26(2):172–176.

Trappe, T. A., White, F., Lambert, C. P., Cesar, D., Hellerstein, M., and Evans, W. J. (2002). Effect of ibuprofen and acetaminophen on postexercise muscle protein synthesis. *Am J Physiol Endocrinol Metab* 282(3):E551–E556.

Tscholl, P., Alonso, J. M., Dollé, G., Junge, A., and Dvorak, J. (2010). The use of drugs and nutritional supplements in top-level track and field athletes. *Am J Sports Med* 38(1):133–140.

Tscholl, P. M., and Dvorak, J. (2012). Abuse of medication during international football competition in 2010 – lesson not learned. *Br J Sports Med* 46(16):1140–1141.

Tscholl, P. M., Junge, A., and Dvorak, J. (2008). The use of medication and nutritional supplements during FIFA World Cups 2002 and 2006. *Br J Sports Med* 42(9):725–730.

Tsitsimpikou, C., Tsiokanos, A., Tsarouhas, K., Schamasch, P., Fitch, K. D., Valasiadis, D., and Jamurtas, A. (2009). Medication use by athletes at the Athens 2004 Summer Olympic Games. *Clin J Sport Med* 19(1):33–38.

van Thuyne, W., and Delbeke, F. T. (2008). Declared use of medication in sports. *Clin J Sport Med* 18 (2):143–147.

Walker, R. J., Fawcett, J. P., Flannery, E. M., and Gerrard, D. F. (1994). Indomethacin potentiates exercise-induced reduction in renal hemodynamics in athletes. *Med Sci Sports Exerc* 26(11):1302–1306.

Warden, S. J. (2005). Cyclooxygenase-2 inhibitors (COXIBs): Beneficial or detrimental for athletes with acute musculoskeletal injuries? *Sports Med* 35(4):271–283.

Warden, S. J. (2009). Prophylactic misuse and recommended use of non-steroidal antiinflammatory drugs by athletes. *Br J Sports Med* 43(8):548–549.

Warden, S. J., Avin, K. G., Beck, E. M., DeWolf, M. E., Hagemeier, M. A., and Martin, K. M. (2006). Low-intensity pulsed ultrasound accelerates and a nonsteroidal anti-inflammatory drug delays knee ligament healing. *Am J Sports Med* 34(7):1094–1102.

Warner, D. C., Schnepf, G., Barrett, M. S., Dian, D., and Swigonski, N. L. (2002). Prevalence, attitudes, and behaviors related to the use of nonsteroidal anti-inflammatory drugs (NSAIDs) in student athletes. *J Adolesc Health* 30(3):150–153.

Wharam, P. C., Speedy, D. B., Noakes, T. D., Thompson, J. M., Reid, S. A., and Holtzhausen, L. M. (2006). NSAID use increases the risk of developing hyponatremia during an Ironman triathlon. *Med Sci Sports Exerc* 38(4):618–622.

Wolfe, M. M., Lichtenstein, D. R., and Singh, G. (1999). Gastrointestinal toxicity of nonsteroidal anti-inflammatory drugs. *N Engl J Med* 340(24):1888–1899.

Woo, W. W., Man, S. Y., Lam, P. K., and Rainer, T. H. (2005). Randomized double-blind trial comparing oral paracetamol and oral nonsteroidal antiinflammatory drugs for treating pain after musculoskeletal injury. *Ann Emerg Med* 46(4):352–361.

World Anti-Doping Agency. (2014). 2014 List of Prohibited Substances and Methods. Available online at https://www.wada-ama.org/en/what-we-do/prohibited-list (accessed 9 September 2014).

Chapter 20

Over-the-counter stimulants

Neil Chester

20.1. Introduction

The term *over-the-counter* (OTC) in relation to pharmaceuticals refers to products used primarily for the treatment of conditions that do not require direct medical attention. These are nonprescription drugs that may be sold over-the-counter at pharmacies or available on general sale off the shelf at various retail outlets, including supermarkets. In recent decades, the classification of many drugs has changed as issues regarding their safety have been clarified. Some prescription drugs have been reclassified and arc now sold over-the-counter and even off-the-shelf, such as ibuprofen. Conversely, some OTC drugs have been withdrawn from the market in many countries following issues surrounding their safety (e.g. phenylpropanolamine).

Whilst there are countless drugs available over-the-counter, it is typically the stimulants that are deemed to be potential performance enhancers in sport. For this reason, there are currently a number of OTC stimulants whose use is prohibited in sport (Table 20.1). Many of these stimulants, known collectively as sympathomimetic amines, are contained in numerous OTC preparations for the treatment of symptoms associated with upper respiratory tract (URT) conditions, such as the common cold, sinusitis, and seasonal rhinitis. In addition, methylxanthines, including caffeine and related substances, are stimulants commonly found in OTC preparations; however, their use is permitted in sport. Products designed specifically to increase alertness and combat drowsiness typically contain methylxanthines. Also, both sympathomimetic amines and methylxanthines are common constituents of products designed to promote weight loss.

From an anti-doping perspective, it would seem that it is the ubiquitous nature of the use of OTC stimulants for therapeutic purposes that poses the most difficult problem in regulating their use. Also, inclusion of specific urinary thresholds and prohibition limited to periods of competition add to the confusion with regards to their legitimate use.

20.2. Upper respiratory tract conditions and exercise

There is evidence to support a causal link between intense exercise and the incidence of URT infection (Nieman *et al.* 1990; Heath *et al.* 1991). In the case of male endurance runners, there appears to be a dose-related effect of exercise training on the risk of URT infection (Heath *et al.* 1991; Nieman *et al.* 1990; Peters and Bateman 1983). This relationship is highlighted by the J-curve model proposed by Nieman *et al.* (1993), whereby the risk of URT infection is reduced below that of sedentary individuals when engaged in

Table 20.1 Over-the-counter stimulants and their status in sport

Stimulant	Permitted*	Prohibited in competition**
Sympathomimetic amines		
Ephedrine		✓
Norephedrine	✓	
Pseudoephedrine		✓
Norpseudoephedrine***		✓
Phenylephrine	✓	
p-Synephrine	✓	
Methylxanthines		
Caffeine	✓	
Theobromine	✓	
Theophylline	✓	

Source: World Anti-Doping Agency (2013a).
* Norephedrine (phenylpropanolamine), phenylephrine, p-synephrine, and caffeine are part of the WADA Monitoring Program.
** Ephedrine, pseudoephedrine, and norpseudoepedrine are prohibited when concentrations in urine are above 10, 150, and 5 µg/ml, respectively.
*** Norpseudoephedrine (cathine) is not available as an OTC stimulant but is commonly detected in urine as a metabolite of pseudoephedrine.

mild- to moderate-intensity exercise training and increased when engaged in high-intensity, high-volume exercise training. However, a direct link between infection and disturbed immune function in athletes has not been fully established. There is evidence that there are important cofactors in the immune response to exercise including diet, lifestyle, and stress (König *et al.* 2000).

20.3. Treatment of upper respiratory tract conditions

Conditions that affect the URT, the symptoms of which can be managed through the use of OTC preparations, include viral or bacterial infections such as the common cold, influenza, pharyngitis, laryngitis, sinusitis, and allergic reactions such as seasonal allergic rhinitis. Symptoms are a consequence of an immune response to the infection or allergic reaction and at the very least are viewed as a nuisance. However, symptoms may be an important part of recovery from infection, and whether symptomatic treatment using OTC preparations affects the recovery time course of URT infection is unclear (Eccles 2005).

The number of OTC medications available for the treatment of symptoms associated with URT conditions is vast. OTC cough, cold, and influenza (flu) preparations available in the United Kingdom during 2012 had a market value of more than £452 million. OTC products available in the United Kingdom for the specific treatment of allergy and hay fever symptoms had a market value totalling more than £88 million in 2012 (Proprietary Association of Great Britain 2013).

The common cold and influenza

Both the common cold and influenza share similar symptoms and are caused by viral infections of the URT. Symptoms typical of cold and flu include pharyngitis, rhinorrhoea, sneezing, nasal congestion, and cough. In addition, flu is characterised by fever, extreme lethargy, and muscle and joint pain. Whilst the symptoms of the common cold gradually present themselves over the first 3 days after infection, the onset of flu symptoms is usually sudden. Both conditions normally last for approximately 5 to 7 days. Headache and sinusitis may also be symptoms.

Although effective vaccines are available to prevent flu, they are generally limited to those who are at specific risk from a bout of flu, such as the elderly and young or those working in environments where the risk of spread of infection is particularly high (e.g. health care professionals and those working in child care). Flu sufferers who have not been immunised or those with the common cold must rely on self-management involving the intake of additional fluids to combat the loss as a consequence of fever. Steam inhalations also help to hydrate the tissues of the URT and reduce congestion. In addition, sufferers may choose to use one of the many OTC preparations available to alleviate the symptoms. Cold and flu medication may contain the following drugs:

- Sympathomimetic amines – to act as decongestants and bronchodilators
- Methylxanthines – to act as bronchodilators
- Analgesics – to relieve pain and act as centrally acting cough suppressants
- Antihistamines – to suppress cough and inhibit sneezing
- Expectorants – to loosen and increase bronchial secretions to enable removal via coughing.

Sinusitis

Sinusitis is an inflammatory condition typically caused by a viral or bacterial infection of the mucosal lining of the paranasal sinuses. It typically presents itself following a URT infection and rhinitis; hence, rhinosinusitis is now considered to be a more accurate name for the condition (Ryan 2008). Rhinosinusitis may be classified as acute or chronic, depending on whether the condition lasts for less than or more than 12 weeks.

A wide range of symptoms are typically experienced, including nasal congestion, nasal discharge, facial discomfort, headache, and hyposmia (limited or no sense of smell). Decongestants, namely sympathomimetic amines, may be used to relieve a blocked nose and ease breathing. Also, analgesics maybe used to relieve headache and facial pain. However, as with other URT conditions, the use of OTC medications simply helps in alleviating the symptoms. Antibiotics may be prescribed if sinusitis is particularly troublesome and persistent.

Allergic rhinitis

Allergic rhinitis is a condition characterised by an allergic hypersensitivity reaction in the nasal mucosa caused by exposure to pollen or other allergens. Symptoms include rhinorrhoea, sneezing, nasal congestion, nasal itching, and itching and watering of the eyes. It affects more than 20 per cent of the UK population (Scadding *et al.* 2008). When the trigger is pollen, the condition is known as seasonal allergic rhinitis or hay fever. Grass pollen is the most common cause of hay fever, with other major allergens including tree pollen, particularly birch, and pollen from weeds such as plantains, mugwort, and docks (Nathan 2002). Allergens that may trigger allergic rhinitis other than plant pollen include fungal spores, fur from cats and dogs, cockroaches, and the house dust mite. Epidemiological data suggest that those suffering from asthma typically suffer from allergic rhinitis (Leynaert *et al.* 1999), with both sharing similar triggers and pathophysiology. Allergic rhinitis is also a risk factor for the development of asthma (Scadding *et al.* 2008). Management of coexisting asthma and allergic rhinitis should be as directed by a physician.

Allergic rhinitis occurs as a consequence of a type 1 hypersensitivity response, whereby exposure to an allergen results in production of specific immunoglobulin E (IgE). The IgE then attaches to mast cells and basophils of the nasal mucosa and conjunctiva of the eye, resulting in sensitisation. Subsequent exposure to the allergen results in an antigen–antibody response, causing basophils and mast cell degranulation and release of inflammatory mediators such as histamine, cytokines, leukotrienes, interleukins, and prostaglandins. Such mediators cause vasodilation and increased permeability of blood vessels that result in local oedema and irritation of nerve endings, thus leading to the characteristic eye and nasal itching.

The goals of treatment of allergic rhinitis include the following (Price *et al.* 2006):

- Unimpaired sleep
- Ability to undertake normal daily activities, including work and school attendance, without limitation or impairment
- Ability to participate fully in sport and leisure activities
- No troublesome symptoms
- No or minimal side effects of treatment.

In addition to reducing the exposure to allergens, treatment includes the use of OTC oral and topical (intranasal and ocular) preparations, which include antihistamines and also sympathomimetics. Oral antihistamines are effective in the treatment of rhinorrhoea, sneezing, nasal itching, and conjunctivitis. Antihistamines limit rhinitis by attaching themselves to the H_1 receptors and acting as antagonists, thus reducing capillary permeability and excessive mucus production. The overall decrease in mucus production complements the effects of sympathomimetics. Both oral and topical sympathomimetic amines, such as phenylephrine and oxymetazoline, may be useful in reducing nasal congestion. Nasal sprays are particularly useful in alleviating severe congestion; however, they should not be used for prolonged periods due to the risk of developing rhinitis medicamentosa (i.e. rebound congestion) and possible mucosal damage (Graf 1997).

20.4. Weight loss

Whilst weight loss products may be useful to the athlete by increasing lean body mass, they are often the domain of those interested in image enhancement, such as the bodybuilder. However, with the levels of obesity increasing and the increased attention on body image, there is a growing market for weight loss products amongst the general public.

Whilst their efficacy is questionable, current OTC weight loss products typically contain herbal extracts that contain a number of active ingredients, including sympathomimetic amines, methylxanthines, and acetylsalicylic acid (aspirin). Such products may act directly via adrenergic receptors to produce thermogenic or lipolytic effects or indirectly via serotonergic pathways in the hypothalamus to bring about appetite suppression (anorectics). The popularity of combining ephedrine, caffeine, and aspirin (i.e. ECA stack) in weight management would appear to be related to the purported synergistic effects of theses three substances. The dampening of the thermogenic effects of sympathomimetics caused by the negative feedback mechanisms is said to be reduced by both methylxanthines and aspirin (Dulloo 1993).

20.5. Relief from fatigue and drowsiness

Fatigue and drowsiness are common conditions experienced in response to poor sleep hygiene and poor work–rest balance. However, chronic fatigue may be symptomatic of a more serious underlying problem, such as depression, diabetes mellitus, hypothyroidism, heart disease, or cancer, and requires medical attention. Whilst there are numerous pharmacological treatments, it is important to assess and address the root cause of the symptoms.

Nevertheless, the treatment of acute fatigue and drowsiness can be successfully managed in the short term through the use of one of numerous OTC products available on the market. Such products generally contain methylxanthines, typically caffeine. Some products have herbal ingredients that contain natural sources of both methylxanthines and sympathomimetic amines. The ingredients are intended to increase alertness and combat drowsiness through activation of the release of central neurotransmitters such as dopamine (sympathomimetic amines) and affecting dopamine transmission by displacement of adenosine at A1 and A2 receptors (methylxanthines).

They are often marketed as energy supplements because they combat symptoms of fatigue and contain high quantities of caffeine. Energy drinks are extremely popular amongst adults and children alike and are a central component of the supplements designed to combat drowsiness. However, there are serious concerns regarding the regulation of these products and consequently the level of caffeine in these drinks, as well as the aggressive marketing campaigns targeted largely at young adults. This has led to significant use of these high-caffeine drinks amongst adolescents and children and increasing numbers of reports of caffeine intoxication following the consumption of such drinks (Reissig *et al.* 2009).

20.6. Sympathomimetic amines

Drugs that mimic the effects of the endogenous mediators of the sympathetic nervous system (i.e. adrenaline and noradrenaline) are referred to as sympathomimetic amines. Sympathomimetic amines work through direct activation of adrenoceptors or indirect activation via the stimulation of release of endogenous catecholamines. The response of any cell or organ to sympathomimetic amines is directly related to the density and proportion of α- and β-adrenoceptors present.

According to Hoffman (2001), the actions of sympathomimetic amines can be classified into the following types:

- Peripheral stimulatory action on vascular smooth muscle in blood vessels supplying the skin, kidneys, mucous membranes, and glandular smooth muscle in salivary and sweat glands
- Peripheral inhibitory action on the smooth muscle of the gut wall, the bronchioles, and the blood vessels supplying the skeletal muscles
- Cardiac excitatory action, inducing increased heart rate and force of contraction
- Metabolic actions, including increased rate of glycogenolysis in the liver and muscles and mobilisation of free fatty acids from adipose tissue
- Endocrine actions, including regulation of the secretion of insulin, renin, and pituitary hormones
- Central nervous system (CNS) actions, including respiratory stimulation, increased wakefulness, psychomotor activity, and reduction in appetite
- Presynaptic actions resulting in the inhibition or facilitation of release of neurotransmitters, such as acetylcholine and noradrenaline.

Not all sympathomimetic amines display all of the actions mentioned to a similar extent.

The profile of effects of each sympathomimetic amine is determined by its relative affinity for the subgroups of adrenoceptors and forms the basis for their classification. Beta$_2$-receptors are located on airway smooth muscle and cause bronchodilation when stimulated. Alpha$_1$-receptors are located on arterial smooth muscle and cause vasoconstriction when stimulated. Consequently, β_2-agonists (e.g. salbutamol) are used as bronchodilators to treat asthma, whilst α_1-agonists (e.g. phenylephrine) are used as vasoconstrictors to treat symptoms of the common cold and associated URT conditions. The primary role of sympathomimetic amines in the treatment of URT conditions is to act as decongestants. When the mucous membranes lining the nose and paranasal sinuses are irritated by infection or allergy, the blood vessels supplying the membrane become enlarged. This leads to fluid accumulation in the surrounding tissue and encourages the production of larger than normal amounts of mucus. Alpha$_1$-agonists cause constriction of the blood vessels, thus reducing the swelling in the lining of the nose and sinuses and acting as decongestants. The most widely available α_1-agonists present in OTC medications include ephedrine, its stereoisomer pseudoephedrine, and phenylephrine. These sympathomimetics pose several potential problems for the sportsperson. First, they can cause significant side effects. Also, the use of both ephedrine and pseudoephedrine is prohibited in competition according to the 2014 World Anti-Doping Agency (WADA 2013a) Prohibited List (Table 20.1).

Potential side effects of sympathomimetic amines

Decongestants, although widely available in OTC preparations, are potent vasoconstrictors. In the United Kingdom, ephedrine is licensed for the treatment of hypotension caused by spinal or epidural anaesthesia and phenylephrine is licensed for the treatment of acute hypotension. Ephedrine, phenylephrine, and pseudoephedrine use is contraindicated in hypertensive patients.

The use of ephedrine has been linked to cardiomyopathy (To et al. 1980) and stroke (Bruno et al. 1993), whilst pseudoephedrine use has also been linked with stroke (Cantu et al. 2003) and temporal coronary artery spasm and myocardial infarction (Weiner et al. 1990). Until fairly recently, phenylpropanolamine (PPA) was a common ingredient of OTC decongestant preparations. However, its use has been linked with hypertensive reactions, cerebral haemorrhage, and psychosis (Gibson and Warrell 1972; Norvenius et al. 1979; Berstein and Diskant 1982; Johnson et al. 1983; Kernan et al. 2000; Cantu et al. 2003). A study by Horwitz et al. (2000) demonstrated an odds ratio for association between haemorrhagic stroke and the use of PPA of 1.23 for cough and cold preparations and 15.92 for appetite suppressants.

According to the US Food and Drug Administration (FDA, 2005) Nonprescription Drugs Advisory Committee, the use of PPA in OTC medications is deemed unsafe. Thus, PPA has been removed from all OTC medications in the United States. However, in the United Kingdom, the Committee on Safety of Medicines, the expert group of the Medicines and Healthcare Products Regulatory Agency (2000) has not recommended a ban on PPA. It considers the evidence of the link between PPA use and haemorrhagic stroke to be weak and largely related to its use as an appetite suppressant – an application not licensed in the United Kingdom. Also, in the United Kingdom the recommended maximum dose for PPA contained in OTC products is lower than that in the United States (100 mg compared to 150 mg). Nevertheless, OTC products containing PPA have tended to be reformulated or withdrawn from the market in the United Kingdom (Arroll 2008).

Table 20.2 Recommended maximal therapeutic doses of common sympathomimetic amines in over-the-counter decongestant preparations

Sympathomimetic	Single dose (mg per 4–6 h)	Daily dose (mg)
Ephedrine	25	100
Phenylephrine	10	40
Pseudoephedrine	60	240

Therefore, from clinical data, it is clear that α_1-agonist sympathomimetic amines can evoke profound systemic cardiovascular side effects when taken orally. Moreover, these effects are both drug specific and dose dependent. The current recommended oral doses for common decongestants are shown in Table 20.2.

There have been numerous reports of the effects of sympathomimetic amines contained in OTC medicines upon cardiovascular parameters. Ephedrine administration (0.8 mg/kg body weight [BW]) was found to increase systolic blood pressure significantly before exercise (Jacobs *et al.* 2003). Doses equivalent to over three to four times the recommended therapeutic dose of pseudoephedrine raised diastolic blood pressure above 90 mm Hg (Drew *et al.*, 1978). These results were in accord with two other studies. Bye *et al.* (1974) reported significant increases in heart rate and systolic blood pressure following relatively high doses of ephedrine (50 mg) and pseudoephedrine (120 mg and 180 mg). Empey *et al.* (1980) found doses of 120 mg and 180 mg produced statistically significant increases in both pulse and systolic blood pressure. However, the increases were deemed to be clinically unimportant because they were considerably less than might be expected to occur in response to either emotion or mild exercise.

Whilst several studies have reported increased cardiovascular stimulation following ingestion of OTC sympathomimetics, it is evident that doses used were at least twice the recommended therapeutic dose. Reports of the effects following the ingestion of sympathomimetics in therapeutic doses have been conflicting. Bye *et al.* (1974) found that a single dose of ephedrine (25 mg) significantly elevated both heart rate and systolic blood pressure. In the same study, a single therapeutic dose of pseudoephedrine (60 mg) significantly elevated only systolic blood pressure, whilst Bright *et al.* (1981) found only a nonsignificant rise in resting heart rate following a single therapeutic dose. Empey *et al.* (1980) reported that ingestion of pseudoephedrine in a therapeutic dose of 60 mg provided maximal nasal decongestion without any cardiovascular or other side effects.

Few researchers have examined the effects of multiple dosing regimens on cardiovascular parameters. Chester (2000; unpublished data) found significant increases in blood pressure following a multiple, therapeutic dosing regimen for pseudoephedrine (i.e. six 60-mg doses over a 36-hour period). Bye *et al.* (1975) reported significant increases in heart rate but not systolic blood pressure after three different dose regimens, one involving two different sustained-release formulations. Prolonged administration of a sustained-release formulation of pseudoephedrine (180 mg twice daily for 2 weeks) increased heart rate and decreased systolic blood pressure.

In terms of action on the CNS, most evidence suggests that OTC sympathomimetics have no stimulatory effect in the relatively low doses used (Bye *et al.* 1975; Kuitunen *et al.* 1984). Bye *et al.* (1974) found that whilst pseudoephedrine lacked any stimulatory effect, even at supratherapeutic doses (180 mg), ephedrine possessed a stimulatory effect at therapeutic doses.

According to Wadler and Hainline (1989), OTC sympathomimetic amines exhibit fewer central stimulatory effects than amphetamines because they are less lipid soluble. Differences in central stimulation are related to differences in lipid solubility within the biological membranes; hence, penetration of the blood–brain barrier determines the ease with which these compounds gain access to central receptors (Lanciault and Wolf 1965).

Danger during endurance exercise has been associated with impaired thermoregulation as a result of the use of sympathomimetic amines. Clearly, the use of stimulants to mask the symptoms of fatigue may enable an individual to continue exercising in a hyperthermic state. Indeed, the deaths of several cyclists during major competition, most notably that of Tom Simpson on Mont Ventoux in the 1967 Tour de France, have been attributed to hyperthermia related to the use of amphetamine (Williams 1974). More recently, in 2003, Major League Baseball player Steve Bechler died as a result of heatstroke; his death was attributed to the use of excessive ephedrine contained in a weight reduction supplement (Charatan 2003). It is likely that hyperthermia is a consequence of increased motor activity and impaired thermoregulation. Although published studies have identified increased thermogenesis (Dulloo and Miller 1986) and a reduction in the drop in core temperature during exposure to low temperature (Vallerand 1993) following administration of ephedrine, no studies have assessed body temperature at comfortable ambient temperatures following the administration of ephedrines.

Reputed ergogenic effects

The sympathetic response involves a myriad of reactions that heighten the capacity of the body to respond to stressful situations. These actions enable an individual to perform physical activity and relate to an increased potential in terms of sports performance.

Amphetamines are structurally related to the OTC sympathomimetics and are possibly the most well known of stimulants prohibited by WADA. Enhanced performance following amphetamine administration may be explained by the fact that amphetamines appear to mask the body's symptoms of fatigue. Both ephedrine and pseudoephedrine are classified as prohibited substances because of their chemical similarity to amphetamines. Therefore, it is assumed that they, like amphetamine, have similar ergogenic properties. However, the literature regarding the effects of common OTC sympathomimetics on sports performance is limited.

Few studies have examined the effects of OTC stimulants on steady-state exercise. Bright et al. (1981) investigated the effects of pseudoephedrine on submaximal treadmill exercise. They concluded that pseudoephedrine in single or double therapeutic doses failed to cause significant cardiovascular and metabolic adjustments in healthy subjects during submaximal exercise. It was likely that any sympathoadrenergic effects that occurred as a result of drug administration were masked during exercise.

Most research that has attempted to elucidate the effects of such drugs on exercise has focused on exercise performance parameters. One of the most appropriate physiological indicators of physical endurance capacity is maximal oxygen consumption (VO_{2max}). An increase in this parameter following drug administration may indicate increased aerobic power and the potential for enhanced aerobic exercise performance. However, Sidney and Lefcoe (1977) found no effect of a therapeutic dose of ephedrine on VO_{2max}. Similarly, Swain et al. (1997) reported no effect of pseudoephedrine and phenylpropanolamine on maximal aerobic capacity following the administration of single or double the therapeutic dose. Clemons and Crosby (1993) examined the effect of a single therapeutic dose of pseudoephedrine prior to performance of a graded exercise test and found no difference in total exercise time to exhaustion.

In relation to time trial performance, Gillies *et al.* (1996) found no improvement in 40-km cycling following administration of double the therapeutic dose of pseudoephedrine. Similarly, Chester *et al.* (2003a) found no improvement in 5-km running performance following a multiple therapeutic dosing regimen of pseudoephedrine (i.e. six 60-mg doses over a 36-hour period). Work involving cycling time trial performance of approximately 30 minutes' duration has provided conflicting results (Pritchard-Peschek *et al.* 2010, 2013, 2014). Whilst Pritchard-Peschek *et al.* (2010) reported an improvement in performance of more than 5 per cent when three times the therapeutic dose of pseudoephedrine was administered when compared to placebo, later studies failed to show any improvement when comparable doses were administered (2.3 and 2.8 mg/kg BW; Pritchard-Peschek *et al.* 2013, 2014). Possible reasons for the disparity were attributed to the use of larger, homogeneous samples leading to lower variability in the data in the later studies. Doses of a similar magnitude (2.5 mg/kg BW) administered prior to more prolonged cycling exercise (approximately 3 hours) similarly had no effect on time trial performance (Betteridge *et al.* 2010).

As with prolonged endurance exercise, data pertaining to shorter duration, more intense exercise are no more convincing. Whilst Hodges *et al.* (2006) concluded that pseudoephedrine administration in greater than the therapeutic dose (i.e. 2.5 mg/kg BW) significantly improves 1,500-m run performance, a study examining 800-m run performance in female collegiate athletes reported no improvement using the same dosing regimen (Berry and Wagner 2012). Using comparable doses of pseudoephedrine (i.e. 180 mg), Gill *et al.* (2000) found a significant increase in peak power output during a 30-s sprint cycle test and maximum torque produced in an isometric knee extension exercise. Nevertheless, following the administration of a lower dose of pseudoephedrine (i.e. 120 mg), no improvements in muscle force production were reported according to a 30-s sprint cycle and maximal voluntary contraction of the muscles associated with dorsiflexion of the ankle and the handgrip exercise (Chu *et al.* 2002).

Whilst there is conjecture regarding the possible ergogenic effects of OTC sympathomimetic amines when administered alone, there is evidence to suggest that in combination with caffeine, pseudoephedrine (Weatherby and Rogerson 2002) and ephedrine (Bell *et al.* 1998, 2002) significantly improves exercise performance. Bell *et al.* (1998) investigated the time to exhaustion during high-intensity cycling exercise following ingestion of such a combination of drugs (5 mg/kg BW caffeine and 1 mg/kg BW ephedrine). Results showed a significant increase in time to exhaustion when compared with trials following placebo ingestion and ingestion of caffeine and ephedrine alone. These results were attributed to increased central nervous system stimulation. There is, however, a paucity of research that assesses the effect of combining caffeine with pseudoephedrine; thus, it requires further examination.

There has been considerable interest in the use of sympathomimetic drugs to promote weight loss by increasing energy expenditure and reducing food intake through appetite suppression. In an animal study performed by Ramsey *et al.* (1998), it was reported that energy expenditure was increased and in some animals, food intake was reduced following the administration of ephedrine and caffeine. Consequently, it was concluded that ephedrine and caffeine treatment could promote weight loss through its action as a thermogenic and anorectic. It appears that ephedrine is effective at increasing thermogenesis and has the potential to reduce body weight in obese individuals (Bukowiecki *et al.* 1982), especially when combined with caffeine or aspirin (Astrup and Toubro 1993). Boozer *et al.* (2001) found significant short-term reduction in weight amongst overweight and obese subjects following supplementation

Table 20.3 Urinary concentration thresholds for specific sympathomimetic amines, above which constitutes an adverse analytical finding

Prohibited substance	Urinary concentration (μg/ml)
Ephedrine	10
Pseudoephedrine	150
Cathine/norpseudoephedrine	5

Source: World Anti-Doping Agency (2013a).

of natural sources of ephedrine and caffeine (ma huang and guarana). However, there have been no studies that have focused on sympathomimetic drug use in nonobese, athletic populations to promote leanness.

Sympathomimetic amine use and WADA regulations

The use of specific sympathomimetic amines – namely ephedrine, pseudoephedrine, and cathine – are restricted by WADA. However, the detection of these substances in urine only constitutes an adverse analytical finding when their concentration is above a specific threshold (Table 20.3).

Prior to 2004, Chester *et al.* (2003b) found that athletes participating at a high level tended to avoid OTC medicines due to the concern that they may contain prohibited substances. Nevertheless, prohibited stimulants contained in readily available OTC products remain a significant proportion of the total number of stimulants accounting for adverse analytical findings (AAFs; Figure 20.1). According to data from the UK Anti-Doping programme

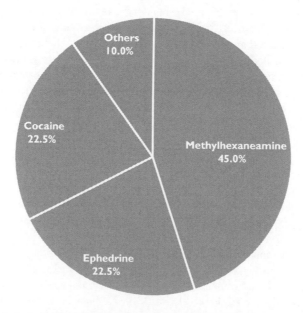

Figure 20.1 Anti-doping rule violations between 2009 and 2013 from the UK Anti-Doping's testing programme relating to the detection of prohibited stimulants (UK Anti-Doping, 2013).

between the years 2009 and 2013, a total of forty AAFs were attributed to stimulant use, of which a quarter involved the detection of ephedrine. On a global scale, during 2012, ephedrine accounted for twelve cases, whilst pseudoephedrine accounted for thirteen and cathine six cases (WADA 2013b).

Because cathine (norpseudoephedrine) is a metabolite of pseudoephedrine, when both are detected in an athlete's sample, the likelihood of cathine's presence being a consequence of pseudoephedrine administration is considered. Consequently, if its presence is above the threshold (or decision limit; see Chapter 4) whilst the concentration of pseudoephedrine is below its respective threshold (Table 20.3), consideration will be given as to whether the threshold has been breached as a consequence of the metabolism of pseudoephedrine (WADA 2013c).

In recent years the number of AAFs attributed to OTC stimulants have been overshadowed by the huge numbers of cases involving methylhexaneamine. Whilst methylhexaneamine, also known as 1,3-dimethylamylamine (DMAA), was originally developed as a nasal decongestant by the pharmaceutical company Eli Lilly, it was withdrawn in 1983 due to concerns regarding its safety (Bussel and Pavlov 2013). Recent doping cases have been as a consequence of the widespread use of preworkout and sliming products that contain the substance, often disguised by pseudonyms such as geranium extract or geranamine on labels. Although the problem has been highlighted due to a number of high-profile cases, there remains a significant number of AAFs involving methylhexaneamine that have been attributed to alleged inadvertent consumption of the substance. Further details on methylhexaneamine and the issues around dietary supplement use can be found in Chapter 21.

The potential for inadvertent doping involving the use of OTC medication would seem high, particularly as evidence suggests that elite athletes have limited knowledge surrounding OTC medication in relation to anti-doping legislation (Mottram et al. 2008). Nevertheless, there is evidence that demonstrates the intention for ephedrine and pseudoephedrine use amongst athletes may be solely for ergogenic purposes (Bents et al. 2004; Bents and Marsh 2006).

Since the introduction of the International Olympic Committee (IOC) prohibited list and drug testing, there have been numerous instances of positive tests for OTC sympathomimetic amines. In the 1972 Munich Olympics, Rick De Mont lost his gold medal in the 400-m freestyle after testing positive for ephedrine. He claimed that he had inadvertently taken ephedrine contained in asthma medication. In 1988, a number of US athletes, including the multi-Olympic champion Carl Lewis, tested positive for ephedrine prior to the Seoul Olympics. They were excused, having claimed that it had been taken inadvertently. In 1994, Diego Maradona was banished from the World Cup after testing positive for a cocktail of ephedrine and ephedrine-related substances. In 2000, the Russian synchronised swimmer Maria Kisseleva was stripped of her European duet title after testing positive for ephedrine. She claimed that it had been given to her by a team doctor to help her lose weight. She was only given a 1-month ban and subsequently won gold in Sydney. More recently, in 2009, the former Sheffield United and Irish International footballer Paddy Kenny received a 9-month ban following a positive test for ephedrine, believed to be as a consequence of using an OTC cold preparation containing ephedrine.

There have also been high-profile cases that have involved positive tests for pseudoephedrine. In 1988 at the Seoul Olympics, the UK and subsequent Olympic 100-m champion Linford Christie tested positive for pseudoephedrine. He was exonerated as he was believed to have taken the drug inadvertently as an ingredient of the Chinese health supplement ginseng. In 2000 at the Sydney Olympics, the IOC demonstrated rather less leniency when Andreea

Răducan, a Romanian gymnast, was stripped of her individual gold medal after testing positive for pseudoephedrine contained in cold medication prescribed by the team doctor. Whilst there was an unsuccessful appeal by Răducan, she did not receive a ban; however, the team doctor was banned from the next two Olympiads. Most recently, at the Sochi Olympics in 2014, the Swedish ice hockey player Nicklas Backstrom tested positive for pseudoephedrine and subsequently missed the gold medal match against Canada. However, as a National Hockey League (NHL) player, he did not serve any sanctions in relation to competition in the NHL because they were not signatories of the World Anti-Doping Code and do not classify pseudoephedrine as a prohibited substance.

In an attempt to reduce the number of positive cases, especially by those athletes using sympathomimetics for legitimate therapeutic reasons, the IOC introduced quantitative levels below which drug detection would not be deemed as a positive case. In recent years, these threshold levels have been revised in an attempt to differentiate between therapeutic use and misuse (Table 20.3). Between the years 2004 and 2010, pseudoephedrine was not classified as a prohibited substance but was part of WADA's Monitoring Program. The Monitoring Program introduced in 2004 enabled WADA to assess the use of particular substances that are open to inadvertent use due to their presence in numerous OTC preparations. Evidence from the programme together with support of its performance-enhancing effects from several scientific studies (Gill *et al*. 2000; Hodges *et al*. 2006) led to the reintroduction of pseudoephedrine on to the Prohibited List. In an attempt to address the extreme intersubject variability in the pharmacokinetics of OTC stimulants as demonstrated in studies by Lefebvre *et al*. (1992), Chester *et al*. (2004), and Strano-Rossi *et al*. (2009), WADA set the threshold of pseudoephedrine at 150 µg/ml. However, further research is needed regarding the pharmacokinetics of OTC stimulants if doping control is to successfully differentiate between therapeutic use and misuse.

20.7. Methylxanthines

Caffeine, theophylline, and theobromine are methylxanthines. In the United Kingdom, both caffeine and theophylline are common constituents of preparations for the treatment of symptoms associated with URT conditions. In addition, caffeine is typically the primary constituent of products designed to relieve fatigue and tiredness, as well as for many OTC weight loss preparations.

There are several commonly accepted mechanisms thought to account for the pharmacological and ergogenic effects of methylxanthines. These mechanisms include the inhibition of cyclic nucleotide phosphodiesterase enzymes that breakdown cyclic adenosine monophosphate (cAMP) and cyclic guanosine monophosphate (cGMP), increased sensitivity of intracellular Ca translocation, and antagonism of adenosine receptors. It is generally accepted that adenosine receptor antagonism is the most important mechanism. Stimulation of the adenosine receptors mediate inhibitory signals, resulting in effects such as suppressed neurotransmission, sedation, pain relief, bronchoconstriction, sodium retention and beta receptor antagonist. As antagonists, methylxanthines block these signals and therefore in effect lead to a stimulatory response. The effectiveness of methylxanthines is directly related to their affinity to the adenosine receptors, of which theophylline and paraxanthine are considered to be the most potent. The significance of this in relation to caffeine is that, following ingestion, caffeine is converted to theobromine, theophylline, and paraxanthine through demethylation in the liver.

Pharmacologically, methylxanthines (typically theophylline) are used for their bronchodilatory effects through inhibition of phosphodiesterase enzymes. However, the relatively high doses required to achieve significant bronchodilation are sufficient to induce side effects such as nausea, vomiting, and headaches, making their use undesirable by patients (Barnes 2006). Their CNS stimulatory properties are widely exploited, especially in products designed to combat fatigue and tiredness. Clearly, this effect has been used extensively in sport and underpins much of the use of caffeine as an ergogenic aid. Other uses of caffeine relate to its positive effect on endurance activity due to its reputed effect on the mobilisation of fatty acids, subsequent fat oxidation, and glycogen sparing. Also, this effect, in addition to its reputed ability to suppress appetite, makes caffeine and other methylxanthines ideal ingredients in weight reduction supplements.

Interest in the effects of caffeine on sports performance has been immense. The ingestion of moderate doses of caffeine (3–6 mg/kg BW) 60 minutes prior to exercise is associated with the enhancement of performance during prolonged, submaximal exercise (Graham and Spriet 1995; Pasman *et al.* 1995) and during high-intensity exercise of short (Jackman *et al.* 1996; Bruce *et al.* 2000) and moderate (MacIntosh and Wright 1995; Bruce *et al.* 2000) duration. Evidence suggesting such an effect on high power output and sprint performance is inconclusive (Collomp *et al.* 1992; Greer *et al.* 1998; Paton *et al.* 2001; Doherty *et al.* 2004). Research into the ergogenic effects of methylxanthines, other than caffeine, has been limited. However, Greer *et al.* (2000) examined the effects of both caffeine and theophylline on a time to exhaustion cycling protocol and concluded that both were ergogenic.

As discussed previously, caffeine is commonly supplemented with sympathomimetic amines (typically ephedrine) in an attempt to heighten its effect on exercise performance. However, whilst the addition of caffeine with ephedrine appears to augment its ergogenic effect, the mechanisms are not completely understood. It is likely that both substances have a complementary effect rather than an additive one.

The attractiveness of caffeine as an ergogenic aid lies not only in the fact that it has been shown to be performance enhancing over a wide range of sporting disciplines, but also because it is relatively safe and readily available. The effects of caffeine on sports performance have been shown to occur following an optimum dose (Graham and Spriet 1995), and this dose is considered to be relatively safe. Nevertheless, as with all drugs, there are side effects and safety issues concerning individuals sensitive to caffeine and those who consume caffeine in large quantities. Side effects may include nausea, insomnia, tachycardia, arrhythmia, and tremor. Further in-depth discussion regarding the use of caffeine in sport and its side effects can be found in Chapter 22.

Whilst caffeine is not classified as a prohibited substance, it remains on the Monitoring Program to enable WADA to monitor its use. Whilst caffeine remains a common constituent of an individual's diet, it is clear that its use as a performance-enhancing drug is increasing. Studies have found athletes using products containing caffeine (Chester and Wojek 2008; Desbrow and Leveritt 2006) with the intention of improving performance. The rise in the energy drink market and the sponsorship of various sports by such drink companies clearly promotes this practice.

20.8. Summary

Sympathomimetic amines and methylxanthines contained in OTC medication have clear therapeutic roles in alleviating the symptoms of URT conditions. In therapeutic doses, these sympathomimetics are typically devoid of adverse side effects and performance-enhancing properties. Even in supratherapeutic doses, research has found it difficult to elucidate the performance-enhancement properties of these drugs. However, pseudoephedrine and ephedrine are both commonly available OTC stimulants and are prohibited in competition. As a consequence of the principle of strict liability, there is a huge responsibility of ensuring that athletes are aware of these stimulants and the products that they are contained in. This responsibility lies firmly with the athletes and their support personnel.

20.9. References

Arroll, B. (2008). Common cold. *British Medical Journal, Clinical Evidence* 6: 1510.

Astrup, A., and Toubro, S. (1993). Thermogenic, metabolic and cardiovascular responses to ephedrine and caffeine in man. *International Journal of Obesity* 17(Suppl 1):S41–S43.

Barnes, P. J. (2006). Theophylline for COPD. *Thorax* 61(9):742–744.

Bell, D. G., Jacobs, I., and Zamecnik, J. (1998). Effects of caffeine, ephedrine and their combination on time to exhaustion during high-intensity exercise. *European Journal of Applied Physiology and Occupational Physiology* 77(5):427–433.

Bell, D. G., McLellan T. M., and Sabiston C. M. (2002). Effect of ingesting caffeine and ephedrine on 10-km run performance. *Medical Science in Sports and Exercise* 34(2):344–349.

Bents, R. T., Tokish, J. M., and Goldberg, L. (2004). Ephedrine, pseudoephedrine, and amphetamine prevalence in college hockey players. *Physician and Sports Medicine* 32(9):30–34.

Bents, R. T., and Marsh, E. (2006). Patterns of ephedra and other stimulant use in collegiate hockey athletes. *International Journal of Sport Nutrition and Exercise Metabolism* 16(6):636–643.

Berry, C., and Wagner, D. R. (2012). Effect of pseudoephedrine on 800 m run times of female collegiate track athletes. *International Journal of Sports Physiology and Performance* 7(3): 237–241.

Berstein, E., and Diskant, B. M. (1982). Phenylpropanolamine: A potentially hazardous drug. *Annals of Emergency Medicine* 11(6):311–315.

Betteridge, S., Mundel, T., and Stannard, S. (2010). The effect of pseudoephedrine on self-paced endurance cycling performance. *European Journal of Sport Science* 10(1):53–58.

Boozer, C. N., Nasser, J. A., Heymsfield, S. B., *et al.* (2001). An herbal supplement containing Ma Huang-Guarana for weight loss: A randomised, double-blind trial. *International Journal of Obesity* 25(3):316–324.

Bright, T. P., Sandage, B. W., and Fletcher, H. P. (1981). Selected cardiac and metabolic responses to pseudoephedrine with exercise. *Journal of Clinical Pharmacology* 21(11–12 Pt 1):488–492.

Bruce, C. R., Anderson, M. E., Fraser, S. F., *et al.* (2000). Enhancement of 2000-m rowing performance after caffeine ingestion. *Medicine and Science in Sports and Exercise* 32(11):1958–1963.

Bruno, A., Nolte, K. B., and Chapin, J. (1993). Stroke associated with ephedrine use. *Neurology* 43 (7):1313–1316.

Bukowiecki, L., Jahjah, L., and Follea, N. (1982). Ephedrine, a potential slimming drug, directly stimulates thermogenesis in brown adipocytes via β-adrenoreceptors. *International Journal of Obesity* 6(4):343–350.

Bussel, I. I., and Pavlov, A. A. (2013). DMAA: Efficacious but is it safe? Available online at http://www.sciencebasedmedicine.org/dmaa-efficacious-but-is-it-safe (accessed 1 March 2014).

Bye, C., Dewsbury, D., and Peck, A. W. (1974). Effects on the human central nervous system of two isomers of ephedrine and triprolidine and their interaction. *British Journal of Clinical Pharmacology* 1(1):71–78.

Bye, C., Hill, H. M., Hughes, D. T. D., *et al.* (1975). A comparison of plasma levels of L(+) pseudo-ephedrine following different formulations, and their relation to cardiovascular and subjective effects in man. *European Journal of Clinical Pharmacology* 8(1):47–53.

Cantu, C., Arauz, A., Murillo-Bonilla, L. M., *et al.* (2003). Stroke associated with sympathomimetics contained in over-the-counter cough and cold drugs. *Stroke* 34(7):1667–1672.

Charatan, F. (2003). Ephedra supplement may have contributed to sportsman's death. *British Medical Journal* 326(7387):464.

Chester, N. (2000). The use of exogenous sympathomimetic amines in sport and exercise. Unpublished PhD Thesis; Liverpool John Moores University.

Chester, N., Mottram, D. R., Reilly, T. *et al*. (2004). Elimination of ephedrines in urine following multiple dosing and the consequences for athletes, regarding doping control. *British Journal of Clinical Pharmacology* 57(1):62–67.

Chester, N., Reilly, T., and Mottram, D. R. (2003a). Physiological, subjective and performance effects of pseudoephedrine and phenylpropanolamine during endurance running exercise. *International Journal of Sports Medicine* 24(1):3–8.

Chester, N., Reilly, T., and Mottram, D. R. (2003b). Over-the-counter drug use amongst athletes and non-athletes. *Journal of Sports Medicine and Physical Fitness* 43(1):111–118.

Chester, N., and Wojek, N. (2008). Caffeine consumption amongst UK cyclist and track and field athletes. *International Journal of Sports Medicine* 29(6):524–528.

Chu, K. S, Doherty, T. J., Parise, G., *et al*. (2002). A moderate dose of pseudoephedrine does not alter muscle contraction strength or anaerobic power. *Clinical Journal of Sports Medicine* 12(6): 387–390.

Clemons, J. M., and Crosby, S. L. (1993). Cardiopulmonary and subjective effects of a 60mg dose of pseudoephedrine on graded treadmill exercise. *Journal of Sports Medicine and Physical Fitness* 33(4):405–412.

Collomp, K., Ahmaidi, S., Chatard, J. C., *et al*. (1992). Benefits of caffeine ingestion on sprint performance in trained and untrained swimmers. *European Journal of Applied Physiology* 64(4):377–380.

Desbrow, B., and Leveritt, M. (2006). Awareness and use of caffeine by athletes competing at the 2005 Ironman Triathlon World Championships. *International Journal of Sport Nutrition and Exercise Metabolism* 16(5):545–558.

Drew, C. D. M., Knight, G. T., Hughes, D. T. D., *et al*. (1978). Comparison of the effects of D-(-)-ephedrine and L-(+)-pseudoephedrine on the cardiovascular and respiratory systems in man. *British Journal of Clinical Pharmacology* 6(3):221–225.

Doherty, M., Smith, P. M., Hughes, M. G., *et al*. (2004). Caffeine lowers perceptual response and increases power output during high-intensity cycling. *Journal of Sports Science* 22(7):637–643.

Dulloo, A. G. (1993). Ephedrine, xanthines and prostaglandin-inhibitors: Actions and interactions in the stimulation of thermogenesis. *International Journal of Obesity* 17(Suppl):S35–S40.

Dulloo, A. G., and Miller, D. S. (1986). The thermogenic properties of ephedrine methylxanthine mixtures: Human studies. *International Journal of Obesity* 10(6):467–481.

Eccles R. (2005). Understanding the symptoms of the common cold and influenza. *Lancet* 5(11):718–725.

Empey D. W., Young G. A., Letley E., *et al*. (1980). Dose-response of the nasal decongestant and cardiovascular effects of pseudoephedrine. *British Journal of Clinical Pharmacology* 9(4):351–358.

Gibson, G. J., and Warrell, D. A. (1972). Hypertensive crisis and phenylpropanolamine. *Lancet* 2 (7775):492–493.

Gill, N. D., Shield, A., Blazevich, A. J., *et al*. (2000). Muscular and cardiorespiratory effects of pseudoephedrine in human athletes. *British Journal of Clinical Pharmacology* 50(3):205–213.

Gillies, H., Derman, W. E., Noakes, T. D., *et al*. (1996). Pseudoephedrine is without ergogenic effects during prolonged exercise. *Journal of Applied Physiology* 81(6):2611–2617.

Graf, P. (1997). Rhinitis medicamentosa: Aspects of pathophysiology and treatment. *Allergy* 52 (40 Suppl): 28–34.

Graham, T. E., and Spriet, L. L. (1995). Metabolic, catecholamine, and exercise performance responses to varying doses of caffeine. *Journal of Applied Physiology* 78(3):867–874.

Greer, F., Friars, D., and Graham, T. E. (2000). Comparison of caffeine and theophylline ingestion: Exercise metabolism and endurance. *Journal of Applied Physiology* 89(3):1837–1844.

Greer, F., McLean, C., and Graham, T. E. (1998). Caffeine, performance, and metabolism during repeated Wingate exercise tests. *Journal of Applied Physiology* 85(4):1502–1508.

Heath, G. W., Ford, E. S., Craven, T. E., *et al*. (1991). Exercise and the incidence of upper respiratory tract infections. *Medicine and Science in Sports Exercise* 23(2):152–157.

Hodges, K., Hancock, S., Currell, K., *et al.* (2006). Pseudoephedrine enhances performance in 1500-m runners. *Medicine and Science in Sports Exercise* 38(2):329–333.

Hoffman, B. B. (2001). Catecholamines, sympathomimetic drugs, and adrenergic receptor antagonists. In J. G. Hardman, L. E. Limbird, and A. G. Gilman (Eds.), *Goodman and Gilman's The Pharmacological Basis of Therapeutics* (10th ed., pp. 215–268). New York, NY: McGraw-Hill.

Horwitz, R. I., Brass, L. M., Kernan, W. M., *et al.* (2000). Phenylpropanolamine and risk of hemorrhagic stroke: Final report of the Yale Hemorrhagic Stroke Project.

Jackman, M., Wendling, P., Friars, D., *et al.* (1996). Metabolic, catecholamine and endurance responses to caffeine during intense exercise. *Journal of Applied Physiology* 81(4):1658–1663.

Jacobs, I., Pasternak, H., and Bell, D. G. (2003). Effects of ephedrine, caffeine, and their combination on muscular endurance. *Medicine and Science in Sports and Exercise* 35(6):987–994.

Johnson, D. A., Etter, H. S., and Reeves, D. M. (1983). Stroke and phenylpropanolamine use. *Lancet*, 2(8356): 970

Kernan, W. N., Viscoli, C. M., Brass, L. M., *et al.* (2000). Phenylpropanolamine and the risk of hemorrhagic stroke. *New England Journal of Medicine* 343(25):1826–1832.

König, D., Grathwohl, D., Weinstock, C., *et al.* (2000). Upper respiratory tract infection in athletes: Influence of lifestyle, type of sport, training effort and immunostimulant intake. *Exercise Immunology Review* 6:102–120.

Kuitunen, T., Karkkainen, S., and Ylitalo, P. (1984). Comparison of the acute physical and mental effects of ephedrine, fenfluramine, phentermine, and prolitane. *Methods and Findings in Experimental and Clinical Pharmacology* 6(5):265–270.

Lanciault, G., and Wolf, H. H. (1965). Some neuropharmacological properties of the ephedrine isomers. *Journal of Pharmaceutical Sciences* 54(6):841–844.

Lefebvre R. A., Surmont, F., Bouckaert, J., *et al.* (1992). Urinary excretion of ephedrine after nasal application in healthy volunteers. *Journal of Pharmacy and Pharmacology* 44(8):672–675.

Leynaert, B., Bousquet, J., Neukirch, C., *et al.* (1999). Perennial rhinitis: An independent risk factor for asthma in nonatopic subjects: Results from the European Community Respiratory Health Survey. *Journal of Allergy Clinical Immunology* 104(2 Pt 1):301–304.

MacIntosh, B. R., and Wright, B. M. (1995). Caffeine ingestion and performance of a 1,500-metre swim. *Canadian Journal of Applied Physiology* 20(2):168–177.

Medicines and Healthcare Products Regulatory Agency. (2000). Phenylpropanolamine and haemorrhagic stroke – update. Available online at http://www.mhra.gov.uk/Safetyinformation/Safety warningsalertsandrecalls/Safetywarningsandmessagesformedicines/CON019551 (accessed 10 September 2014).

Mottram, D. R., Chester, N., Atkinson, G., *et al.* (2008). Athletes' knowledge and views on over-the-counter medication. *International Journal of Sports Medicine* 29(10):851–855.

Nathan, A. (2002). How to treat hay fever and associated allergic conditions in the pharmacy. *Pharmaceutical Journal* 268:575–578.

Nieman, D. C., Johanssen, L. M., Lee, J. W., *et al.* (1990). Infectious episodes in runners before and after the Los Angeles Marathon. *Journal of Sports Medicine and Physical Fitness* 30(3):316–328.

Nieman, D. C., Henson, D. A., and Gusewitch, G. (1993). Physical activity and immune function in elderly women. *Medicine and Science in Sports and Exercise* 25(7):823–831.

Norvenius, G., Widerlov, E., and Lönnerhölm, G. (1979). Phenylpropanolamine and mental disturbance. *Lancet* 2(8156–8157):1367–1368.

Pasman, W. J., van Baak, M. A., Jeukendrup, A. E., *et al.* (1995). The effect of different dosages of caffeine on endurance performance time. *International Journal of Sports Medicine* 16(4):225–230.

Paton, C. D., Hopkins, W. G., and Vollebregt, L. (2001). Little effect of caffeine ingestion on repeated sprints in team-sport athletes. *Medicine and Science in Sports and Exercise* 33(5):822–825.

Peters, E. M., and Bateman, E. D. (1983). Ultramarathon running and upper respiratory tract infections. *South African Medical Journal* 64(15):582–584.

Price, D., Bond, C., Bouchard, J., *et al.* (2006). International Primary Care Respiratory Group (IPCRG) Guidelines: Management of allergic rhinitis. *Primary Care Respiratory Journal* 15(1):58–70.

Pritchard-Peschek, K. R., Jenkins, D. G., Osborne, M. A. *et al.* (2010). Pseudoephedrine ingestion and cycling time trial performance. *International Journal of Sports Nutrition, Exercise and Metabolism* 20(2):132–138.

Pritchard-Peschek, K. R., Jenkins, D. G., Osborne, M. A., *et al.* (2014). The dose-response relationship between pseudoephedrine ingestion and exercise performance. *Journal of Science and Medicine in Sport*, 17(5):531–534.

Pritchard-Peschek, K. R., Osborne, M. A., Slater, G. J., *et al.* (2013). Pseudoephedrine and preexercise feeding: Influence on performance. *Medicine, Science, Sport and Exercise* 45(6):1152–1157.

Proprietary Association of Great Britain. (2013). Annual review 2013. Available online at http://www.pagb.co.uk/publications/pdfs/annualreview2013.pdf (accessed 2 March 2014).

Ramsey, J. J., Colman, R. J., Swick, A. G., *et al.* (1998). Energy expenditure, body composition and glucose metabolism in lean and obese rhesus monkeys treated with ephedrine and caffeine. *American Journal of Clinical Nutrition* 68(1):42–51.

Reissig, C. J., Strain, E. C., and Griffiths, R. R. (2009). Caffeinated energy drinks: A growing problem. *Drug and Alcohol Dependence* 99(1–3):1–10.

Ryan, D. (2008). Management of acute rhinosinusitis in primary care: Changing paradigms and the emerging role of intranasal corticosteroids. *Primary Care Respiratory Journal* 17(3):148–155.

Scadding, G. K., Durham, S. R., Mirakian, R., *et al.* (2008). BSACI guidelines for the management of allergic and non-allergic rhinitis. *Clinical and Experimental Allergy* 38(1):19–42.

Sidney, K. H., and Lefcoe N. M. (1977). The effects of ephedrine on the physiological and psychological responses to submaximal and maximal exercise in man. *Medicine and Science in Sports and Exercise* 9(2):95–99.

Strano-Rossi, S., Leone, D., de la Torre, X., *et al.* (2009). The relevance of the urinary concentration of ephedrines in anti-doping analysis: Determination of pseudoephedrine, cathine, and ephedrine after administration of over-the-counter medications. *Therapeutic Drug Monitoring* 31(4):520–526.

Swain, R. A., Harsha, D. M., Baenziger, J., *et al.* (1997). Do pseudoephedrine or phenylpropanolamine improve maximum oxygen uptake and time to exhaustion? *Clinical Journal of Sport Medicine* 7 (3):168–173.

To, L. B., Sangster, J. F., Rampling, D., *et al.* (1980). Ephedrine-induced cardiomyopathy. *Medical Journal of Australia* 2(1):35–36.

UK Anti-Doping (2013). The results of the UK Anti-Doping's national programme. Available online at http://www.ukad.org.uk/anti-doping-rule-violations/facts-and-figures (accessed 13 March 2014).

US Food and Drug Association. (2005). Phenylpropanolamine-containing drug products for over-the-counter human use; Tentative final monographs. Available online at http://www.gpo.gov/fdsys/pkg/FR-2005-12-22/html/E5-7646.htm (accessed 13 March 2014).

Vallerand, A. L. (1993). Effects of ephedrine/xanthines on thermogenesis and cold tolerance. *International Journal of Obesity* 17(Suppl 1):S53–S56.

Wadler, G. I., and Hainline, B. (1989). *Drugs and the Athlete*. Philadelphia, PA: F.A. Davis.

Weatherby, R. P., and Rogerson, S. (2002). Caffeine potentiation of the performance enhancing effects of pseudoephedrine. In *Proceedings of the Sixth IOC World Congress on Sport Sciences* (p. 110). St. Louis, MO: IOC World Congress on Sport Science.

Weiner, I., Tilkian, A. G., and Palazzolo, M. (1990). Coronary artery spasm and myocardial infarction in a patient with normal coronary arteries: Temporal relationship to pseudoephedrine ingestion. *Catheterization and Cardiovascular Diagnostics* 20(1):51–53.

Williams, M. H. (1974). *Drugs and Athletic Performance*. Springfield, IL: Charles C. Thomas.

World Anti-Doping Agency. (2013a). The 2014 Prohibited List international standard. Available online at https://www.wada-ama.org/en/what-we-do/prohibited-list (accessed 9 September 2014).

World Anti-Doping Agency. (2013b). 2012 anti-doping testing figures report. Available online at https://wada-main-prod.s3.amazonaws.com/resources/files/WADA-2012-Anti-Doping-Testing-Figures-Report-EN.pdf (accessed 9 September 2014).

World Anti-Doping Agency. (2013c). WADA Technical Document – TD2013DL. Available online at https://wada-main-prod.s3.amazonaws.com/resources/files/WADA-TD2013DL-Decision-Limits-for-the-Confirmatory-Quantification-Threshold-Substances-2.0-EN.pdf (accessed 9 September 2014).

Chapter 21

Sports supplements and herbal preparations

Neil Chester

21.1. Introduction

Even as a book entitled *Drugs in Sport*, it is beyond remit to review, in detail, all supplements that might be used by athletes for the purpose of enhancing performance and maintaining health. Indeed, many supplements that are pharmacological in nature are covered elsewhere in this book. Countless other supplements are available to the athlete but are not considered to be an issue with respect to doping (i.e. they are not present on the World Anti-Doping Agency [WADA] Prohibited List); these are reviewed extensively in other texts. Interested readers are directed to the reviews on nutritional supplements published in the *British Journal of Sports Medicine* (Volumes 43–47) for further information relating to specific supplements.

The use of products labelled as sports supplements does bring with it a number of important challenges from an anti-doping perspective. Indeed, inadvertent doping is a real and serious problem for athletes, their entourages, and anti-doping organisations alike. The regulation of the sports supplements industry is not as comprehensive as that surrounding the pharmaceutical industry; therefore, in recent years, many issues have come to light as a consequence of the contamination, adulteration, and mislabelling of supplements. In addition, the use of herbal supplements, in which the active ingredients are often unclear or unknown, may put an athlete at risk of contravening anti-doping rules.

Whilst strict liability remains WADA's guiding principle, the significance of inadvertent doping cannot be underestimated. Indeed, a positive test can have a huge impact on an athlete's career. Therefore, a major challenge remains in terms of limiting the chances of an anti-doping rule violation (ADRV) occurring as a consequence of supplement use.

This chapter examines the use of supplements in sport and discusses the challenges to athletes, their support staff, and anti-doping organisations in allowing legitimate use, yet preventing indiscriminate use and ensuring that WADA is both credible and operational.

21.2. What are sports supplements?

Sports supplements may encompass a wide range of dietary interventions that may be used to maintain health and promote exercise performance. Supplements may be characterised into three broad categories:

- Medication, such as over-the-counter (OTC) products used to alleviate symptoms or treat an illness or long-term conditions (see Chapter 20)
- Health-related products, including micronutrients, which may supplement the diet with nutrients that may be required due to the demands of the sport or a poor diet
- Ergogenic aids, which are designed to enhance sports performance.

Clearly, the latter category is particularly broad and may encompass many of the performance- and image-enhancing drugs (PIEDs) outlined throughout this book. However, it also includes numerous supplements that are generally accepted in sport due to their availability in the diet (albeit in smaller amounts) or natural presence in the body.

Whilst ergogenic aids, particularly those not typically classified as PIEDs, are the focus of this chapter, it is clear that this category of dietary supplements is positioned in a grey area from an anti-doping perspective. There has been considerable debate surrounding ergogenic aids, particularly when a new product hits the market, in terms of its safety and legitimacy as a 'legal' ergogenic aid.

21.3. Why do athletes use supplements?

Athletes may consider using a wide range of supplements according to their particular health status, training status, and the demands of their particular sport. The following factors have been highlighted by Mottram (2011) as potential reasons for their use:

* To substitute for a poor-quality diet
* To provide additional nutrients to support the demands of training and competition
* To help alleviate illness or injury or aid in its recovery
* To facilitate recovery from training and competition
* To provide ergogenic advantage during training or competition.

Clearly, supplements play an important part in effective sports nutrition. Good nutrition is often compromised by the constraints of everyday living, heavy training, and competition schedules. Supplements can therefore ensure that the diet maintains its balance of macronutrients and micronutrients consumed in the required amounts in a timely manner, thus ensuring optimal exercise performance and recovery.

A major focus of many athletes' sports supplement regimens is direct improvement in performance, which might involve consumption prior to or even during a competition or training session. These supplements are specific to the demands of the exercise in terms of the intensity and duration of effort and the nature of the activity (i.e. whether it incorporates significant skill-based elements and decision making). In combination with an event-specific regimen, a postevent, recovery supplement plan is typically used to enhance recovery and adaptation from a competition or training session.

In addition to the seemingly rational justification for supplement use, athletes may simply consider their use because competitors or training partners are using them. Also, the drive to be successful will typically result in athletes turning to a variety of supplements, with the belief that they will offer the improvement required to succeed. In addition, within professional sport, the demands to succeed are also shared amongst an athlete's support staff. Therefore, additional pressure to use supplements is placed on athletes by their entourage and possibly by sports supplement companies who may sponsor athletes or sports teams.

21.4. The prevalence of supplement use

It is clear from a sales perspective that sports supplements have grown in popularity over recent years. Indeed, a consumer research report stated that the UK sports nutrition market was worth £260 million in 2012 (Euromonitor International 2013). The growth in sales of sports supplements is evidenced by their widespread availability throughout mainstream retail outlets, including supermarkets as well as the internet. It is clear that sports supplement use, once the domain of the competitive athlete, is now widespread across recreational athletes and sedentary individuals alike.

Whilst drug use in sport is practiced in a covert manner, unsurprisingly there is less reticence in terms of discussing supplement use amongst athletes. Numerous studies have attempted to provide an accurate estimation of supplement use amongst athletes, with varied success. Figures on the scope and extent of supplement use vary widely. It has been suggested that between 40 and 100 per cent of athletes use supplements, often as multiple regimens and at higher than normal doses (Baume *et al.* 2007).

At the Sydney Olympics in 2000, Corrigan and Kazlauskas (2003) recorded the declarations of supplement use by the 2,758 athletes who were drug tested at the games. At least seventeen different classes of supplements were reported, with the most frequently cited being multivitamins (1,116), vitamin C (810), creatine (316), and amino acids (190). At the Athens Olympics in 2004, Tsitsimpikou *et al.* (2009) again used athlete declarations during doping control tests to examine medication and supplements use. Just over 75 per cent of athletes declared use of medication and supplements, with food supplements the most common (45 per cent of respondents), followed by vitamins (43 per cent) and proteins/ amino acids (14 per cent).

A study by Tscholl *et al.* (2008) examined the use of medication and supplement use amongst players at the Fédération Internationale de Football Association World Cup in 2002 and 2006. Supplement use by players prior to each match was recorded from reports by each team physician. Of all supplements, 43 per cent were categorised as medications, whilst 57 per cent were nutritional supplements. Again, the most common nutritional supplements were vitamins (41 per cent) followed by minerals (21 per cent) and amino acids (11 per cent).

Sundgot-Borgen *et al.* (2003) investigated the use of selected supplements within Norwegian elite athletes compared with a control group. A similar percentage of female athletes (54 per cent) and controls (52 per cent) reported using one or more supplements, whereas more male athletes (51 per cent) than controls (32 per cent) used supplements. In the athlete group, the main supplements used were minerals (males 26 per cent; females 42 per cent), amino acids (males 12 per cent; females 3 per cent), and creatine (males 12 per cent; females 3 per cent).

Nieper (2005) found that 62 per cent of UK junior international track-and-field athletes were using supplements, with an average of 2.4 products per athlete, and that males used ergogenic aids more often than females. Multivitamins and minerals were the most popular products used. Whilst 25 per cent reported using supplements for ergogenic purposes, the main reasons for their use were for health (45 per cent) and to enhance the immune system (40 per cent).

Erdman *et al.* (2006) surveyed Canadian high-performance athletes and found that 88 per cent reported using dietary supplements during the previous 6 months, with an average of 3.08 supplements per user. Sport drinks (22 per cent), sport bars (14 per cent), multivitamins and minerals (14 per cent), protein supplements (9 per cent), and vitamin C (6 per cent) were the most frequently reported supplements used. Protein supplements were significantly more likely to be used by athletes at the highest performance level.

21.5. The risks associated with supplement use

As mentioned, the sports supplement market is particularly buoyant and is currently experiencing rapid growth. Manufacturers are capitalising on the perceived need by many individuals to supplement their diet for the demands of exercise training and competition. Whilst many products are deemed to be rather innocuous, the safety associated with high doses and their long-term use is often unknown. Unlike therapeutic drugs, nutritional supplements are not required to have strong scientific and clinical evidence concerning their safety and efficacy before being allowed to be sold to the public (Clarkson 1996). They are not subject to the same independent, scientific scrutiny as regulated medicines (Herbert 1999; Maughan 2005).

In addition to the concerns associated with long-term use and relatively high doses of particular supplements, there has also been concern regarding their use as a gateway to the future use of illicit performance enhancers. Several researchers have attempted to elucidate the relationship between supplement use and possible use of prohibited substances in the future (Backhouse *et al.* 2013). Understandably, this link remains under debate but it does pose the question if, by advocating or encouraging ergogenic aids, we are normalising their use and blurring the lines between acceptable supplementation and doping.

Whilst evidence shows that the minority of athletes use prohibited substances to enhance sport performance (see Chapter 25), there is clear evidence of widespread supplement use. Debate in terms of the legitimacy and the ethics surrounding the use of particular sports supplements remains; however, the ambitious yet responsible athlete will use whatever is deemed to be acceptable and ensure prohibited PIEDs are avoided. Nevertheless, whilst this course of action might have been acceptable in the past, the significant risks associated with supplement use have become clear recently. Numerous ADRVs have been attributed to the use of seemingly innocuous sports supplements, and research studies have revealed the real issue of supplement contamination and potential adulteration.

Indeed, whilst sports supplements manufacturers exploit the innate competitiveness of those participating in sport, some products can fall into a 'grey area' in relation to doping and contravening the spirit of sport. Many products may contain additional active ingredients from herbal extracts or synthetically synthesised pharmaceuticals. It is therefore essential that athletes and their support personnel are fully aware of the ingredients contained in any supplements used to ensure that they limit the chances of falling foul of the anti-doping regulations. WADA upholds a strict liability policy whereby athletes are responsible for any prohibited substance found in their blood or urine. Ignorance or negligence is not considered to be an acceptable justification for a positive test result.

As part of this chapter, several herbal supplements are reviewed to highlight the link between what might be deemed to be natural, safe supplements and potentially hazardous doping agents (Section 21.6). The major concern with herbal supplements is that there are no assurances in terms of their content (and the exact quantity) of active ingredients. Also, many herbs have been found to contain high quantities of heavy metals (e.g. mercury, lead) as a consequence of the level of soil contamination in countries where the herbs are grown, such as China (Mueller and Hingst 2013).

Athletes are also asked to be vigilant and keep their drink bottles with them at all times to avoid the possibility of sabotage by fellow competitors. Whilst evidence to support this practice is lacking, it would seem plausible that sabotage might be a possible option for an extremely motivated athlete when pressure to outperform his or her competitor(s) is critical.

Contamination

Unlike the pharmaceuticals market, the sports supplements market is not closely regulated. As a result, many products have been found to be affected by contamination due to poor manufacturing and quality control procedures. Inadvertent contamination may occur through contamination of the raw materials used or cross-contamination during the manufacturing process of sports supplements. Clearly, safety is a major issue when the label and packaging do not reflect the contents of a particular product.

Research carried out over recent years has demonstrated how real the problem of supplement contamination actually is. Between 10 and 25 per cent of products tested were found to be contaminated (Baume *et al.* 2007). Many of these contaminants are liable to result in an adverse analytical finding during drug testing. Two sources of contamination have been proposed (Burke 2004):

- Cross-contamination due to poor manufacturing practice
- Undeclared additions of active ingredients to supplements in order to increase their efficacy.

Whilst the first source would appear to be true contamination that could be alleviated through improved manufacturing procedures, the second source would seem to describe adulteration of sports supplements.

The main contaminants in supplements have been shown to be stimulants, such as ephedrine, anabolic androgenic steroids (AAS), and their precursors, often referred to as prohormones (Baume *et al.* 2007). Prohormones are legally available as sports supplements and aggressively marketed as having enormous potential to increase muscle growth and strength (Geyer *et al.* 2008). The most common are the precursors of testosterone and nandrolone, including 4-androstenedione, 4-androstenediol, 5-androstenediol (precursors of testosterone); 19-norandrostenedione and 19-norandrostenediol (precursors of nortestosterone); and dehydroepiandrosterone (Yonamine *et al.* 2004).

An international study found that from a total of 634 products purchased from shops and the internet, a significant proportion (almost 15 per cent) of supplements contained AAS and related substances (including prohormones) that were not declared on their packaging. Also, the extent of contaminated supplements varied among countries, with the Netherlands (25.8 per cent), Austria (22.7 per cent), the United Kingdom (18.8 per cent), and the United States (18.8 per cent) all reporting higher contamination than the average (Geyer *et al.* 2004).

A similar study was conducted on 103 dietary supplements purchased from the internet (Baume *et al.* 2006). The products were screened for the presence of stimulants, anabolic steroids, and their precursors and metabolites. Results showed that approximately one in five supplements were contaminated with substances not declared on the label, all of which would have resulted in an adverse analytical finding if an athlete had used these products prior to a drug test.

A study by Russell *et al.* (2013) performed a prohibited drug screening on 114 products obtained from the largest sports supplement companies in Europe. Supplements were chosen randomly and included a wide range of products, none of which was part of a routine drug screen programme. Results found that 10 per cent of products were contaminated with prohibited substances, including AAS and stimulants, with a total of twenty prohibited substances identified. Despite the increased awareness of contamination issues related to sports supplements, this research highlights that the problem remains a real issue.

Athletes should be aware that WADA-accredited laboratories can detect prohibited substances and their metabolites at much lower concentrations (parts per billion, µg/l) than the levels detectable by the majority of supplement manufacturers (parts per million, mg/l;

Mottram 2011). In reality, this means that supplement companies may abide by manufacturing guidelines from a general health and safety perspective, yet still produce supplements that might put an athlete at risk of a positive drug test.

The contamination of sports supplements is not only an issue with regards to prohibited substances but also concerning the purity of products and the cleanliness of the manufacturing process. Indeed, contaminants in addition to prohibited substances, including broken glass and animal faeces, have been discovered (Maughan *et al*. 2011).

Adulteration, counterfeiting, and mislabelling

As mentioned, there may be a more sinister motivation behind the presence of a prohibited substance in a sports supplement. Adulteration of sports supplements during the manufacturing process may provide enhanced ergogenic properties to otherwise innocuous products through the addition of a prohibited substance. Substitution of one active ingredient for another (i.e. counterfeiting) is not uncommon in the manufacture of products from the illicit market (Graham *et al*. 2009).

Mislabelling is another major issue associated with the adulteration of products. Research has shown that not only do products sometimes contain substances not stated on the label, but also that they might contain substances in different quantities (Van Thuyne *et al*. 2006).

Accuracy and quality of information and advice concerning sports supplements

Heavy advertising through magazines and the internet has allowed unrestricted access to a wide range of supplements (Baume *et al*. 2007). Manufacturers may make exaggerated claims regarding the ergogenic properties of their products (Beltz and Doering 1993). Such claims are rarely substantiated by sound scientific data in peer-reviewed journals (Nieman and Pedersen 1999).

Athletes often self-prescribe supplements but may seek advice from a variety of sources. Coaches were found to be the main advisors on supplement use for male (58 per cent) and female (52 per cent) elite Norwegian athletes (Sundgot-Borgen *et al*. 2003). Erdman *et al*. (2007) also reported that athletes found coaches to be a valuable source of advice in terms of supplement use (41 per cent of respondents); however, family and friends (52.7 per cent) and teammates (44 per cent) were considered most valuable. In a survey by Nieper (2005), 72 per cent of respondents claimed to have access to a sports dietician but tended to underutilise this resource. Subjects indicated that coaches (65 per cent) had the greatest influence on their supplement use, with doctors (25 per cent) and sports dieticians (30 per cent) being less important.

Considering the specific dangers that have been highlighted with respect to the indiscriminate use of sports supplements from both an anti-doping and health and safety perspective, there is a need to ensure that accurate information is readily available. Regulation is needed in terms of limiting the unrealistic claims made by sports supplements companies. Advertising should also be sensitive to a potential young market to ensure that children are not intentionally influenced by the marketing of sports supplements. It is also necessary to educate not only athletes but their entourages in the safe use of supplements.

21.6. Herbal supplementation

Herbs may contain many active ingredients, and the exact quantities and contents are seldom labelled. Whilst herbal products contain active ingredients, they are classified as food supplements rather than drugs, and they undergo less stringent quality control procedures prior to their sale. Most herbal supplements have not been subject to extensive scientific scrutiny and rigorous clinical trials. This poses a significant problem in terms of the safety of herbal supplement use. The major risks of taking herbal supplements include the purity of the ingredients and the possibility of contamination, as well as possible interactions among the ingredients and among other supplements consumed simultaneously. Athletes should therefore exercise extreme caution when contemplating the use of natural/herbal supplements.

Whilst it is beyond the scope of this book to provide a comprehensive review of the countless herbal supplements available, it is pertinent to highlight two distinct groups of herbs that athletes may contemplate using: herbal stimulants and so called 'natural testosterone boosters'. Many supplements aimed at the weight loss market contain herbal ingredients that are natural sources of stimulants related to ephedrine and caffeine. Also, a recent area of growth in the sports supplements industry is the development of the pre-workout supplement. These supplements are aimed at individuals who might require a boost by way of a stimulant to enhance performance during a training session. Another area of growth in the supplements market is in products designed to enhance muscle bulk. Whilst there are many examples of supplements that contain prohormones in an attempt to enhance testosterone levels and subsequent muscle gains (see Chapter 5), there are also several herbs termed *natural testosterone boosters* that have reputed benefits in promoting muscle growth.

Natural testosterone boosters

Supplements promoted as testosterone boosters typically contain prohormones; however, natural testosterone boosters include several herbs that allegedly increase circulating testosterone via other mechanisms. Clearly, enhanced testosterone levels offer the potential for increased muscle bulk and function.

Tribulus terrestris

Tribulus terrestris is one of the most commonly used natural testosterone boosters. It is promoted as a supplement to produce gains in lean muscle mass and strength. These gains are claimed to occur in response to increased luteinising hormone and subsequent increases in testosterone. Whilst the mechanisms by which *Tribulus* might exert its effects have not been elucidated, it is believed to be in response to steroidal saponins contained in the herb (Ganzera *et al.* 2001).

Despite its widespread use, there has been limited research into its reputed ergogenic effects. Studies that have examined supplementation have failed to report any significant effects in terms of gains in lean body mass and muscular strength (Antonio *et al.* 2000; Poprzecki *et al.* 2005; Rogerson *et al.* 2007). Whilst anti-doping organisations would actively discourage the use of *Tribulus* due to the many claims made surrounding its efficacy, Rogerson *et al.* (2007) investigated whether *Tribulus* use might increase an individual's testosterone/epitestosterone (T:E) ratio and thus lead to the possible failure of a drug test. However, the T:E ratio was not altered following 5 weeks of supplementation with *Tribulus*.

Eurycoma longifolia Jack

Eurycoma longifolia Jack (EL) is a popular herb in the countries of Southeast Asia and is commonly known as Tongkat Ali in Malaysia (Chen *et al.* 2012). In Asian countries, it is used for its reputed health benefits pertaining to a wide range of conditions (Chen *et al.*, 2012).

However, its potential effect on sexual function and anabolic effect on skeletal muscle has created interest in terms of its use as an ergogenic aid. Although there are no studies that have examined the prevalence of its use, it is now starting to infiltrate the sports supplement market in the West.

The mechanisms behind the efficacy of EL have not been elucidated. However, the phyto-chemical eurycomanone, a quassinoid, is deemed to provide testosterone-boosting properties. It has been reported that eurycomanone is able to enhance testosterone levels in an animal model by aromatase inhibition in Leydig cells, thus reducing the conversion of testosterone to estradiol (Low *et al.* 2013).

Studies have also examined the potential of EL as an ergogenic aid in terms of increasing muscle mass and improving exercise performance. Preliminary data have been provided by Hamzah and Yusuf (2003), which revealed improvements in muscle strength and muscle size following five weeks of supplementation with EL (150 mg/day) in combination with resistance training. Similarly, George *et al.* (2013) reported improvements in muscle strength following EL supplementation (300 mg/day) without resistance training. Research is required to further examine the effects of EL on exercise performance and provide information on potential mechanisms, particularly from an anti-doping perspective.

Herbal stimulants

There are a large number of products available for weight reduction, combating drowsiness, relieving fatigue, and enhancing sports performance – all containing a variety of herbal stimulants. Typically, herbal stimulants contain caffeine and related methylxanthines, of which the most common are coffee and tea. Herbal stimulants may also contain ephedrine and related sympathomimetic amines.

Guarana

Guarana is a South American plant whose seeds contain caffeine (2.5–5 per cent), theophylline and theobromine in small amounts, and large amounts of tannins (Carlini 2003). Guarana is widely available as a constituent of numerous OTC supplements designed to suppress appetite, relieve tiredness, and enhance sports performance. The effects of guarana are mediated largely through its active ingredients caffeine and theophylline via the mechanisms outlined in Chapter 22.

There has been limited research into the efficacy of guarana supplementation in humans. Research examining the effects of herbal supplements containing guarana and ma huang has shown significant fat reduction and weight loss in humans (Boozer *et al.* 2001). Research using animal models has shown that guarana reduced fatigue in mice subjected to forced swimming and increased memory in rats (Espinola 1997). Supplementation of doses of caffeine equivalent to that contained in the guarana extract did not show any improvement in performance. It has been suggested that phytochemicals other than methylxanthines (e.g. tannins) contained in guarana may be responsible for the observed improvements in performance (Espinola 1997).

Ephedra sinica (ma huang)

Ma huang is the name in Chinese medicine given to the plant species *Ephedra sinica*. *Ephedra sinica* is a natural source of ephedrine, pseudoephedrine, norephedrine, and norpseudoephedrine.

Ephedra sinica is typically an ingredient in weight loss preparations as a consequence of ephedrine's thermogenic and anorectic properties. Ma huang typically contains up to 24 mg of ephedrine and related sympathomimetics per unit dose (Bucci 2000). Limited research has examined the use of ma huang as an ergogenic aid. Whilst it is likely that it offers the same ergogenic benefits as its isolated constituents, further work is necessary to elucidate the effects of consuming combined sympathomimetics in herbal form.

Citrus aurantium

Weight loss products often marketed as 'ephedra free' typically contain *Citrus aurantium* (Seville orange or bitter orange extract) as a substitute for ephedra. The peel of bitter orange is known as zhi shi in traditional Chinese medicine and is used in the treatment of gastrointestinal complaints, such as indigestion and constipation. The principal active ingredients of *Citrus aurantium* include the sympathomimetics synephrine (~6 per cent) and octopamine (Haller *et al.* 2005).

Synephrine acts at the α_1-adrenergic receptors, leading to vasoconstriction and increased blood pressure (Bui *et al.* 2006). Evidence from animal models suggests that octopamine activates lipolysis via the β_3-adrenoreceptors of adipocytes, thus accounting for *Citrus aurantium*'s purported thermogenic effect in humans (Carpene *et al.* 1999). However, β_3-adrenoreceptor agonists are less active in human adipocytes (Fugh-Berman and Myers 2004); therefore, it is likely that any positive effect on weight loss may be attributed to the effects on appetite suppression. However, 'ephedra-free' weight loss products not only contain *Citrus aurantium* but also other herbs, such as guarana and green tea, which are all rich in methylxanthines. This combination of sympathomimetics and methylxanthines is thought to produce marked effects in weight loss.

Whilst 'ephedra-free' products are deemed to be safer than their ephedra counterparts, there has been limited research examining their safety. It is possible that the combined effects of synephrine and caffeine may be similar to the reported effects from ephedrine and caffeine, including hypertension, myocardial infarction, and stroke. Haller *et al.* (2005) demonstrated significant cardiovascular stimulation following the administration of a supplement containing synephrine, octopamine, and caffeine. However, no effect on blood pressure was found following administration of a supplement containing only synephrine (46.9 mg). Bui *et al.* (2006) has shown increases in heart rate and systolic and diastolic blood pressure in young, healthy adults following a single 900-mg dose of a *Citrus aurantium* (6 per cent synephrine) supplement. It is also ironic that the term *ephedra free* is used to highlight the fact that the supplement does not contain ephedrine, which is a prohibited substance, yet *Citrus aurantium* is a source of octopamine (albeit in small amounts), which is also a prohibited substance (WADA 2013b).

21.7. Anti-doping violations involving the use of sports supplements

It is not uncommon for any athlete who tests positive for a prohibited substance to claim that it was an inadvertent offence and likely to be due to supplement contamination, adulteration, or sabotage. Whilst several of the claims that reach the headlines appear implausible, many may be considered true. Despite such claims, there are few athletes who avoid sanctions due to the principle of 'strict liability.'

Nandrolone

Around the turn of the twenty-first century, a number of high-profile cases involved athletes who had tested positive for the AAS nandrolone. In most cases, athletes claimed that they had ingested the steroid in a contaminated nutritional supplement, an assertion that was considered to be plausible (Ayotte 1999).

A tennis player, Greg Rusedski, tested positive for nandrolone in July 2003, claiming it was a result of taking contaminated electrolyte supplement pills that the Association of Tennis Professionals (ATP) had been giving out to tennis players through its trainers. A number of other tennis players similarly tested positive for nandrolone between September 2002 and May 2003. Many of these players were below the cut-off level that was in place for testing purposes and were therefore not sanctioned. Greg Rusedski and another six players were above the cut-off level, but they were exonerated by the ATP. The ATP Anti-Doping Tribunal acknowledged that it could not prosecute a case when it had created the situation itself by the action of its trainers distributing contaminated supplements.

Subsequently, the ATP commissioned an anti-doping expert to investigate the source of the nandrolone, but they found no trace of nandrolone in approximately 500 pills tested. The conclusion was ambiguous (Mottram 2011):

> While the circumstantial evidence points to nandrolone-related contamination of the electrolyte-replacement products as the source … there is insufficient evidence to prove that the electrolytes were the cause of the test results. Similarly there is not sufficient evidence to prove they were not the cause.

Methylhexaneamine

The numerous doping cases involving methylhexaneamine in recent years have clearly highlighted the serious issues around the supplement industry from an anti-doping and health and safety perspective. Table 13.1 demonstrated the significant number of adverse analytical findings involving methylhexaneamine. Indeed, according to the WADA 2012 anti-doping testing figures, 46 per cent of adverse analytical findings involving stimulants were attributed to methylhexaneamine, which accounted for 320 occurrences worldwide (WADA 2013a).

Methylhexaneamine (2-amino-4-methylhexane; 1,3-dimethylamylamine; DMAA) was first manufactured synthetically by the pharmaceutical company Eli Lilly and marketed as a vasoconstrictor under the name Forthane (Zhang *et al*. 2012). Despite its removal as a pharmaceutical in 1970, DMAA has recently been reintroduced as a constituent of numerous sports supplements promoted as fat burners and preworkout aids (Mueller and Hingst 2013). The growth in this sector of the sports supplements market, demonstrated by the increased use of DMAA-containing products, coincided with its addition as a nonspecified stimulant to the WADA Prohibited List in 2010. Subsequently, a plethora of adverse analytical findings have been attributed to DMAA contained in such products.

What is particularly interesting in the case of DMAA is that its presence in sports supplements was disguised as a natural herb ingredient on the label of these products. Indeed, each of these products made reference to an ingredient known as geranium stem, geranium oil extract, or geranamine. Reference to a natural herb ingredient allowed manufacturers to market their products as a dietary supplement despite their containing a pharmacological active ingredient. Whist reference material quoted a research study that claimed the ingredient was a natural constituent of geranium oil, this finding has been disputed. Studies examining geranium oil have concluded that DMAA is not an active constituent (Zhang *et al.* 2012) and that products that are labelled with geranium oil but contain DMAA have been adulterated (Lisi *et al.* 2011).

Despite the numerous doping cases involving DMAA, the most disturbing aspect of these sports supplements are the reports of several fatalities attributed to their use. The tragic case of Claire Squires highlights the huge health risk that sports supplements pose. As a recreational athlete, Claire Squires' death due to acute cardiac failure in the 2012 London Marathon was attributed to extreme exertion and the use of a DMAA-containing supplement (William 2013). In August 2012, the Medicines and Healthcare Products Regulatory Agency (2012) issued a statement that all DMAA-containing products should be removed from the UK market due to concerns regarding their safety. However, judging by recent positive tests involving DMAA, its use continues to be a problem in elite sport (UK Anti-Doping 2013).

21.8. Safeguarding athletes against inadvertent doping through supplement use

It is essential to consider a proactive approach in terms of limiting the possibility of a positive drug test and the potential harm caused by the use of a sports supplement.

Are supplements necessary?

Clearly, a key question that needs to be considered is whether supplements confer any advantage to the athlete. In a review by Deldicque and Francaux (2008), it was stated that several types of supplements have demonstrated improved sport performance at a higher levels than that expected with a well-balanced diet. Nevertheless, the evidence base for the efficacy of many supplements is not robust. Indeed, due to the lucrative nature of the sports supplements industry, there are numerous products marketed that do not have strong scientific research to support their use.

Product testing

It is clear that it is not only unrealistic to expect athletes to avoid sport supplements, but it may also put them at a distinct disadvantage against their competitors. Indeed, there are several reasons why supplements may be helpful to the athlete (Section 21.3). Whilst that might not include the use of the latest product offered on the internet, it is clear that even a somewhat responsible athlete can risk a doping offence through the use of a seemingly ordinary supplement. For this reason, a widespread product testing scheme has been developed to safeguard athletes.

Numerous manufacturers subscribe to supplement testing programmes known as Informed Sport, whereby each batch of a specified product is analysed for the presence of substances contained on the WADA Prohibited List. A negative result provides confidence to both the athlete and the manufacturer that a registered product is safe to use without the repercussions of a doping offence.

The Informed Sport supplement testing programme involves testing of products to ISO 17025 standards. This is an internationally recognised standard for analytical laboratories, which ensures that testing is performed to the required high standards and that the limits of detection relating to a contaminant is in line with WADA-accredited laboratory testing.

In addition, the programme includes an assessment of each stage involved in the manufacture of a product, from the source of raw materials to packaging and storage of products. Analysis of raw materials for possible contaminants is an important stage in terms of ensuring the safety of a product. Only when all analytical tests (including batch testing) report negative results can companies use the Informed Sport logo to market their products.

There are, however, limitations with such a testing programme. Indeed, a 100 per cent guarantee that the use of a registered product will not result in a positive drugs test cannot be given. Because WADA does not provide a definitive list of all substances that are prohibited, it is not possible to test products for all prohibited substances. Also, by its very nature, batch testing cannot be completely reliable because only a very small sample of all products are tested. Therefore, there is always the likelihood of products 'slipping through the net.'

Recommendations for athletes

Current recommendations from anti-doping organisations are that athletes should avoid the use of supplements. Clearly, this recommendation allows WADA to uphold its strict liability policy. A more practical solution is that, when supplements are used, they should only be those from reputable manufacturers that test their products for the presence of prohibited substances.

Whilst the risk of supplement contamination is genuine, athletes may safeguard themselves against the possibility of a doping offence by taking the following precautions:

- Perform a needs analysis. Do you need to supplement the diet?
- Consult a nutritionist and/or the scientific literature to determine the efficacy of a supplement.
- Be wary of products that appear to be too good to be true, as manufacturers are likely to be making false claims.
- Exercise caution when considering the use of products that are described as natural and contain herbal ingredients.
- Read the label on all products. Consult an anti-doping organisation for advice with respect to the status of any unknown ingredients.
- Only use products from reputable manufacturers that subscribe to a supplement testing programme.
- Be wary of purchasing products from the internet or independent sport supplements shops.
- Keep sight of your personal feeding bottle at all times during training and competition.

Athletes not only risk jeopardising their reputation and career but also their health if they do not ensure a responsible approach to supplement use. Clearly, athletes intent on using supplements need to be vigilant with respect to the validity of the source of their products.

21.9. References

Antonio, J., Uelmen, J., Rodriguez, R., and Earnest, C. (2000). The effects of *Tribulus terrestris* on body composition and exercise performance in resistance-trained males. *International Journal of Sport Nutrition and Exercise Metabolism* 10(2): 208–215.

Ayotte, C. (1999). Nutritional supplements and doping controls. *New Studies in Athletics* 14:37–42.

Backhouse, S. H., Whitaker, L., and Petroczi, A. (2013). Gateway to doping? Supplement use in the context of preferred competitive situations, doping attitude, beliefs and norms. *Scandinavian Journal of Medicine and Science in Sports* 23(2):244–252.

Baume, N., Hellemans, L., and Saugy, M. (2007). Guide to over-the-counter sports supplements for athletes. *International Sports Medicine Journal* 8(1):2–10.

Baume, N., Mahler, N., Kamber, M., *et al*. (2006). Research of stimulants and anabolic steroids in dietary supplements. *Scandinavian Journal of Medical Science in Sports* 16(1):41–48.

Beltz, S. D., and Doering, P. L. (1993). Efficacy of nutritional supplements used by athletes. *Clinical Pharmacy* 12(12):900–908.

Boozer, C. N., Nasser, J. A., Heymsfield, S. B., *et al*. (2001). An herbal supplement containing Ma Huang-Guarana for weight loss: A randomised, double-blind trial. *International Journal of Obesity* 25(3):316–324.

Bucci, L. R. (2000). Selected herbals and human exercise performance. *American Journal of Clinical Nutrition* 72(Suppl):624S–636S.

Bui, L. T., Nguyen, D. T., and Ambrose, P. J. (2006). Blood pressure and heart rate effects following a single dose of bitter orange. *Annals of Pharmacotherapy* 40(1):53–57.

Burke, L. M. (2004). Contamination of supplements: An interview with Professor Ron Maughan. *International Journal of Sport Nutrition and Exercise Metabolism* 14(4):493–496.

Carlini, E. A. (2003). Plants and the central nervous system. *Pharmacology and Biochemistry and Behaviour* 75(3):501–512.

Carpene, C., Galitzky, J., Fontana, E., *et al*. (1999). Selective activation of β_3-adrenoceptors by octopamine: Comparative studies in mammalian fat cells. *Naunyn-Schmiedeberg's Archives of Pharmacology* 359(4):310–321.

Chen, C. K., Muhamad, A. S., and Ooi, F. K. (2012). Herbs in exercise and sports. *Journal of Physiological Anthropology* 31(4):1–7.

Clarkson, P. M. (1996). Nutrition for improved sport performance: Current issues on ergogenic aids. *Sports Medicine* 21(6):393–401.

Corrigan, B., and Kaslauskas, R. (2003). Medication use in athletes selected for doping control at the Sydney Olympiad (2000). *Clinical Journal of Sports Medicine* 13(1):33–40.

Deldicque, L., and Francaux, M. (2008). Functional food for exercise performance: Fact or foe? *Current Opinions in Clinical Nutrition and Metabolic Care* 11(6):774–781.

Erdman, K. A., Fung, T. S., and Reimer, R. A. (2006). Influence of performance level on dietary supplementation in elite Canadian athletes. *Medicine and Science in Sports and Exercise* 38(2): 349–356.

Erdman, K. A., Fung, T. S., Doyle-Baker, P. K., *et al*. (2007). Dietary supplementation of high performance Canadian athletes by age and gender. *Clinical Journal of Sports Medicine* 17(6):458–464.

Espinola, E. B., Dias, R. F., Mattei, R., *et al*. (1997). Pharmacological activity of Guarana (Paullinia cupana Mart.) in laboratory animals. *Journal of Ethnopharmacology* 55(3):223–229.

Euromonitor International. (2013). Sports nutrition in the United Kingdom. Available online at http://www.euromonitor.com/sports-nutrition-in-the-united-kingdom/report (accessed 1 March 2014).

Fugh-Bernam, A., and Myers, A. (2004). Citrus aurantium, an ingredient of dietary supplements marketed for weight loss: Current status of clinical and basic research. *Experimental Biology and Medicine* 229(8):698–704.

Ganzera, M., Bedir, E., and Khan, I. A. (2001). Determination of steroidal saponins in Tribulus terrestis by reversed-phase high performance liquid chromatography and evaporative light scattering detection. *Journal of Pharmaceutical Sciences* 90(11):1752–1758.

George, A., Liske, E.., Chen, C. K., and Ismail, S. B. (2013). The Eurycoma longifolia freeze-dried water extract-physta does not change normal ratios of testosterone to epitestosterone in healthy males. *Journal of Sports Medicine and Doping Studies* 3(2):1–6.

Geyer, H., Parr, M. K., Mareck, U., *et al*. (2004). Analysis of non-hormonal nutritional supplements for anabolic androgenic steroids: Results of an international study. *International Journal of Sports Medicine* 25(2):124–129.

Geyer, H., Parr, M. K., Koehler, K., *et al*. (2008). Nutritional supplements cross-contaminated and faked with doping substances. *Journal of Mass Spectrometry* 43(7):892–902.

Graham, M. R., Ryan, P., Baker, J. S., *et al*. (2009). Counterfeiting in performance and image-enhancing drugs. *Drug Testing and Analysis* 1(3):135–142.

Haller C. A., Benowitz, N. L., and Jacob, P. (2005). Hemodynamic effects of ephedra-free weight-loss supplements in humans. *American Journal of Medicine* 118(9):998–1003.

Hamzah, S., and Yusuf, A. (2003). The ergogenic effects of Tongkat Ali (Eurycoma longifolia): A pilot study. *British Journal of Sports Medicine* 37(Abstract 007):465–466.

Herbert, D. L. (1999). Recommending or selling nutritional supplements enhances potential legal liability for sports medicine practitioners. *Sports Medicine Alert* 5(11):91–92.

Lisi, A., Hasick, N., Kazlauskas, R., and Goebel, C. (2011). Studies of methylhexaneamine in supplements and geranium oil. *Drug Testing and Analysis* 3(10–11):873–876.

Low, B. S., Choi, S.-B., Abdul Wahab, H., *et al*. (2013). Eurycomanone, the major quassinoid in Eurycoma longifolia root extract increases spermatogenesis by inhibiting the activity of phosphodi-esterase and aromatase in steroidogenesis. *Journal of Ethnopharmacology* 149(1):201–207.

Maughan, R. J. (2005). Contamination of dietary supplements and positive drug tests in sport. *Journal of Sports Sciences* 23(9):883–889.

Maughan, R. J., Greenhaff, P. L., and Hespel, P. (2011). Dietary supplements for athletes: Emerging trends and recurring themes. *Journal of Sport Sciences* 29(S1):S57–S66.

Medicines and Healthcare Products Regulatory Agency. (2012). MHRA to remove popular sports supplement used by international athletes from the market. Available online at http://www.mhra .gov.uk/NewsCentre/Pressreleases/CON180711 (accessed 1 March 2014).

Mottram, D. R. (2011). Supplement use in sport. In D. R. Mottram (Ed.), *Drugs in Sport* (5th ed.). London, UK: Routledge.

Mueller, K., and Hingst, J. (2013). *The athlete's guide to sports supplements*. Champaign, IL: Human Kinetics.

Nieman, D. C., and Pedersen, B. K. (1999). Exercise and immune function: Recent developments. *Sports Medicine* 27(2):73–80.

Nieper, A. (2005). Nutritional supplement practices in UK junior national track and field athletes. *British Journal of Sports Medicine* 39(9):645–649.

Poprzecki, S., Zebrowska, A., Cholewa, J., *et al*. (2005). Ergogenic effects of *Tribulus terrestris* supplementation in men. *Journal of Human Kinetics* 13:41–50.

Rogerson, S., Riches, C., Jennings, C., *et al*. (2007). The effect of five weeks of *Tribulus terrestris* supplementation on muscle strength and body composition on muscle strength and body composition during preseason training in elite rugby league players. *Journal of Strength and Conditioning Research* 21(2):348–353.

Russell, C., Hall, D., and Brown, P. (2013). HFL Sport Science European supplement contamination survey. Available online at http://informed-sport.com/sites/default/files/HFL%20Sport%20Science%20 2013%20European%20Supplement%20Contamination%20Survey.pdf (accessed 1 March 2014).

Sundgot-Borgen, J., Berglund, B., and Torstveit, M. K. (2003). Nutritional supplements in Norwegian elite athletes: Impact of international ranking and advisors. *Scandinavian Journal of Medical Science in Sports* 13(2):138–144.

Tscholl, P. M., Junge, A., and Dvorak, J. (2008). The use of medication and nutritional supplements during FIFA World Cups 2002 and 2006. *British Journal of Sports Medicine* 42(9):725–730.

Tsitsimpikou, C., Tsiokanos, A., Tsarouhas, K., *et al*. (2009). Medication use by athletes at the Athens 2004 Summer Olympic Games. *Clinical Journal of Sports Medicine* 19(1):33–38.

UK Anti-Doping. (2013). UK National Anti-Doping Programme. Available online at http://www.ukad .org.uk/assets/uploads/Files/2013_14_Q1_report_updated.pdf (accessed 1 March 2014).

Van Thuyme, W., Van Eenoo, P., and Delbeke, F. T. (2006). Nutritional supplements: Prevalence of use and contamination with doping agents. *Nutrition Research Reviews* 19(1):147–158.

William, H. (2013). Amphetamine-like drug was factor in death of London Marathon runner Claire Squires. Available online at http://www.independent.co.uk/news/uk/home-news/amphetaminelike-drug-was-factor-in-death-of-london-marathon-runner-claire-squires-8472689.html (accessed 1 March 2014).

World Anti-Doping Agency. (2013a). 2012 anti-doping testing figures report. Available online at https://wada-main-prod.s3.amazonaws.com/resources/files/WADA-2012-Anti-Doping-Testing-Figures-Report-EN.pdf (accessed 9 September 2014).

World Anti-Doping Agency. (2013b). The 2014 Prohibited List international standard. Available online at https://www.wada-ama.org/en/what-we-do/prohibited-list (accessed 9 September 2014).

Yonamine, M., Garcia, P. R., and de Moraes Moreau, R. L. (2004). Non-intentional doping in sports. *Sports Medicine* 34(1):697–704.

Zhang, Y., Woods, R. M., Breitbach, Z. S., and Armstrong, D. W. (2012). 1,3-Dimethylamylamine (DMAA) in supplements and geranium products: Natural or synthetic? *Drug Testing Analysis* 4(12):986–990.

Chapter 22

Caffeine

Neil Chester

22.1. Introduction

Caffeine is a phytochemical found in a wide variety of plant species distributed throughout the world. Its most common sources are coffee, tea, and cocoa. The incorporation of caffeine into various over-the-counter (OTC) medications implies that it has a useful therapeutic role. Indeed, it is a key constituent in numerous OTC medications for relief from pain and upper respiratory tract conditions, including the common cold and influenza. Because it is a constituent of a large number of commonly available beverages and foodstuffs (Table 22.1) and its use is generally unregulated and accepted throughout the world, caffeine is believed to be one of the most widely used drugs.

Caffeine has great appeal as an ergogenic aid, with extensive scientific research supporting its performance-enhancing properties over a wide range of sporting activities. It is commonly employed by many individuals for its psychotropic properties to increase wakefulness, alertness, and concentration. However, despite the widespread use of caffeine as a performance-enhancing drug, there remains conjecture regarding the exact mechanisms behind these properties.

As a consequence of caffeine's widespread consumption and limited side effects at low to moderate doses, together with the fact that it is extremely difficult – if not impossible – to differentiate via a drug test between habitual consumption and use for the purpose of enhancing performance, the World Anti-Doping Agency (WADA) removed caffeine from its Prohibited List in 2004. However, although not prohibited, caffeine has been part of the WADA Monitoring Program since its inception on 1 January 2004. Evidence gathered from the programme would potentially support or oppose the reintroduction of caffeine to the Prohibited List.

Within society as a whole, there appears to have been a general increase in the consumption of caffeine in recent years as a consequence of the growth in café culture and an expansion of the caffeinated drinks market targeted at the young, among other reasons. In sport, the use of caffeine as an ergogenic aid appears to have increased as well, following its removal from the Prohibited List. Yet, as a consequence of a general acceptance of caffeine use in society, there remains almost an unwillingness to accept or appreciate its negative side effects and the ethical implications of its use as an ergogenic aid in organised sport.

22.2. Pharmacology of caffeine

Chemically, caffeine is classified as a methylxanthine and is closely related to two other naturally occurring methylated xanthines: theophylline and theobromine (Figure 22.1).

Table 22.1 Caffeine content of selected beverages and over-the-counter (OTC) products

Beverage/OTC product	Caffeine content (mg)
Coffee	
Ground	105*
Instant	54*
Decaffeinated (instant)	2*
Decaffeinated (ground)	6*
Tea	
Black	40*
Decaffeinated	1*
Soft drinks	
Coca-Cola (355 ml)	34.5**
Pepsi Cola (355 ml)	38**
Dr. Pepper (355 ml)	41**
Sports drinks	
Lucozade Sport with caffeine boost (500 ml)	80
Energy drinks	
Red Bull (250 ml)	80
Relentless (500 ml)	160
Red Bull Energy Shot (100 ml)	133
Lucozade Alert (250 ml)	80
OTC cold and flu medication	
Benylin Cold and Flu Max strength	25/capsule
Beechams Powders	50/sachet
Do-Do Chesteze***	50/tablet
Lemsip Max Cold and Flu	25/capsule
OTC pain relief medication	
Anadin Extra	45/tablet
Askit Powders	110/sachet
Panadol Extra	65/tablet
OTC products for the relief of tiredness	
Pro-Plus	50/tablet

* Average caffeine levels according to the Food Standards Agency (2004).
** Caffeine levels according to Ressig *et al.* (2009).
*** Do-Do Chesteze also contains theophylline (100 mg) and ephedrine (18.31 mg).

Caffeine (1,3,7-trimethylxanthine) is a trimethylated xanthine, whilst theophylline and theobromine are dimethylated xanthines. Pharmacologically, theophylline is considered to be the most potent of the naturally occurring methylxanthines with theobromine, a constituent of cocoa, being the least potent (Undem and Lichtenstein 2001).

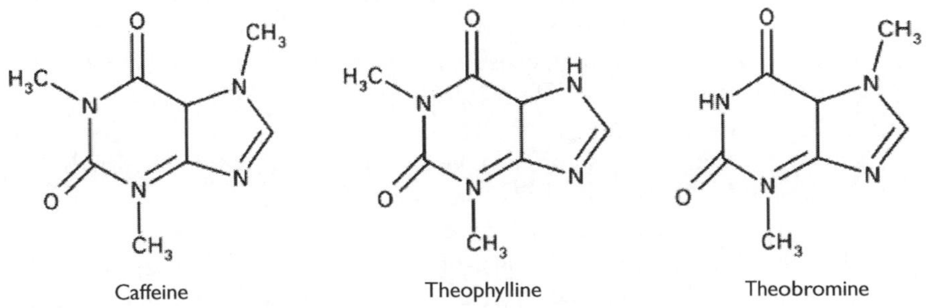

Caffeine   Theophylline   Theobromine

Figure 22.1 Chemical structure of naturally occurring methylxanthines.

Caffeine is rapidly absorbed via the gastrointestinal tract and reaches peak plasma concentrations between 30 and 60 minutes after oral ingestion (Sawynok and Yaksh 1993). Due to its lipophilic properties, caffeine is distributed widely around the body, easily crossing the blood–brain barrier and placenta. The half-life of caffeine in healthy individuals is approximately 4 hours (Lelo et al. 1986a), and it is metabolised extensively through demethylation into paraxanthine (80 per cent), theobromine (11 per cent), and theophylline (4 per cent) by chytochrome P450 enzymes in the liver (Lelo et al. 1986b).

Caffeinated chewing gum is a recent addition to the marketplace. It offers an advantage over traditional methods of caffeine administration/consumption in terms of the speed of absorption. Whilst bioavailability is similar to other methods, chewing gum allows rapid absorption into the circulation via the buccal mucosa, thus bypassing first-pass metabolism and limiting the risk of gastrointestinal side effects (Paton et al. 2010).

22.3. Mechanisms of action of caffeine

Whilst it is accepted that caffeine has marked pharmacological, physiological, and performance-enhancing effects, some conjecture remains regarding the exact mechanisms involved. However, the principal mechanism by which caffeine exerts its effects is believed to be as an adenosine receptor antagonist. It is the only mechanism that is believed to occur at caffeine concentrations in the magnitude of those experienced following typical caffeine consumption (Fredholm 1995).

Adenosine is a modulator of various physiological processes, both in the central nervous system (CNS) and in the peripheral tissues via adenosine receptors. Adenosine receptors are located in most tissues, including the brain, heart, smooth muscle, adipocytes, and skeletal muscle. The effects of adenosine are therefore widespread. Adenosine receptors, located on the cell membrane and coupled to G-proteins, can be divided into four subtypes: A_1, A_{2A}, A_{2B}, and A_3. Stimulation of A_1 receptors typically initiates inhibitory responses through a reduction in cyclic adenosine monophosphate (AMP) and stimulation of potassium channels. Inhibition of calcium flux is also believed to occur following A_1 receptor activation (Shimada and Suzuki 2000). Activation also inhibits noradrenergic, dopaminergic, serotonergic, and acetylcholinergic neurotransmission. The A_{2A} receptors are linked to dopaminergic neurons, and stimulation of these receptors appears to be involved in the inhibition of dopaminergic neurotransmission. The A_{2B} receptors are believed to be low-affinity receptors serving a modulating role, whilst A_3 receptors are believed to be sparsely distributed in the CNS (Graham 1997).

Caffeine, which is similar in structure to adenosine, has the most affinity to the A_1 and A_{2A} receptors. Also, its ability to cross the blood–brain barrier means that it readily affects the CNS. Because adenosine has largely an inhibitory effect, caffeine, as an adenosine receptor antagonist, therefore has a stimulatory effect. The complex nature of caffeine's actions relates to the ubiquitous nature of adenosine receptors and the fact that it is able to operate via the receptors in both a direct or indirect manner.

Despite the importance of adenosine receptor antagonism in characterising the effects of caffeine, other related mechanisms are believed to play a role. Inhibition of cyclic nucleotide phosphodiesterase, which leads to increased cyclic AMP and increased sensitivity of calcium translocation, are considered to be key mechanisms.

Caffeine's ability to inhibit cyclic nucleotide phosphodiesterase enzymes is significant because it results in increased intracellular levels of cyclic AMP and cyclic guanosine monophosphate (GMP). These molecules act as secondary messengers, enabling signal-response pathways to be enhanced. Cyclic AMP is involved in the signal-response pathway that activates inactive hormone-sensitive lipase and stimulates lipolysis in adipose tissue. Increased sympathetic nervous system activity also results in enhanced intracellular cyclic AMP levels, leading to increased lipolysis. These mechanisms fit neatly with the positive effects of caffeine associated with endurance exercise performance and the proposed glycogen-sparing hypothesis. However, such mechanisms are not considered to account primarily for the enhanced endurance that follows caffeine consumption. Indeed, research has found improvements without significant increases in circulating adrenaline and free fatty acids (FFAs) or a reduction in the respiratory exchange ratio (Graham and Spriet, 1991, 1995).

The ability of caffeine to effect calcium translocation in the muscle may contribute directly to performance enhancement during physical exercise. Increases in intracellular calcium have been observed with caffeine. Caffeine seems to interfere with excitation-contraction coupling. Caffeine activates the release of calcium from the sarcoplasmic reticulum, which binds with troponin and activates the myofilaments, leading to contraction. Whilst this has been demonstrated *in vitro* using high caffeine doses, the ability to show similar effects using doses comparable with those taken by humans has proved difficult (Tarnopolsky 2008).

Because the ability to combat fatigue may relate directly to maintenance of electrolyte homeostasis, caffeine may have a direct impact as a consequence of its reported effect on potassium levels. Lindinger *et al.* (1993) reported that plasma potassium increased to a lesser extent during exercise following caffeine administration. The significance of this finding is that fatigue is associated with suppression in resting membrane potential and therefore less motor unit activation and force production. This may occur as a result of loss of potassium from the myocyte, thus increasing plasma potassium levels, or less release of calcium from the sarcoplasmic reticulum. The lower plasma potassium levels observed following caffeine administration may be a consequence of increased plasma clearance or a lower efflux from the active muscle. It has been hypothesised that caffeine works directly or indirectly via adrenaline to stimulate muscle sodium/potassium ATPase and subsequent potassium uptake (Lindinger *et al.* 1993, 1996).

22.4. Performance-enhancing properties of caffeine

As an ergogenic aid, caffeine is used extensively across many sports in an attempt to increase alertness and perception, mask the symptoms of fatigue, spare energy substrates, and increase muscle force production and endurance. Whilst these effects following caffeine administration have not been demonstrated unequivocally, there is widespread support amongst the athletic and scientific community alike.

The effects of caffeine administration on performance show great inter-individual variation. Individuals who display limited ergogenic effects following caffeine ingestion are often termed *nonresponders*. The factors that are likely to contribute to this variation may relate to the source of caffeine ingested, the dose and timing of ingestion, and individual characteristics relating to caffeine habituation and metabolism. The effects of caffeine have been shown to be most prominent amongst individuals who do not consume caffeine on a regular basis as opposed to habitual consumers (Bell and McLellan 2002).

Whilst there is no evidence to support a dose–response relationship in terms of caffeine and performance, there appears to be an optimum dose above which adverse side effects may prevail and potentially be detrimental to performance. Positive improvements in performance have been shown following relatively low doses of caffeine (i.e. 2.1 mg/kg body weight [BW];

Kovacs *et al.* 1998). However, the optimum dose for performance enhancement is believed to be between 3 and 6 mg/kg BW (Spriet 2002). Higher doses of caffeine (i.e. 9 mg/kg BW) have shown no further improvements in performance (Graham and Spriet 1991; Pasman *et al.* 1995).

To aid sports performance, caffeine is typically ingested 1 hour before competition. However, whilst caffeine is rapidly absorbed, it is metabolised relatively slowly and remains at high concentrations in the circulation for several hours. There is a suggestion that its metabolic action (i.e. peak FFA levels) may peak at 3 hours after exercise and therefore may incur the greatest effect on endurance exercise performance (Nehlig and Debry 1994). However, because caffeine-induced lipolysis is not deemed to be a central mechanism in improved endurance exercise, such a proposal is unlikely to significantly influence performance.

Interestingly, although coffee is considered to be the most widespread source of caffeine, its use as an ergogenic aid has been questioned. Whilst pure caffeine ingestion enhanced endurance performance, Graham *et al.* (1998) found no effect following caffeine ingestion in the form of coffee. It was suggested that some constituents of coffee may interfere with caffeine and its ergogenic properties (Graham 2001). Nevertheless, other studies have refuted this claim and have demonstrated ergogenic effects following caffeine ingestion as a constituent of coffee (Wiles *et al.* 1992; Hodgson *et al.* 2013). In practice, an issue in administering caffeine through coffee relates to the difficulty in standardising the dose of caffeine consumed.

There has been limited research into the effects of other methylxanthines on sports performance. Theophylline is considered to be the most potent of the naturally occurring methylxanthines. However, Morton *et al.* (1989) found no effects on VO_{2max}, muscular performance (strength, power, and endurance) and psychomotor performance following the administration of 10–13 mg/kg BW per day of theophylline over a 4-day period. Conversely, Greer *et al.* (2000) examined the effects of both caffeine and theophylline and found both enhanced endurance cycling performance.

Most research has tended to focus on the impact of acute caffeine supplementation on competitive events. Whilst there is a clear rationale for assessing the ergogenic effects of caffeine during competition, it may be pertinent to examine the effects of caffeine supplementation during a training regimen. It is realistic to speculate that the use of caffeine as a training aid would have a significant impact on subsequent competitive performance.

Endurance exercise

Research by Costill *et al.* (1978) demonstrated significant increases in endurance cycling performance following moderate doses of caffeine. This research paved the way for the huge interest in caffeine as a performance-enhancing substance in endurance exercise. It was proposed that caffeine promoted FFA mobilisation through increased catecholamine release. Glycogen sparing was believed to occur as a consequence of greater FFA utilisation by the exercising muscles due to increased availability of circulating FFA. It is now understood that this is not the sole mechanism, nor is it the most important. In most instances, exercise performance is not limited by muscle glycogen. Whilst caffeine is clearly able to affect muscle fuel supply, this mechanism does not account for the many ergogenic effects experienced during endurance and short-term exercise alike.

Nonetheless, the ergogenic effects of caffeine on endurance performance would appear to be unquestionable. Caffeine ingestion (3–13 mg/kg BW) has been shown to improve time to exhaustion using exercise protocols at 80–85 per cent VO_{2max} (Graham and Spriet 1995;

Pasman *et al.* 1995). Similarly, in more ecologically valid time-trial protocols, endurance performance lasting between 30 and 60 min has shown improvements following doses of caffeine between 3 and 6 mg/kg BW (Kovacs *et al.* 1998; Bridge and Jones 2006; Laurence *et al.* 2012). Performance of short-term endurance exercise has also shown improvements following caffeine ingestion. In rowing, caffeine ingestion (6–9 mg/kg BW) has significantly enhanced 2000-m time-trial performance (Anderson *et al.* 2000; Bruce *et al.* 2000). In swimming, 1500-m time-trial performance was enhanced following caffeine ingestion (6 mg/kg BW; MacIntosh and Wright 1995).

Anaerobic exercise

Whilst the effects of caffeine on endurance exercise have been widely documented, there has been relatively less attention placed upon the effects of caffeine supplementation on short-term, high-intensity exercise. The studies that have been conducted are not conclusive in their support for caffeine as an aid to anaerobic exercise performance.

Very few studies have examined the effects of caffeine on sport-specific sprinting performance. Collomp *et al.* (1992) assessed whether caffeine ingestion (250 mg) had any impact on 100-m freestyle swimming. In trained swimmers, swimming velocity significantly increased under caffeine conditions. As part of a protocol to simulate rugby union, Stuart *et al.* (2005) examined the effects of caffeine (6 mg/kg BW) on 20- and 30-m sprints; they found improvements in mean performance.

Maximal accumulated oxygen deficit (MAOD), an indirect measure of anaerobic capacity, has been employed to examine the effects of caffeine on anaerobic performance (Doherty 1998; Bell *et al.* 2001). Doherty (1998) found that caffeine ingestion (5 mg/kg BW) improved time to exhaustion in a running protocol by 14 per cent, whilst Bell and colleagues (2001) reported significant improvements in both time to exhaustion and MAOD using a cycling protocol under caffeine conditions (5 mg/kg BW).

The Wingate test has also been used to assess potential improvements in anaerobic performance in response to caffeine supplementation (Collomp *et al.* 1991; Kang *et al.*, 1998; Beck *et al.* 2006; Greer *et al.* 2006). However, only Kang and colleagues (1998) demonstrated enhanced performance. Following caffeine doses of 2.5 and 5 mg/kg BW, significant improvements were reported in total, peak, and mean power during a 30-s Wingate test.

It has been speculated that if caffeine's effects are mediated by the CNS, then any effects in competition may be masked by the heightened arousal experienced in competition (Davis and Green 2009). It is clear that further research is required to establish the ergogenic value of caffeine on anaerobic performance.

Resistance exercise

In light of the reputed effects of caffeine on contractile properties of muscle and on central mechanisms such as motivation, it would seem extremely feasible that caffeine would have a positive impact upon resistance exercise. Despite several studies examining the ergogenic properties of caffeine on such exercise, there appears to be no conclusive evidence to support its use.

Commonly used methods to assess muscular strength include the determination of one repetition maximum (1 RM), isokinetic peak torque, or force produced during an isometric maximal voluntary contraction (MVC). Beck *et al.* (2006) reported a significant increase in bench-press 1 RM but no increase in leg-press 1 RM following caffeine ingestion. Astorino *et al*. (2008), however, found no increase in bench-press or leg-press 1 RM following caffeine ingestion (6 mg/kg BW). In a study by Bond *et al*. (1986), the effects of caffeine ingestion (5 mg/kg BW) on isokinetic knee flexor and extensor strength were examined. There were no significant differences in peak torque across a range of speeds (30, 150, and 300 deg/s) between caffeine and placebo trials. In elite athletes, Jacobson *et al*. (1992), however, reported greater peak torque for knee flexors at speeds of 30, 150, and 300 deg/s and for knee extensors at speeds of 30 and 300 deg/s following caffeine consumption (7 mg/kg BW). Similarly, a study by Duncan *et al*. (2014) demonstrated a significant effect of caffeine ingestion (6 mg/kg BW) over placebo on peak torque during isokinetic knee extension exercise across three speeds (30, 150, and 300 deg/s) with an augmented effect, with increases in angular velocity. Kalmar and Cafarelli (1999) reported a significant increase in MVC following caffeine administration (6 mg/kg BW), whilst Tarnopolsky and Cupido (2000) found no ergogenic value of caffeine in relation to MVC.

Several studies have examined muscular endurance using repetitions of exercises at a percentage of 1 RM until volitional fatigue. Beck *et al*. (2006) found no significant effect of caffeine on bench-press and leg-press exercises (80 per cent 1 RM) to failure. Using a similar protocol (60 per cent 1 RM until failure), Astorino *et al*. (2008) reported nonsignificant increases in muscular endurance following caffeine ingestion in the order of 11 and 12 per cent for bench-press and leg-press exercises, respectively. Muscular endurance has been assessed in other studies through sustained isometric contractions. Caffeine has shown positive effects on isometric knee extensions (50 per cent MVC) in doses of 6 mg/kg BW (Kalmar and Cafarelli 1999; Plaskett and Cafarelli 2001; Meyers and Cafarelli 2005).

Intermittent exercise

Team games, such as football and rugby, are characterised by aerobic exercise interspersed with repeated, intermittent bouts of high-intensity anaerobic exercise. The ability to assess physiological performance has proved extremely difficult within these sports. Of those researchers that have attempted to assess intermittent exercise, few have been successful in recreating the demands of a game.

The Yo-Yo intermittent recovery test developed by Bangsbo *et al*. (2008) was developed to simulate the activity pattern of sports such as football. Applying this test to an intervention study involving caffeine supplementation (6 mg/kg BW) showed an enhancement in fatigue resistance over placebo (Mohr *et al*. 2011). Schneiker *et al*. (2006) examined the effect of caffeine supplementation (6 mg/kg BW) on a repeated sprint protocol consisting of two 36-min halves (18 × 4-s sprints and 2-min active recovery between each sprint). Performance, with respect to the total amount of sprint work and mean power output, was enhanced under caffeine conditions. However, Paton *et al*. (2001) investigated the effects of caffeine ingestion (6 mg/kg BW) on a repeated 20-m sprint protocol (10 × 20-m sprint with 10-s recovery following each sprint) and found no effect on performance or fatigue.

The difficulty in assessing physiological performance has led many researchers to focus on physiological function or skill performance. Stuart *et al*. (2005) examined the effects of caffeine (6 mg/kg BW) on a battery of tests chosen to simulate the physical and skill demands of a rugby union match. Whilst improvements in most tests were evident, performance of tackle speed and reduction in fatigue in 30-m sprint speed were performance measures that had been particularly enhanced by caffeine supplementation. Foskett *et al*. (2009)

demonstrated improvements in passing accuracy and jump performance amongst football players participating in a simulated soccer-specific activity following caffeine ingestion (6 mg/kg BW). Such research highlights clearly the multifaceted effects of caffeine and its ability to enhance not only physiological performance but also cognitive function and psychomotor performance.

Cognitive function

Caffeine is used extensively by the wider population to increase alertness in a variety of situations, such as conditions of sleep deprivation, at nighttime, during the postlunch dip, and during periods of long working hours, such as studying or prolonged driving. There is a large body of evidence to support the use of caffeine as a cognitive performance enhancer, especially in conditions of low arousal. It has been shown to increase cognitive function, such as alertness and mood state (Penetar *et al.* 1993), as well as vigilance, learning, and memory (Lieberman *et al.* 2002), under conditions of sleep deprivation.

Effects on mood and motor performance are believed to be related to caffeine's affinity to A_{2A} receptors and stimulation of dopaminergic neurotransmission. The positive effect of caffeine on mood has been demonstrated via reports of lower anxiety and increased contentedness, self-confidence, and motivation following ingestion (Lieberman *et al.* 1987).

Decreased reaction time typically demonstrates improved selective attention and efficient information processing. The positive effect of caffeine on cognitive performance tasks has been demonstrated with reaction time (Smit and Rogers 2000) and choice reaction time (van Duinen *et al.* 2005).

Whilst much of the research has centred on enhancement of generic behavioural characteristics following caffeine ingestion, they are clearly transferable to sport. However, it may be difficult to assess the effects on more complex tasks within a sporting context because the heightened state of arousal that is typical of competition may mask any effects likely by caffeine ingestion.

22.5. Caffeine combinations

The coadministration of nutritional and pharmacological substances to enhance performance is common. Combinations of caffeine with additional supplements, including carbohydrate and sympathomimetic amines, may further enhance sports performance.

Whilst ingestion of carbohydrate supplements during exercise is common amongst endurance athletes, the introduction of caffeine as an ingredient of such supplements (i.e. sports drinks, gels) is relatively new and has no doubt increased following caffeine's removal from the WADA Prohibited List. A study examining the ingestion of a sports drink (a carbohydrate-electrolyte solution) with added caffeine (2.1, 3.2, and 4.5 mg/kg BW) during a 1-h cycling time trial led to an improvement in performance (Kovacs *et al.* 1998). Similarly, Cox *et al.* (2002) reported improved time-trial performance following 2 h of steady-state cycling amongst subjects who coingested carbohydrate and caffeine during exercise in the form of Coca-Cola (3 × ~1.5 mg/kg BW). Caffeine in low doses (~1.5–3 mg/kg BW) ingested with carbohydrate during exercise would therefore appear to have ergogenic benefits.

In work by Pederson *et al.* (2008), the coingestion of carbohydrate with high doses of caffeine (8 mg/kg BW) after exhaustive exercise resulted in significantly greater muscle glycogen resynthesis during the 4 hours postexercise when compared with carbohydrate ingestion alone. According to the authors, the rate of glycogen resynthesis (~60 mmol/kg dry weight per h) was deemed to be the highest that has been observed in humans under physiological conditions. Whilst further research is required, caffeine may play a key role in nutritional strategies designed to promote optimal recovery.

Caffeine in combination with sympathomimetic amines is often employed in weight reduction therapy. Caffeine with ephedrine is a particularly common combination used for its thermogenic and anorectic properties. Boozer et al. (2001) found significant weight reduction in obese individuals following supplementation with natural sources of caffeine and ephedrine (guarana and ma huang). Indeed, several products marketed as herbal weight loss supplements typically contain caffeine from guarana, a plant from South America whose seeds contain caffeine, theophylline, and theobromine (Espinola et al. 1997). These products also contain natural sources of sympathomimetics, such as ephedrine and synephrine in the form of ma huang and *Citrus aurantium*, respectively. Both caffeine and ephedrine are also commonly combined with acetylsalicylic acid (aspirin) for its weight reduction properties (Astrup and Toubro 1993). Whilst the mechanisms behind the weight-reducing effects of such drug combinations are not clearly understood, both caffeine and aspirin are believed to work synergistically with the thermogenic effects of ephedrine (Dulloo 1993).

In addition to weight loss, research in recent years has supported the use of caffeine in combination with ephedrine or pseudoephedrine directly as a performance-enhancing aid (Bell et al. 1998, 2002; Weatherby and Rogerson 2002). Bell et al. (1998) demonstrated a significant improvement in time to exhaustion using a cycling protocol (85 per cent VO_{2max}) following caffeine (5 mg/kg BW) and ephedrine (1 mg/kg BW) supplementation over placebo and supplementation of caffeine alone. Ephedrine (0.8 mg/kg BW) and caffeine (4 mg/kg BW) in combination have also shown improvements in a 10-km run time trial whilst wearing fighting order weighing approximately 11 kg (Bell et al. 2002). There is limited support for the combination of caffeine with pseudoephedrine; nevertheless, Weatherby and Rogerson (2002) reported an improvement in short-duration, supramaximal cycling exercise following the supplementation of 300 mg of caffeine with 120 mg of pseudoephedrine. Whilst the combination of caffeine with ephedrines appears to boost performance-enhancing properties, there is clearly a need for further research to elucidate the performance-enhancing mechanisms.

22.6. Therapeutic actions of caffeine

The inclusion of methylxanthines in many OTC medications is as a bronchodilator or an analgesic adjuvant. Theophylline is largely incorporated into cold and flu preparations due to its role as a bronchodilator, whilst caffeine is typically incorporated into pain relief medication as an adjuvant to aspirin or acetaminophen (paracetamol). Evidence suggests that combining a peripheral-acting analgesic such as acetaminophen with caffeine provides pain relief that is typical of the relief experienced when combined with a centrally acting analgesic (Laska et al. 1984). Therefore, the side effects of a centrally acting analgesic can be avoided and it precludes the need to take high doses of aspirin and paracetamol. Research has suggested that these effects are mediated by central amplification of cholinergic neurotransmission (Ghelardini et al. 1997). However, the mechanisms behind these properties of caffeine are not clearly understood. Indeed, some studies have questioned the analgesic adjuvant properties of caffeine (Zhang and Li Wan Po 1996, 1997).

22.7. Adverse side effects of caffeine

Plasma caffeine concentrations above 15 μg/ml can result in toxic symptoms such as tachycardia, arrhythmia, and tremor. Concentrations greater than 80 μg/ml are considered to be fatal (Riesselmann *et al.* 1999). Despite the widespread availability and consumption of products containing caffeine, there are relatively few reports of caffeine intoxication. Nevertheless, in a review by Banerjee *et al.* (2014), eight adult cases of fatal intoxication within a 10-year period (1999–2009) were highlighted within the state of Maryland. Whilst no deaths were attributed to overconsumption of caffeine-containing foods in that report, a recent case in the United Kingdom involved the death of a 40-year-old man following the consumption of twelve caffeinated sweets believed to amount to almost 1 g of caffeine (Bradley 2013). Cirrhosis of the liver was believed to have been a confounding factor in the man's death because it would result in reduced metabolism of caffeine and thus lead to an accumulation in the circulation.

The safety of caffeine consumption in relation to the cardiovascular system has long been a contentious issue. Dietary caffeine intake has been linked with cardiovascular mortality and morbidity (James 2004). Rosenberg *et al.* (1988) suggested that consumption of caffeinated coffee increases the risk of myocardial infarction. Also, research has shown a positive relationship between coffee consumption and elevations in systolic blood pressure (Jee *et al.* 1999). However, there is a considerable body of evidence that opposes these conclusions. A large prospective study by Grobbee *et al.* (1990) found no association with coffee consumption and increased risk of coronary heart disease or stroke. Indeed, low to moderate caffeine consumption in the form of coffee may even have cardioprotective effects, attributed to the antioxidants present in coffee (Cornelis and El-Sohemy 2007).

The most noticeable side effects of caffeine are those pertaining to the CNS. Whilst caffeine is ingested for its positive effects on cognitive function, excessive doses may cause numerous side effects. Insomnia, headache, nervousness, restlessness, tremors, and irritability are examples of side effects following high-dose administration of caffeine. Chronic consumption of caffeine can lead to dependence and tolerance as the body upregulates the number of adenosine receptors. Withdrawal symptoms are frequently experienced upon abrupt cessation of its consumption. According to Reeves *et al.* (1997), acute caffeine withdrawal can cause distress and symptoms of nausea, nervousness, tachycardia, arrhythmia, and insomnia. Interestingly, the symptoms experienced during withdrawal are similar to those following excessive caffeine consumption. Silverman *et al.* (1992) demonstrated that withdrawal symptoms, including a drop in mood, increased anxiety, fatigue, and headache, can also be experienced in low to moderate caffeine consumers. Indeed, Evans and Griffiths (1999) confirmed that withdrawal and physical dependence can occur at low doses and following a short period of exposure (i.e. 3 consecutive days).

Frequent urination is a commonly stated symptom of caffeine ingestion. Excessive fluid loss through urination may result in diuresis and a reduction in plasma volume. However, such concerns would appear to be unfounded. Whilst mild diuresis was demonstrated following administration of caffeinated drinks, there were no significant changes in urine and plasma osmolarity, sweat rate, or plasma volume (Wemple *et al.* 1997).

Groups that are believed to be particularly sensitive to caffeine include pregnant women, infants, and children. Caffeine consumption is deemed to be particularly problematic due to the extended half-life of caffeine within pregnant women and infants and the high doses of caffeine, in relation to body weight, that are consumed by children. The half-life of caffeine is extended during pregnancy by approximately twofold when compared with nonpregnant women (Knutti *et al.*, 1981). This is significant because it extends the time at which caffeine can exert its effects and increases the potential for toxicity. Caffeine also freely crosses the placenta and passes into breast milk (Undem and Lichtenstein 2001). Further evidence has linked caffeine consumption in pregnant women with low birth weight (Cade 2008).

Caffeine is often mistakenly associated with poor iron absorption. Whilst the consumption of tea and coffee has been shown to negatively affect dietary iron absorption (Morck *et al.* 1983; Hurrell *et al.* 1999), this has not been attributed to caffeine intake. Tea and coffee contain polyphenols that can bind to iron, making it difficult to absorb. A recommendation to avoid such beverages at mealtimes is particularly important for people at risk of iron deficiency.

22.8. Caffeine use and WADA regulations

In 1984, caffeine was included in the International Olympic Committee Prohibited List and a urinary concentration threshold of 15 µg/ml was set in an attempt to combat inadvertent positive drug tests following normal/acceptable caffeine intake. In 1985, this threshold was reduced to 12 µg/ml, and caffeine remained on the Prohibited List until 2004. In 2004, WADA produced its first Prohibited List and specific stimulants such as caffeine and pseudoephedrine were removed, and, with phenylephrine, were included in the Monitoring Program.

The purpose of the Monitoring Program is to examine specific substances with the aim of identifying potential misuse (WADA 2009). This data may be used as evidence to support the reintroduction of substances back to the Prohibited List (WADA 2003). As a consequence, the consumption of caffeine was allowed in sport without restriction. However, the motivation behind the removal of caffeine from the Prohibited List remains unclear. According to the Prohibited List committee, there was concern with regards to whether caffeine levels in the urine were a good determinant of misuse due to the high degree of intersubject variability in urine caffeine levels (WADA 2003). It would appear that the premise behind the Monitoring Program is to avoid the frustration and adverse publicity associated with an inadvertent positive drug test caused by legitimate use of therapeutic OTC medication or acceptable social consumption of caffeine. This would suggest that whilst caffeine has been removed from the Prohibited List, WADA is not advocating its use as a performance-enhancing supplement. Unfortunately, this message has not been clearly voiced.

Undoubtedly, with the advent of the Monitoring Program, there was the potential for caffeine use to increase markedly within sport. However, laboratory data do not support this (Van Thuyne and Delbeke, 2006). Analysis of urinary caffeine levels before and after the removal of caffeine from the Prohibited List showed that the overall percentage of positive samples remained the same. Surprisingly, overall urinary caffeine concentrations actually dropped after 2004. Following the examination of samples in relation to sport, only cycling and powerlifting showed an increase in urinary caffeine concentrations. Del Coso *et al.* (2011), in their examination of 20,686 doping control urine samples between 2004 and 2008, found only 0.6 per cent exceeding the former urinary threshold, with endurance sports demonstrating the highest use.

With a view to examining the motives of caffeine use pre- and post-2004, Chester and Wojek (2008) surveyed 480 track and field athletes and cyclists. It was revealed that use of caffeine for performance-enhancing purposes was high, especially amongst the elite, and that this had increased post-2004. Further work assessing the impact of the changes to the Prohibited List in 2004 was carried out by Desbrow and Leveritt (2006). Almost 90 per cent of competitors questioned at the 2005 Ironman Triathlon World Championships intended to use caffeine prior to or during the competition.

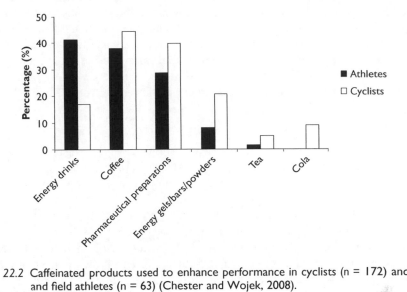

Figure 22.2 Caffeinated products used to enhance performance in cyclists (n = 172) and track and field athletes (n = 63) (Chester and Wojek, 2008).

The sports supplements market, whilst considered a niche market, has attempted to profit from the reclassification of caffeine in elite sport. Caffeine has been added to numerous products in an attempt to increase their efficacy as ergogenic supplements. Evidence of the use of caffeinated energy gels, bars, and powders in addition to more traditional sources of caffeine (i.e. coffee, energy drinks, pharmaceutical preparations) amongst track-and-field athletes and cyclists has been shown by Chester and Wojek (2008; Figure 22.2).

Central to the caffeinated sports supplements market is the caffeinated energy drinks market. This market has grown exponentially in recent years, with UK consumption believed to have more than doubled between the years 2006 and 2012. In 2012, consumption of caffeinated energy drinks was estimated at 276 million litres (British Soft Drinks Association 2013). The primary consumers are thought to be those under 35 years of age and predominantly male.

An investigation into the consumption of caffeinated energy drinks amongst college students from the United States found that 51 per cent of participants regularly consume an average of one energy drink per month (Malinauskas *et al.* 2007). The reasons put forward for their consumption was to increase alertness following insufficient sleep (67 per cent), to increase energy (65 per cent), and to consume with alcohol for social reasons (54 per cent). Side effects were regularly reported, such as headaches (22 per cent) and heart palpitations (19 per cent). Energy drinks were attributed to 6 per cent of total caffeine intake by children and adolescents in the United States in 2009–2010 (Branum *et al.* 2014).

There is concern regarding the excessive use of caffeinated energy drinks, which has been compounded by reports of several deaths throughout Europe linked with such misuse (Dhar *et al.* 2005). The sale of high-caffeine energy drinks is banned in a number of countries, such as France and Denmark, which have imposed a statutory limit of 150 μg/ml of caffeine in soft drinks (Finnegan 2003). James (2012) argued that widespread regulation should be considered involving the following measures: improved labelling of products with high caffeine content, restrictions placed on advertising of such products, taxation of high caffeine-containing products, and age restrictions on their sale.

Clearly, only a small proportion of the caffeinated energy drinks market relates to their use in sport. Nevertheless, the expansion in the caffeinated energy drinks market coupled with a 6.4 per cent growth in sales from coffee retail outlets in the United Kingdom in 2013 to over £6.2 billion in turnover (Algebra Strategies Ltd 2013, cited by Eversham 2014) would suggest a significant increase in the consumption of caffeine across the general population. Undoubtedly, a rise in caffeine consumption throughout society is likely to affect both the social use and ergogenic use of caffeine by those participating in sport.

22.9. Summary

Caffeine is arguably the most commonly used performance-enhancing drug in the world due to its wide-ranging effects and its appeal to athletes across a broad spectrum of sports. Despite caffeine's clear performance-enhancing properties, it still provokes great interest amongst the scientific community. Whilst significant improvements in numerous sporting activities have been shown following moderate dosing with caffeine, there remains some conjecture with respect to the mechanisms behind these effects.

Although the use or consumption of caffeine is generally accepted, if not embraced, within most cultures of the world, it still commands attention from health authorities. With recent growth in coffee sales and the exponential growth in the caffeinated energy drinks market, attention has been placed on caffeine consumption amongst children. Particular concern relates to the aggressive marketing techniques of such drink companies and their effect on consumption amongst children. From a sporting perspective, it may be difficult to reconcile the anti-doping message whilst caffeine, an established performance-enhancing drug, is condoned and even actively promoted within many sporting bodies.

22.10. References

Anderson, M. E., Bruce, C. R., Fraser, S. F. *et al.* (2000). Improved 2000 meter rowing performance in competitive oarswomen after caffeine ingestion. *International Journal of Sports Nutrition and Exercise Metabolism* 10(4): 464–475.

Astorino, T. A., Rohmann, R. L., and Firth, K. (2008). Effect of caffeine ingestion on one-repetition maximum muscular strength. *European Journal of Applied Physiology* 102(2):127–132.

Astrup, A., and Toubro, S. (1993). Thermogenic, metabolic and cardiovascular responses to ephedrine and caffeine in man. *International Journal of Obesity* 17(Suppl 1):S41–S43.

Banerjee, P., Ali, Z., Levine, B., and Fowler, D. R. (2014). Fatal caffeine intoxication: A series of eight cases from 1999 to 2009. *Journal of Forensic Science* 59(3):865–868.

Bangsbo, J., Laia, F. M., and Krustrup, P. (2008). The Yo-Yo intermittent recovery test: A useful tool for evaluation of physical performance in intermittent sports. *Sports Medicine* 38(1):37–51.

Beck, T. W., Housh, T. J., Schmidt, R. J., *et al.* (2006). The acute effects of caffeine-containing supplement on strength, muscle endurance and anaerobic capabilities. *Journal of Strength and Conditioning Research* 20(3):506–510.

Bell, D. G., Jacobs, I., and Ellerington, K. (2001). Effect of caffeine and ephedrine on anaerobic exercise performance. *Medicine and Science in Sports and Exercise* 33(8):1399–1403.

Bell, D. G., Jacobs, I., and Zamecnik, J. (1998). Effects of caffeine, ephedrine and their combination on time to exhaustion during high-intensity exercise. *European Journal of Applied Physiology and Occupational Physiology* 77(5):427–433.

Bell, D. G., and McLellan, T. M. (2002). Exercise endurance 1, 3 and 6 h after caffeine ingestion in caffeine users and non-users. *Journal of Applied Physiology* 93(4):1227–1234.

Bell, D. G., McLellan, T. M., and Sabiston, C. M. (2002). Effect of ingesting caffeine and ephedrine on 10-km run performance. *Medicine and Science in Sports and Exercise* 34(2):344–349.

Bond, V., Gresham, K., McRae, J., *et al.* (1986). Caffeine ingestion and isokinetic strength. *British Journal of Sports Medicine* 20(3):135–137.

Boozer, C. N., Nasser, J. A., Heymsfield, S. B., *et al.* (2001). A herbal supplement containing Ma Huang-Guarana for weight loss: A randomised, double-blind trial. *International Journal of Obesity* 25(3):316–324.

Bradley, S. (2013). Dad John Jackson died from caffeine overdose after eating sweet shop mints. Available online at http://www.birminghammail.co.uk/news/local-news/dad-john-jackson-died-caffeine-6170091 (accessed 28 February 2014).

Branum, A. M., Rossen, L. M., and Schoendorf, K. C. (2014). Trends in caffeine intake among U.S. children and adolescents. *Pediatrics* 133(3):386–393.

Bridge, C. A., and Jones, M. A. (2006). The effect of caffeine on 8 km run performance in a field setting. *Journal of Sport Sciences* 24(4):433–439.

British Soft Drinks Association. (2013). The 2013 UK soft drinks report. Available online at: http://www.britishsoftdrinks.com/write/MediaUploads/Publications/2013UKsoftdrinksreport.pdf (accessed 11 September 2014).

Bruce, C. R., Anderson, M. E., Fraser, S. F., *et al.* (2000). Enhancement of 2000 m rowing performance after caffeine ingestion. *Medicine and Science in Sports and Exercise* 32(11):1958–1963.

Cade, J. (2008). Maternal caffeine intake during pregnancy and risk of fetal growth restriction: A large prospective observational study. Available online at http://www.foodbase.org.uk/results.php?f_category_id=&f_report_id=273 (accessed 11 September 2014).

Chester, N., and Wojek, N. (2008). Caffeine consumption amongst British athletes following changes to the 2004 WADA Prohibited List. *International Journal of Sports Medicine* 29(6):524–528.

Collomp, K., Ahmaidi, S., Audran, M., *et al.* (1991). Effects of caffeine ingestion on performance and anaerobic metabolism during the Wingate test. *International Journal of Sports Medicine* 12(5):439–443.

Collomp, K., Ahmaidi, S., Chatard, J. C., *et al.* (1992). Benefits of caffeine ingestion on sprint performance in trained and untrained swimmers. *European Journal of Applied Physiology* 64(4):377–380.

Cornelis, M. C., and El-Sohemy, A. (2007). Coffee, caffeine and coronary heart disease. *Current Opinion in Clinical Nutrition and Metabolic Care* 10(6):745–751.

Costill, D. L., Dalsky, G. P., and Fink, W. J. (1978). Effects of caffeine ingestion on metabolism and exercise performance. *Medicine and Science in Sports* 10(3):155–158.

Cox, G. R., Desbrow, B., Montgomery, P. G., *et al.* (2002). Effect of different protocols of caffeine intake on metabolism and endurance performance. *Journal of Applied Physiology* 93(3):990–999.

Davis, J. K., and Green, J. M. (2009). Caffeine and anaerobic performance ergogenic value and mechanisms of action. *Sports Medicine* 39(10):813–832.

Del Coso, J., Munoz, G., and Munoz-Guerra, J. (2011). Prevalence of caffeine use in elite athletes following its removal from the World Anti-Doping Agency list of banned substances. *Applied Physiology, Nutrition and Metabolism* 36(4):555–561.

Desbrow, B., and Leveritt, M. (2006). Awareness and use of caffeine by athletes competing at the 2005 Ironman Triathlon World Championships. *International Journal of Sports Nutrition and Exercise Metabolism* 16(5):545–558.

Dhar, R., Stout, C. W., Link, M. S., *et al.* (2005). Cardiovascular toxicities of performance enhancing substances in sports. *Mayo Clinic Proceedings* 80(10):1307–1315.

Doherty, M. (1998). The effects of caffeine on the maximal accumulated oxygen deficit and short-term running performance. *International Journal of Sports Nutrition* 8(2):95–104.

Dulloo, A. G. (1993). Ephedrine, xanthines and prostaglandin-inhibitors: Actions and interactions in the stimulation of thermogenesis. *International Journal of Obesity* 17(Suppl):S35–S40.

Duncan, M. J., Thake, C. D., and Downs, P. J. (2014). The effect of caffeine ingestion on torque and muscle activity during resistance exercise in men. *Muscle and Nerve*, Epub ahead of print.

Espinola, E. B., Dias, R. F., Mattei, R., *et al.* (1997). Pharmacological activity of guarana (*Paullinia cupana* Mart.) in laboratory animals. *Journal of Ethnopharmacology* 55(3):223–229.

Evans, S. M., and Griffiths, R. R. (1999). Caffeine withdrawal: A parametric analysis of caffeine dosing conditions. *Journal of Pharmacology and Experimental Therapeutics* 289(1):285–294.

Eversham, E. (2014). Branded coffee shop sales up 9.3% in 2013. Available online at http://www.bighospitality.co.uk/Trends-Reports/Branded-coffee-shop-sales-up-9.3-in-2013 (accessed 5 March 2014).

Finnegan, D. (2003). The health effects of stimulant drinks. *Nutrition Bulletin* 28(2):147–155.

Food Standards Agency. (2004). Survey of caffeine levels in hot beverages. Available online at http://www.food.gov.uk/science/research/surveillance/food-surveys/fsis2004branch/fsis5304 (accessed 5 September 2014).

Foskett, A., Ali, A., and Gant, N. (2009). Caffeine enhance cognitive function and skill during simulated soccer activity. *International Journal of Sports Nutrition and Exercise Metabolism* 19(4):410–423.

Fredholm, B. B. (1995). Adenosine, adenosine receptors and the actions of caffeine. *Pharmacology and Toxicology* 76(2):93–101.

Ghelardini, C., Galeotti, N., and Bartolini, A. (1997). Caffeine induces central cholinergic analgesia. *Naunyn Schmiedebergs Archives of Pharmacology* 356(5):590–595.

Graham, T. E. (1997). The possible actions of methylxanthines on various tissues. In T. Reilly and M. Orme (Eds.), *Proceedings of the Estelle Foundation Symposium: The clinical pharmacology of sport and exercise* (vol. 7, pp. 257–270). Amsterdam, the Netherlands: Elsevier.

Graham, T. E. (2001). Caffeine and exercise: Metabolism, endurance and performance. *Sports Medicine* 31(11):785–807.

Graham, T. E., Hibbert, E., and Sathasivam, P. (1998). Metabolic and exercise endurance effects of coffee and caffeine ingestion. *Journal of Applied Physiology* 85(3):883–889.

Graham, T. E., and Spriet, L. L. (1991). Performance and metabolic responses to a high caffeine dose during prolonged exercise. *Journal of Applied Physiology* 71(6):2292–2298.

Graham, T. E., and Spriet, L. L. (1995). Metabolic, catecholamine and exercise performance responses to various doses of caffeine. *Journal of Applied Physiology* 78(3):867–874.

Greer, F., Friars, D., and Graham, T. E. (2000). Comparison of caffeine and theophylline ingestion: Exercise metabolism and endurance. *Journal of Applied Physiology* 89(5):1837–1844.

Greer, F., Morales, J., and Coles, M. (2006). Wingate performance and surface EMG frequency variables are not affected by caffeine ingestion. *Applied Physiology Nutrition and Metabolism* 31(5):597–603.

Grobbee, D. E., Rimm, E. B., Giovannucci, E., *et al.* (1990). Coffee, caffeine and cardiovascular disease in men. *New England Journal of Medicine* 323(15):1026–32.

Hodgson, A. B., Randell, R. K., and Jeukendrup, A. E. (2013). The metabolic and performance effects of caffeine compared to coffee during endurance exercise. *PLoS One* 8(4):e59561.

Hurrell, R. F., Reddy, M., and Cooke, J. D. (1999). Inhibition of non-haem iron absorption in man by polypenolic-containing beverages. *British Journal of Nutrition* 81(4):289–295.

Jacobson, B. H., Weber, M. D., Claypool, L., *et al.* (1992). Effects of caffeine on maximal strength and power in elite male athletes. *British Journal of Sports Medicine* 26(4):276–280.

James, J. E. (2004). Critical review of dietary caffeine and blood pressure: A relationship that should be taken more seriously. *Psychosomatic Medicine* 66(1):63–71.

James, J. E. (2012). Death by caffeine: How many caffeine-related fatalities and near misses must there be before we regulate? *Journal of Caffeine Research* 2(4):149–152.

Jee, S. H., He, J., Whelton, P. K., *et al.* (1999). The effect of chronic coffee drinking on blood pressure: A meta-analysis of controlled clinical trials. *Hypertension* 33(2):647–652.

Kalmar, J. M., and Cafarelli, E. (1999). Effects of caffeine on neuromuscular function. *Journal of Applied Physiology* 87(2):801–808.

Kang, H., Kim, H., and Kim, B. (1998). Acute effects of caffeine intake on maximal anaerobic power during the 30s Wingate cycling test. *Journal of Exercise Physiology Online* 1.

Knutti, R., Rothweiler, H., and Schlatter, C. (1981). Effect of pregnancy on the pharmacokinetics of caffeine. *European Journal of Clinical Pharmacology* 21(2):121–126.

Kovacs, E. M. R., Stegen, J. H. C. H., and Brouns, F. (1998). Effects of caffeinated drinks on substrate metabolism, caffeine excretion and performance. *Journal of Applied Physiology* 85(2):709–715.

Laska, E. M., Sunshine, A., Mueller, F., *et al.* (1984). Caffeine as an analgesic adjuvant. *JAMA: Journal of the American Medical Association* 251(13):1711–1718.

Laurence, G., Wallman, K., and Guelfi, K. (2012). Effects of caffeine on time trial performance in sedentary men. *Journal of Sport Sciences* 30(12):1235–1240.

Lelo, A., Birkett, D. J., Robson, R. A., *et al.* (1986a). Comparative pharmacokinetics of caffeine and its primary demethylated metabolites paraxanthine, theobromine and theophylline in man. *British Journal of Clinical Pharmacology* 22(2):177–182.

Lelo, A., Miners, J. O, Robson, R. A., *et al.* (1986b). Quantitative assessment of caffeine partial clearances in man. *British Journal of Clinical Pharmacology* 22(2):183–186.

Lieberman, H. R., Tharion, W. J., Shukitt-Hale, B., *et al.* (2002). Effects of caffeine, sleep loss and stress on cognitive performance and mood during US Navy SEAL training. *Psychopharmacology* 164(3)(:250–261.

Lieberman, H. R., Wurtman, R. J., Emde, R. J., *et al.* (1987). The effects of low doses of caffeine on human performance and mood. *Psychopharmacology* 92(3):308–312.

Lindinger, M. I., Graham, T. E., and Spriet, L. L. (1993). Caffeine attenuates the exercise-induced increase in plasma [K$^+$] in humans. *Journal of Applied Physiology* 74(3):1149–1155.

Lindinger, M. I., Willmets, R. G., and Hawke, T. J. (1996). Stimulation of Na+, K+-pump activity in skeletal muscle by methylxanthines: evidence and proposed mechanisms. *Acta Physiologica Scandinavica* 156(3):347–353.

MacIntosh, B. R., and Wright, B. M. (1995). Caffeine ingestion and performance of a 1,500-metre swim. *Canadian Journal of Applied Physiology* 20(2):168–177.

Malinauskas, B. M., Aeby, V. G., Overton, R. F., *et al.* (2007). A survey of energy drink consumption patterns amongst college students. *Nutrition Journal* 6:35.

Meyers, B. M., and Cafarelli, E. (2005). Caffeine increases time to fatigue by maintaining force and not by altering firing rates during submaximal isometric contractions. *Journal of Applied Physiology* 99(3):1056–1063.

Mohr, M., Nielsen, J. J., and Bangsbo, J. (2011). Caffeine improves intermittent exercise performance and reduces muscle interstitial potassium accumulation. *Journal of Applied Physiology* 111(5): 1372–1379.

Morck, T. A., Lynch, S. R., and Cook, J. D. (1983). Inhibition of food iron absorption by coffee. *American Journal of Clinical Nutrition* 37(3):416–420.

Morton, A. R., Scott, C. A., and Fitch, K. D. (1989). The effects of theophylline on the physical performance and work capacity of well-trained athletes. *Journal of Allergy and Clinical Immunology* 83(1):55–61.

Nehlig, A., and Debry, G. (1994). Caffeine and sports activity: A review. *International Journal of Sports Medicine* 15(5):215–223.

Pasman, W. J., van Baak, M. A., Jeukendrup, A. E., *et al.* (1995). The effect of different dosages of caffeine on endurance performance time. *International Journal of Sports Medicine* 16(4):225–230.

Paton, C. D., Hopkins, W. G., and Vollerbregt, L. (2001). Little effect of caffeine ingestion on repeated sprints in team-sport athletes. *Medicine and Science in Sports and Exercise* 33(5):822–825.

Paton, C. D., Lowe, T., and Irvine, A. (2010). Caffeinated chewing gum increases repeated sprint performance and augments increases in testosterone in competitive cyclists. *European Journal of Applied Physiology* 110(6):1243–1250.

Pedersen, D. J., Lessard, S. J., Coffey, V. G., *et al.* (2008). High rates of muscle glycogen resynthesis after exhaustive exercise when carbohydrate is coingested with caffeine. *Journal of Applied Physiology* 105(1):7–13.

Penetar, D., McCann, U., Thorne, D., *et al.* (1993). Caffeine reversal of sleep deprivation effects on alertness and mood. *Psychopharmacology* 112(2–3):359–365.

Plaskett, C. J., and Cafarelli, E. (2001). Caffeine increases endurance and attenuates force sensation during submaximal isometric contractions. *Journal of Applied Physiology* 91(4):1535–1544.

Reeves, R. R., Struve, F. A., and Patrick, G. (1997). Somatic dysfunction increase during caffeine withdrawal. *Journal of the American Osteopathic Association* 97(8):454–456.

Reissig, C. J., Strain, E. C., and Griffiths, R. R. (2009). Caffeinated energy drinks – a growing problem. *Drug and Alcohol Dependence* 99(1–3):1–10.

Riesselmann, B., Rosenbaum, F., Roscher, S., *et al*. (1999). Fatal caffeine intoxication. *Forensic Science International* 103(1):S49–S52.

Rosenberg, L., Palmer, J. R., Kelly, J. P., *et al*. (1988). Coffee drinking and nonfatal myocardial infarction in men under 55 years of age. *American Journal of Epidemiology* 128(3):570–578.

Sawynok, J., and Yaksh, T. L. (1993). Caffeine as an analgesic adjuvant. A review of pharmacology and mechanisms of action. *Pharmacological Reviews* 45(1):43–85.

Schneiker, K. T., Bishop, D., Dawson, B., *et al*. (2006). Effects of caffeine on prolonged intermittent-sprint ability in team-sport athletes. *Medicine and Science in Sports and Exercise* 38(3):578–585.

Shimada, J., and Suzuki, F. (2000). Medicinal chemistry of adenosine receptors in brain and periphery. In H. Kase, P. J. Richardson, and P. Jenner (Eds.), *Adenosine receptors and Parkinson's disease* (pp. 31–48). Oxford, UK: Elsevier.

Silverman, K., Evans, S. M., Strain, E. C., *et al*. (1992). Withdrawal syndrome after the double-blind cessation of caffeine consumption. *New England Journal of Medicine* 327(16):1109–1114.

Smit, H. J., and Rogers, P. J. (2000). Effects of low doses of caffeine on cognitive performance, mood and thirst in low and higher caffeine consumers. *Psychopharmacology* 152(2):167–173.

Spriet, L. L. (2002). Caffeine. In M. S. Bahrke and C. E. Yesalis (Eds.), *Performance-enhancing substances in sport and exercise* (pp. 267–278). Champaign, IL: Human Kinetics.

Stuart, G. R., Hopkins, W. G., Cook, C., *et al*. (2005). Multiple effects of caffeine on simulated high-intensity team sport performance. *Medicine and Science in Sports and Exercise* 37(11):1998–2005.

Tarnopolsky, M. (2008). Effect of caffeine on the neuromuscular system – potential as an ergogenic aid. *Applied Physiology Nutrition and Metabolism* 33(6):1284–1289.

Tarnopolsky, M., and Cupido, C. (2000). Caffeine potentiates low frequency skeletal muscle force in habitual and nonhabitual caffeine consumers. *Journal of Applied Physiology* 89(5):1719–1724.

Undem, B. J., and Lichtenstein, L. M. (2001). Drugs used in the treatment of asthma. In J. G. Hardman, L. E. Limbird, and A. G. Gilman (Eds.), *Goodman and Gilman's the pharmacological basis of therapeutics* (10th ed., pp. 733–754). New York, NY: McGraw-Hill.

Van Duinen, H., Lorist, M. M., and Zijdewind, I. (2005). The effect of caffeine on cognitive task performance and motor fatigue. *Psychopharmacology* 180(3):539–547.

Van Thuyne, W., and Delbeke, F. T. (2006). Distribution of caffeine levels in urine in different sports in relation to doping control before and after the removal of caffeine from the WADA Doping List. *International Journal of Sports Medicine* 27(9):745–750.

Weatherby, R. P., and Rogerson, S. (2002). Caffeine potentiation of the performance enhancing effects of pseudoephedrine. *Medicine and Science in Sports and Exercise* 34(5):110.

Wemple, R. D., Lamb, D. R., and McKeever, K. H. (1997). Caffeine vs caffeine-free sports drinks: Effects on urine production at rest and during prolonged exercise. *International Journal of Sports Medicine* 18(1):40–46.

Wiles, J. D., Bird, S. R., Hopkins, J., and Riley, M. (1992). Effect of caffeinated coffee on running speed, respiratory factors, blood lactate and perceived exertion during 1500-m treadmill running. *British Journal of Sports Medicine* 26(2):116–120.

World Anti-Doping Agency. (2003). Policy into practice. Available online at https://wada-main-prod.s3.amazonaws.com/resources/files/PlayTrue_2003_3_Policy_Into_Practice_EN.pdf (accessed 11 September 2014).

World Anti-Doping Agency. (2009). World Anti-Doping Code. Available online at https://elb.wada-ama.org/en/resources/the-code/2009-world-anti-doping-code#.VBILJsstDX4 (available 11 September 2014).

Zhang, W. Y., and Li Wan Po, A. (1996). Analgesic efficacy of paracetamol and its combination with codeine and caffeine in surgical pain—a meta-analysis. *Journal of Clinical Pharmacy and Therapeutics* 21(4):261–282.

Zhang W. Y., and Li Wan Po, A. (1997). Do codeine and caffeine enhance the analgesic effect of aspirin? A systematic overview. *Journal of Clinical Pharmacy and Therapeutics* 22(2):79–97.

Medical and pharmaceutical aspects of major event organisation

Chapter 23

Medical services for international games

Mark Stuart

23.1. Introduction

Providing a medical service at international multisport events, such as Olympic, Paralympic, and Commonwealth Games, is a truly unique challenge on a scale unrivalled by any other sporting event. Not only must the medical services cater to the highly specialised therapeutic needs of up to 15,000 athletes during the course of these events, but they must also supply the needs of accredited support staff, team officials, medical units, press and broadcast teams, volunteer workforce, and spectators.

For the London 2012 Olympic and Paralympic Games, approximately 250,000 accredited people were under the care of the games medical services and could access free treatment if required. In addition, first-aid and emergency medical support was available for an estimated 9 million spectators while they were at the competition venues. Over 53,000 medical encounters for 32,000 people were recorded during the period of both the Olympic and Paralympic Games, which occurred across all of the medical facilities provided by the Organising Committee. Around 30 per cent of these medical encounters were athletes (LOCOG 2012).

The operational period for medical services at London 2012 was from the opening of the athlete villages on 9 July to their closing after the Paralympic Games on 12 September – a period of 70 days. Polyclinics were open daily from 7am to 11pm, with two shifts and emergency cover outside these hours. In addition to services within the athlete villages, medical cover extended to 145 medical rooms located across all competition and training venues.

23.2. The games polyclinic

Within the athlete village at every Olympic, Paralympic, and Commonwealth Games is a purpose-built medical centre known as the polyclinic. This is the main medical facility for athletes and team officials. Medical services offered in the polyclinic are comprehensive and include emergency medical services, sports medicine, general practice, medical imaging, dentistry, eye services (ophthalmologists, opticians, and optometrists), physiotherapy, massage therapy, hydrotherapy, podiatry, pathology, medical records, interpreter services, doping control, gender verification, and pharmacy.

All of these medical services are provided free to the athletes and team officials for the duration of the games and are staffed by a dedicated team of expert volunteers. The polyclinic is busiest early in the morning and late at night, which coincides with athletes' training and competition schedules.

The Games polyclinic provides an environment unlike any other regular medical practice. On admission, an athlete has immediate access to state-of-the-art diagnostic and treatment equipment and a multidisciplinary team with expertise in sports medicine. It is a unique environment where fast and comprehensive care can be provided. For example, within a single visit, an athlete might have a specialist sports medicine consultation, ultrasound or magnetic resonance imaging (MRI) scan interpreted by a radiographer, physiotherapy or nursing intervention, and counseling on his or her prescribed medicine by the polyclinic pharmacists.

At all Games, the polyclinic has close connections with nearby hospitals where patients are referred if they require longer-term or intensive care. At the London 2012 Games, three designated hospitals were appointed in central London for this purpose if required. A total of 532 referrals to designated hospitals were made over the period of the Olympic and Paralympic Games from the games medical services (LOCOG 2012).

In Beijing, there were twenty-one official Olympic hospitals. If an athlete, official, or Olympic family member was admitted, their care was coordinated through a 'green passage' process, which meant a speedy and priority service was provided. The designated Olympic hospitals were also able to provide the Olympic pharmacies with any medicines not stocked in the village as needed.

23.3. Examples of games polyclinics

For the London 2012 Olympic and Paralympic Games, there were three polyclinics – one for each of the athlete villages: Stratford (near the Olympic Park), Eton Dorney (rowing and canoe sprint athlete village), and Weymouth (sailing athlete village). The main polyclinic in London was based in a new-build facility destined to be a primary care facility after the Games for the local community. The internal design was adapted to accommodate the specialist services required for treatment and care of athletes during the event. The London 2012 Polyclinic services were considered to be of an extraordinarily high standard.

One of the most complex installations in the London polyclinic was the imaging equipment. There were two MRI scanners, one X-ray commuted tomography scanner (CT), one digital X-ray, and two ultrasound machines. Given the size and sensitivity of the machines, the MRI and CT scanners were positioned in demountable buildings outside the front entrance of the polyclinic.

The physical therapy section of the London polyclinic required a large area because of the high volume of consultations and the amount of equipment it contained, including a full rehabilitation gymnasium, ice bath area, and hydrotherapy pool. This department was the busiest service during the games, with thousands of athletes accessing these services. The London 2012 Games were the first to introduce chiropractors and osteopathy to the range of medical services available, which proved to successfully complement the physiotherapy and sport massage services.

Similarly, the polyclinic in the Beijing 2008 Olympic Village contained a fully stocked pharmacy, six dental surgeries, two MRI machines, optometry services dispensing hundreds of pairs of glasses, an emergency medicine department, counseling services, a physiotherapy unit with dozens of treatment beds, and – for the first time in an Olympic polyclinic – an acupuncture and moxibustion clinic.

At the Sydney 2000 Games, approximately 20,000 visits over a 1-month period were recorded for the polyclinic in the athletes' village. There were 3,619 physician consultations, 2,884 physiotherapy treatments, and 5,622 visits to the pharmacy, making the pharmacy one of the busiest medical services at the Games. In Atlanta in 1996, 2,474 athletes and Olympic staff were assessed in the polyclinic (New South Wales Health Department, 2000).

Dental and eye services are always in high demand at international games. The polyclinic services provide an opportunity for athletes from countries with limited access to medical resources to access routine and screening services for dental and optical treatment; the provision of these services is considered an obligation of the host city.

There were eight dental surgeries in operation for London 2012 and five for Beijing 2008; at both games, these were constantly busy. A total of 2,541 dental consultations were recorded during the London 2012 Olympic period, compared with 910 consultations at the Atlanta 1996 Olympics (LOCOG 2012).

Optometry services are similarly busy: 2,258 pairs of spectacles were issued over the period of both the Olympic and Paralympic Games at London 2012, mainly to athletes and team officials. In comparison, 620 pairs of spectacles and 50 sets of contact lenses were issued in Atlanta (LOCOG 2012).

The Sochi 2014 Olympic Winter Games had three polyclinics to serve the medical requirements of 2,850 athletes from 89 countries, as well as their accompanying team members, such as coaches and medical staff. One polyclinic served the residents of the Coastal Olympic Village; the Endurance Village and Alpine Villages were in the mountains – each with its own polyclinic. The polyclinics in Sochi had good connections with a number of designated hospitals, with a number of helicopters on standby to take injured athletes from mountain venues to nearby hospitals with emergency departments.

23.4. Medical workforce

Staffing Olympic and Paralympic medical services is a huge logistical operation. The organising committees of these events will appoint a planning and management team up to 5 years prior to the games. The medical division will usually be divided into specialist departments. For London in 2012, the medical services comprised a number of planning workstreams under the areas of pharmacy, sports medicine, primary care, physiotherapy, emergency medicine, dentistry, optometry, podiatry, and medical imaging. During the Games, a huge team of medical volunteers run the service, and an extensive recruitment campaign starts at least a year prior to the Games.

For the London 2012 Olympic and Paralympic Games, a total of approximately 4,500 medical volunteers provided specialist care at thirty-five Olympic venues – similar numbers ran the Sydney 2000 medical service. For the Atlanta 1996 Olympics, 4,000 medical volunteers were recruited. In Athens in 2004, approximately 400 specialist doctors, 400 nurses, and 400 physiotherapists made up the core of the local medical team (LOCOG 2012).

In addition to the local medical workforce, more than 1,000 doctors and hundreds of visiting medical professionals who travel with the teams will also reside in the athlete village. They also will access the Games medical services to treat members of their own team.

23.5. Education and training for the medical workforce

Training for the medical workforce is a massive undertaking, particularly given the volume and range of professions represented within the games medical division. For most Olympic and Paralympic Games, this is usually delivered in three stages:

- *Stage 1 – General orientation:* This training provides an introduction to the games, an orientation of the structure and remit of the organising committee, and outlines the tasks ahead for the organisers. For London 2012, this orientation was delivered to 70,000 volunteers across all departments of the organising committee.

- *Stage 2 – Role-specific training:* Role-specific training is specific to the various roles within the medical services team. It introduces the specific and unique professional requirements of working as a medical professional at the games.
- *Stage 3 – Venue-specific training:* Venue-specific training is site-specific training for the volunteer medical workforce, and it is usually delivered at the polyclinics within the athlete villages. This gives volunteers an opportunity to experience their Games-time work environment and the clinical facilities that will be available to them during their time at work.

23.6. Interpreter services

The availability of a comprehensive interpreter service at the polyclinic ensures that medical staff can communicate effectively with their patients. This is especially important when athletes are being dispensed drugs with restrictions in sport, where they must know the notification procedures and consequences of taking such drugs.

23.7. Medical services at sporting venues

At every Olympic sporting venue, specific medical facilities are provided for athletes and spectators. At the main Olympic stadium, there may be two main athlete medical rooms near the field of play stocked with equipment and medicines for sports injuries and emergency situations. There will also be a number of spectator medical rooms on each tier or level of the stadium, and additional medical stations in the public areas immediately outside the venue. For the London 2012 Olympic Games, medical services were provided at thirty-five spectator competition venues, forty-one training venues, and fifty-five noncompetition venues (such as official hotels) across eight cities of the United Kingdom.

In Beijing, the medical stations in the Olympic Park area contained a comprehensive selection of drugs for spectator use. These included insulin, glyceryl trinitrate, cardiac emergency drugs, asthma inhalers, and intravenous fluids. Single doses of drugs were administered to spectators, who would be referred to a designated hospital if further treatment was required.

The nature of the sporting event also determines how the medical services are delivered and the types of drugs that are available for athlete use. For sailing and rowing, medical boats closely follow the competition, and motorbikes carry supplies for the road cycling and marathon events. During the Olympic Games, the equestrian events carry the most risk of serious trauma injuries; along the 5.7-km route for the Olympic cross-country events in Hong Kong in 2008, twenty-four medical teams were stationed at any one time. Each medical team was equipped with a suitcase containing over thirty emergency drugs and a variety of medical equipment suitable for trauma.

For the mountain venues of the Sochi 2014 Olympic Winter Games, mobile medical teams used snowmobiles for transport and doctors on skis carrying first-response equipment were positioned along some of the long ski slope courses. Helicopter landing sites were also created at various parts of the mountain close to the courses to enable fast access to medical care if required.

23.8. Summary

In summary, medical services for international games are a complex and integral part of delivering these huge events safely. The design and planning of medical services are undertaken many years prior to the games and involve creating new facilities and coordinating local and national healthcare services across the host country. Medical facilities at events range from portable medical kits and medical clinics at competition venues to comprehensive hospital-style polyclinic facilities within the athlete villages.

Games-wide medical services ensure that everyone either competing, working, or watching the Games has access to the full spectrum of medical care when required, ranging from simple first-aid to lifesaving emergency care.

23.9. Bibliography

Brennan, R. J., Keim, M. E., Sharp, T. W., *et al.* (1997). Medical and public health services at the 1996 Atlanta Olympic Games: An overview. *Medical Journal of Australia* 167(11–12):595–598.

Clements, A. (2003). Medical support for the greatest show on Earth. *British Travel Health Association Journal* 5:52–54.

Eaton, S. B., Woodfin, B. A., Askew, J. L., *et al.* (1997). The polyclinic at the 1996 Atlanta Olympic Village. *Medical Journal of Australia* 167(11–12):599–602.

LOCOG (2012). London Organising Committee of the Olympic and Paralympic Games. Internal communications and reports. Unpublished data.

New South Wales Health Department. (2000). *NSW health services for the Sydney 2000 Olympic and Paralympic Games*. Sydney, Australia: NSW Health Department.

Stiel, D., Trethowan, P., and Vance, N. (1997). Medical planning for the Sydney 2000 Olympic and Paralympic Games. *Medical Journal of Australia* 167(11–12):593–594.

Sydney Organising Committee of the Olympic Games (SOCOG), Olympic Co-ordination Authority (2001). *Official report of the XXVII Olympiad*. Sydney, Australia: SOCOG.

Chapter 24

Pharmacy services for international games

Mark Stuart

24.1. Introduction

Pharmacy services are an important and integral part of medical services for athletes, team officials, and spectators at international games. These services cover the provision of medicines across all areas of the event, including competition and training venues, hotels, and athlete villages. Pharmacy services are integral to all services across the games, and each polyclinic will have a registered pharmacy premises.

Pharmacy planning for Olympic and Paralympic Games usually starts 4 years out from the event, with a chief pharmacist and an expert planning team appointed to design the service. The chief pharmacist position often carries statutory responsibilities for the games according to the drug regulatory laws of the host country.

Pharmacists are at the front line when it comes to drug use and supply to athletes at Olympic Games. In this specialist environment, pharmacists require an advanced level of sport-specific pharmacological and clinical knowledge in order to effectively contribute to the health care of the athlete. They are also responsible for supporting anti-doping during the games by implementing robust systems of supply of drugs to athletes and by the provision of expert information to athletes on drugs banned in sport and their permitted alternatives.

An extensive array of complex clinical, professional, legal, and regulatory issues related to medicine use must be considered by organising committees in their planning of an event as complex and on such a huge scale as the Olympic Games. As part of the games medical department, pharmacy services are responsible for ensuring that the necessary medicine management and clinical governance frameworks are in place to provide an excellent standard of pharmacy service for both athletes and spectators.

24.2. Scope of the games pharmacy service

The primary remit of the team responsible for pharmacy services is to design and oversee a safe, efficient, and accurate dispensary service and to plan a system of supply, storage, and management of medicines for use at competition and training venues. This includes the design of systems to manage a range of drugs used for emergency medicine, including controlled drugs that are carried and used by doctors at the various competition venues. Drug distribution systems between the polyclinic pharmacies and the competition venues are generally designed such that one model of logistics and operation can be replicated across all venues, irrespective of the events taking place.

In collaboration with the other medical departments of the organising committee, the pharmacy team is also responsible for facilitating the selection of medicines stocked in the

Table 24.1 Scoping considerations for Olympic and Paralympic pharmacy services

Provide medicine requirements of athletes, officials, spectators, media, and Olympic families

Provide fully stocked polyclinic pharmacies in the athlete villages and satellite pharmacies

Supply medicines for other departments in the polyclinic, including

- Dentistry
- Physiotherapy
- Podiatry
- Imaging
- Emergency rooms

Supply and manage medicines at competition venues in the following areas:

- Athlete field-of-play medical stations
- Spectator medical stations within stadia
- Medical and first-aid areas in spectator precincts outside the venues

Supply emergency drugs for the field-of-play and crowd doctors

Provide an independent retail pharmacy for press and broadcast

Provide veterinary pharmacy services for equestrian events

Facilitate local purchase of stock drugs if required by visiting team doctors

Monitor that drugs issued to athletes comply with WADA regulations

Provide an international medicine information service from the polyclinic pharmacy for visiting team doctors on:

- International medicines
- Drugs prohibited in sport

Provide training and information for medical volunteers and citywide pharmacies on drugs prohibited in sport

Consider a response plan for medicine access during disaster scenarios

---

polyclinic pharmacies and those that are available in athlete and spectator medical rooms at the competition venues. This list of drugs is compiled to form the games formulary, and a printed pharmacy guide is then produced and distributed to all health care professionals working at the games.

An overview of the scoping considerations for Olympic and Paralympic pharmacy services is presented in Table 24.1.

24.3. The London 2012 pharmacy services

For at the 2012 Olympic Games in London, pharmacy services were one of seven specialty clinical areas of the Olympic and Paralympic medical services and were responsible for providing the medicine needs for 11,200 athletes of twenty-six Olympic sports across thirty-four competition venues, followed by 4,200 athletes of twenty Paralympic sports across twenty-one competition venues. In addition, the pharmacy services covered the medicine needs of around 250,000 accredited people, and also an estimated 9 million spectators while they were attending events.

There were three athlete villages, each containing a fully stocked pharmacy to provide the medicine requirements of accredited athletes, team officials, Olympic and Paralympic families, and other residents of the villages. The pharmacies operated in a similar style to a hospital outpatient dispensary and were the coordinating points of medicines supply for the athlete and spectator medical facilities at all Olympic and Paralympic venues.

The pharmacy in the athlete village in Stratford, London, was situated in a purpose-built polyclinic located in the athletes' residential area. The pharmacies in the Weymouth Sailing Village and Eton Dorney Rowing Village were situated in temporary facilities within the residential areas of these villages.

The operational period of the service was from the opening of the Olympic Villages on 9 July 2012 until the closure of the Paralympic Villages on 12 September 2012. The service to spectators covered 17 days of Olympic competition and 11 days of Paralympic competition.

There was huge enthusiasm from pharmacists and pharmacy technicians across the United Kingdom to work as a volunteer at the Games. More than 1,200 people applied for the roles and 100 volunteers were recruited to form the pharmacy team. During the course of both the Olympic and Paralympic Games, a total of 5,200 prescriptions were dispensed through the three polyclinic pharmacies.

A different model of staffing was applied to the pharmacy services for the Sochi 2014 Olympic Winter Games. Three full-time pharmacists were permanently stationed at each of the three pharmacies for the duration of the Olympic and Paralympic Games. This model ensured an efficient transfer of knowledge across the Games period, and ensured a continuity of service across the games period.

24.4. Role of pharmacists during the games

The primary role of the games pharmacist is to provide a safe, efficient, and accurate pharmacy service. Their role involves clinical screening, dispensing, and providing clinical advice, especially about drugs used in sports medicine.

As well as looking after the athletes' therapeutic sports medicine requirements, the doctors and pharmacists are also responsible for ensuring that the athletes do not inadvertently take a prohibited substance. In the international games environment, athletes rely heavily on the knowledge and advice of pharmacists, doctors, and other medical staff for information on drugs banned in sport, particularly for drugs that are prescribed for the first time in the polyclinic at the games.

Pharmacists must be familiar with the list of prohibited substances and the regulations for the provision of drugs that have a restricted status. They must also be aware of drugs that require prior notification through the Therapeutic Use Exemption (TUE) procedure in order to advise athletes appropriately.

There are very tight procedures and a specific Olympic prescription form to ensure that the athletes do not fall foul of a doping offence. Strict systems of dispensing prohibited drugs are in place to ensure that drugs issued to athletes comply with the World Anti-Doping Agency (WADA) regulations. This involves meticulous scrutiny of prescribing new drugs to athletes that require TUEs.

24.5. Education for games pharmacy workforce

The provision of pharmacy services requires pharmacy volunteers to have knowledge and skills in a variety of areas beyond normal professional duties, particularly with respect to the provision of medicines to athletes, including knowledge of prohibited drugs and the pharmacology of specific drugs used routinely in sports medicine. Intensive and specialist training on drugs in sport is provided for pharmacists and other health care professionals working in the Games environment, which is delivered in the year before the start of the Games.

For the London 2012 Games, a major education programme was specifically developed for the pharmacy and broader medical workforce in collaboration with a leading national pharmacy education institution. The strategy was to also provide an education and training programme that would provide a post-Games legacy for the profession of pharmacy, both nationally and internationally.

The programme was delivered as an online e-learning programme containing three sections:

1   Doping and anti-doping in sport
2   Pharmacy services and support in sport and fitness
3   Medical services at international sporting events.

The primary objective for the programme was to provide a body of knowledge to support the role of pharmacist and pharmacy technician volunteers at the 2012 Games. All of the pharmacy volunteers were required to undertake the package and to pass the associated assessment as a prerequisite for acceptance of a place on the pharmacy team.

For the Sochi 2014 Winter Games, a training programme was delivered by the International Olympic Committee Medical Commission to the pharmacists during the opening week of service. This programme covered Games-specific issues such as the TUE application process and the process for dispensing a prohibited drug to an athlete if the need arose.

24.6. Support for local health care services

An additional responsibility of the Games medical and pharmacy services is to ensure that health care professionals in the host city have the necessary information at hand should an athlete seek advice or treatment outside of the athlete village environment.

For the Manchester 2002 Commonwealth Games, an education programme containing information about drugs in sport was delivered to pharmacies and emergency departments within the vicinity of the games. For the Beijing 2008 Games, all medical staff working in the city received training to equip them with knowledge about the drugs restricted in sport. Similarly, for the London 2012 Games, local and national pharmacy organisations worked together to distribute information for community and hospital pharmacies to support them during the games should they need to provide care to a competing athlete.

24.7. Medicine governance

Comprehensive policies and standard operating procedures are required at international games. These policies and procedures are in place to ensure a safe and standardised approach to medicine management by all members of the pharmacy team, as well as to comply with pharmacy laws of the host country and the recommendations of governing organisations, such as the International Olympic Committee.

For the London 2012 Games, these policies and procedures were developed in collaboration with national pharmacy organisations and professional and regulatory bodies. The policies and procedures covered all aspects of pharmacy services, such as the following:

•   The storage and supply of medicines at competition venues
•   Prescribing and dispensing procedures

- Issuing WADA-prohibited drugs
- Accessing international medicine information.

24.8. The games formulary and medicine handbook

The main focus of medical treatment at international games is to provide care for newly acquired injuries or diseases rather than treating or diagnosing existing complaints; this is reflected in the list of drugs available for prescribing in the polyclinic. The range of medicines stocked in the pharmacy needs to reflect those known and used by the global medical community, as well as those frequently used in the host country.

The formulary is compiled to reflect the specific drug needs of all the medical specialties, including sports medicine, dentistry, physiotherapy, podiatry, optometry, and massage therapies. A consultation process is usually undertaken with experts in sports medicine and with clinical representatives of the various polyclinic medical departments.

For games such as Commonwealth or Olympic Games, a list of around 200 different drugs is available for prescribing within the athlete village by local and visiting team doctors. A smaller list of essential medicines for urgent care is also available for doctors to administer from the medical rooms at competition venues.

For the London 2012 Games, a range of different sets of drugs were provided, depending on the setting. These various sets included the following:

- Drugs with a sport focus for athlete medical rooms
- Drugs with a general and first-aid focus for spectator medical rooms
- Emergency drug sets to be carried by crowd doctors
- First-aid drugs for inclusion in first responders' medical kits.

The only variable was in the number of the drug packs at each venue, which depended on the size of the venue and numbers of athletes and spectators using the venue.

Most athletes who are taking long-term medicine for pre-existing conditions will generally bring enough of their own supplies to last them for the period when they are away from home. There is therefore less emphasis in the formulary on drugs for long-term or chronic conditions or those associated with geriatric or paediatric medicine. A limited supply of the most common but necessary medicines used by the general population, such as antihypertensive drugs, are kept, but are only likely to be used for the purpose of assisting a team official or spectator who has left his or her regular drugs at home.

Drugs and diagnostic agents required by the other polyclinic departments such as dentistry, optometry, podiatry, and imaging are also included on the formulary and are issued by the pharmacy to these departments during the Games.

At every Games, a medicine handbook is published, which contains the list of drugs on the formulary and also lists the status of each drug according to the WADA list of prohibited substances. This handbook serves as a primary reference for both local and international prescribing doctors. It also contains specific advice to team doctors about how they access medicines for their team and the prescribing procedures specific to the host country.

Drugs for Winter versus Summer Games

Planning for a pharmacy at a Winter Olympic Games must take into account unique environmental factors, such as freezing temperatures and high altitude, and the medical conditions that can result.

At the 2002 Salt Lake City Winter Olympics, there were approximately 11,000 people, including spectators, treated at thirty-five medical stations located throughout the venues. There were around 2,000 medical encounters in the Olympic Village Polyclinic. The majority of cases were influenza and respiratory infections, but forty-three cases of altitude sickness and sixteen cases of frostbite were treated. The relatively moderate altitude of the mountain venues for the Turin 2006 and Sochi 2014 Winter Olympic Games meant that drugs to treat altitude-related conditions were not considered to be essential for inclusion.

Tropical and international medicine

With athletes and support staff from more than 200 countries living in close proximity in the athlete village, the risk of intercontinental disease transmission exists. The medical services must consider having access to drugs for conditions that may not necessarily be endemic or common in the host country.

At the 1996 Atlanta Games, eight cases of malaria were reported, and there was one case of an athlete with malaria and thrombocytopenia who required hospitalisation. There were also three cases of hepatitis and one case of filariasis. Several athletes requested human immunodeficiency virus tests, with no positive results.

At the Manchester Games, a purpose-built observation ward in the polyclinic was used for overnight observation of an athlete with malaria, with the pharmacy promptly obtaining the appropriate antimalarial treatment. This four-bed ward in the polyclinic would be used to quarantine an athlete from the rest of the team should an infectious disease be diagnosed. At the Melbourne 2006 Commonwealth Games, there was one case of malaria – a condition that is rarely seen in Australia.

Rigorous reporting systems are in place to notify public health authorities of suspected medical conditions that might pose a threat to public health.

Traditional medicines

The Beijing 2008 Olympics were the first games where traditional medicines were available from the polyclinic. The Beijing and Hong Kong Olympic Village pharmacies stocked four traditional Chinese medicines: ren dan and huoxiang zhengqi for heatstroke, tiger balm ointment for the relief of insect bites, and golden throat lozenges, a popular Chinese remedy for sore throats.

Although these traditional medicines were available from the Olympic pharmacy, they were not dispensed to athletes routinely. This was primarily because WADA recommends caution to athletes about the use of herbal preparations, whose composition cannot always be guaranteed.

24.9. Medicine information services

The polyclinic pharmacy is the primary point for medicine information during the games. Pharmacists are often requested to identify foreign drugs and to provide information on the status of medicines in relation to the WADA rules.

Access to robust medicine information resources are required to ensure that pharmacy staff can access safe and accurate information on both local and international medicines. In addition, the provision of a medicine information service is required to support the local and visiting team doctors in their practice in the host country. Comprehensive international drug references are always available in the games pharmacy to assist in identifying foreign drug names and determine specific constituents of combination drug products.

At the London 2012 Games, a 24-hour on-call medicine information service was provided for all visiting health care professionals via the polyclinic pharmacy by an existing national medicine information service.

At Olympic and Commonwealth Games, WADA also usually runs an athlete outreach education centre within the athlete village. This programme teaches athletes about the principles of drug-free sport and the testing procedures that they will inevitably encounter at international games.

A common question asked at the pharmacy by athletes is about whether their nutritional supplements are banned. Most athletes at international games take a variety of supplements, which are often recommended by coaches and team nutritionists. The advice that must be given to athletes by pharmacists is one of caution, as there have been cases where prohibited substances have been found in commonly available nutritional supplements.

24.10. Patterns of drug use

Elite athletes at international games are in peak physical condition, and are possibly the fittest and healthiest people on Earth. The patterns of therapeutic drug use at these events are therefore very different from those seen in the average community.

The athletes are most focused in the days before the start of competition. For most, participation at the event will be the culmination of years of intense training and the highlight of their sporting career. Their anxiety about maintaining perfect health in the days before competition is understandably high, and obsession for a perfect physical state is reflected in the initial demands of the medical services.

At Olympic Games, medical services begin about 2 weeks before the opening ceremony when the athlete village opens and the athletes start arriving, until a few days after the closing ceremony. Drug usage commonly peaks just before the opening ceremony and continues until the end of the first week of competition. After this time, there is typically a gradual decline in dispensed prescriptions until the closing ceremony and, then a dramatic drop in drug usage occurs as the athletes start to leave the village. Conversely, the demand for physiotherapy, magnetic resonance imaging, and ultrasound imaging services increases over the course of the games as injuries in athletes become more prevalent.

During the London 2012 Games, a total of 5,200 prescriptions representing 6,849 individual items were dispensed from the polyclinic pharmacies over the Olympic and Paralympic period. Similar to previous Games, the vast majority of items prescribed were for acute conditions. The most commonly prescribed drugs during the 2012 Games are shown in Table 24.2.

In Manchester in 2002, antibiotic prescriptions accounted for the majority of the prescriptions dispensed before the start of the competition period. After the opening ceremony, the daily number of antibiotic prescriptions dropped considerably. This trend might be explained by the possible inappropriate overprescribing of antibiotics for either prophylactic measures or very mild respiratory symptoms. The high level of antibiotic prescriptions very early at these games illustrates the immediate focus of sports medicine at this level. There can be pressure on prescribers from athletes and coaches to act in some way on the most minor of symptoms to ensure they do not hinder performance. In addition, athletes may be less likely to seek medical attention before their event than after competition.

Table 24.2 Most commonly prescribed medicines during the London 2012 Olympic Games period

Medicine	Number of pre-scriptions	Percent of total prescriptions dispensed
Paracetamol 500-mg tablets	456	10.95%
Ibuprofen 400-mg tablets	162	3.89%
Diclofenac sodium 50-mg gastroresistant tablets	132	3.17%
Ibuprofen 200-mg tablets	96	2.30%
Strepsils lozenges	96	2.30%
Amoxicillin 500-mg capsules	87	2.09%
Hydrocortisone 1% cream	79	1.90%
Amoxicillin 250-mg capsules	78	1.87%
Xylometazoline 0.1% nasal spray	77	1.85%
Cetirizine 10-mg tablets	73	1.75%
Loratadine 10-mg tablets	72	1.73%
Omeprazole 20-mg gastroresistant capsules	63	1.51%
Diclofenac 1% gel	60	1.44%
Diclofenac sodium 75-mg modified-release tablets	57	1.37%

Anti-inflammatory drugs are by far the most commonly prescribed class of drugs for athletes over the course of the games. Diclofenac has long been the drug most prescribed to athletes at Olympic Games, accounting for about half of all the prescriptions for anti-inflammatory drugs.

The use of injectable local anaesthetics and corticosteroids is common for the treatment of sporting injuries affecting the joints. Prescriptions for drugs such as lignocaine and methyl-prednisolone are commonly dispensed for severe injuries, where they are injected intra-articularly for treatment of acute pain and inflammation. These drugs can be subject to abuse because of their ability to enable otherwise injury-free athletes to exert themselves past natural pain limits. Such use contravenes sporting ethics and can put athletes at risk of more serious injury.

Antifungal drugs usually account for a significant number of prescriptions at international sporting events. The use of shared training and changing facilities accounts for a high rate of fungal infections, such as 'athlete's foot.' The incidence of fungal infections varies with the seasons. Games held in warmer, tropical climates would typically see a higher demand for antifungal drugs. There was a greater proportion of antifungal drugs prescribed at the Sydney 2000 Games than at the much cooler Manchester 2002 Commonwealth Games.

Local factors can also present unique demands for particular medicines. At the Sydney 2000 Olympics, seasonal allergies were common amongst athletes given that the Games were held in spring. At the Manchester 2002 Games, a plague of biting insects at the shooting venue meant that antihistamines, topical corticosteroids, and anti-itch preparations had to be quickly provided to athletes and spectators. At the Melbourne 2006 Commonwealth Games, approximately fifteen athletes presented at the polyclinic with irritated eyes caused by smoke and ash from the fireworks inside the stadium during the opening ceremony – soothing anti-inflammatory eyedrops were prescribed to them.

For the Sochi 2014 Olympic Winter Games, a total of 1,405 prescriptions were dispensed across the three Olympic Villages. Only 26 per cent of these were dispensed to athletes, and the rest were mostly dispensed to the workforce. Most of the larger teams attending the games brought significant pharmacy supplies with them.

24.11. Prescribing procedures

Prescribing and dispensing of drugs in the games polyclinic is undertaken with great caution to ensure that the prescription falls within the WADA rules. A unique prescription form is always used at Olympic Games, which differs from regular prescription orders by the type of information that the International Olympic Committee specifies must be recorded. Doctors must document the athlete's unique games accreditation number and country. If a prohibited drug is prescribed, approval for a TUE must be obtained and shown to the pharmacy at the time of dispensing; the signatures from the athlete, doctor, and pharmacist are obtained to indicate the informed consent of the athlete.

As an additional precaution, the pharmacy in the polyclinic will have a bespoke dispensing system, which alerts the pharmacist if a prohibited substance is being supplied. The pharmacist can then ensure that the athlete completes the necessary documentation and obtains the appropriate authorisation from the Games medical commission to use the drug.

If a WADA-prohibited drug is considered to be necessary for the treatment of an athlete, the doctor and pharmacist must inform the athlete about the consequence of taking the drug. The athlete must then sign the prescription to acknowledge an understanding of the treatment being prescribed. Prohibited drugs require notification to the Games medical commission, using a TUE form, before the athlete competes.

As an additional precaution, all prohibited drugs are labelled as such at the time of dispensing. They are often also stored separately from drugs that are permitted, further minimising the risk of dispensing them incorrectly.

Failure to submit a TUE form declaring the therapeutic use of a prohibited drug could result in a doping violation should the athlete test positive for these substances. However, any drug is permitted to be administered to an athlete for treatment in an emergency or life-threatening situation.

Prescribing by team doctors

Each team present at international games usually has at least one accompanying doctor. The laws of the host country will often govern the rights that visiting doctors have in relation to prescribing and supply of drugs to the athletes they are looking after.

For the Sydney Olympics, 1,109 visiting team doctors were given prescribing rights in Australia for the period of the Games. A similar arrangement was in place for the London 2012 Games. This enabled the visiting doctors to prescribe drugs from the Games formulary for members of their own team only.

In Manchester 2002, such prescribing rights were not allowed by UK law at the time, so all prescriptions had to be written by doctors registered in the United Kingdom. Similarly, at the 1996 Commonwealth Games in Kuala Lumpur, only prescriptions written by doctors registered with the Malaysian Medical Council were honoured; team doctors were advised to procure temporary registration for the period of these Games with the Malaysian Medical Council.

All visiting team doctors for the Sochi 2014 Games were given temporary registration in Russia to prescribe to members of their own delegation.

24.12. Quality testing of drugs

For the Beijing 2008 Olympic Games – and for the first time in Games history – the Chinese government went to significant lengths to ensure the quality of medicines used in the Beijing

Olympic Polyclinic. Quality control testing of all batches of drugs used at the Games was undertaken.

The expected quantity of medicines to be used for the Olympic and Paralympic period was estimated, and then three times this amount was sent for sample testing to ensure that the composition complied with strict pharmacopoeia standards. This was in addition to the standard Chinese quality assurance testing that the drugs had already passed. The testing ensured that the therapeutic qualities of the drugs were correct and that there were no contaminants in each batch.

24.13. Importation of drugs for team use

Most teams will bring complete medical kits with them, which will include significant amounts of medicines and injury rehabilitation equipment. All teams will have allocated space within the athlete village to set up their own medical clinics and are provided with secure storage for medicines. Approximately 80 per cent of all teams at the Sydney 2000 Games bought their own medical teams and drug supplies with them.

Guidance is always given to the participating countries by the games organisers about the legal procedures for importing large quantities of drugs for therapeutic use. The team doctors are usually required to submit detailed lists of imported medicines to the medical services at the Games, government customs, and importation authorities. The importation of performance-enhancing drugs and other controlled substances such as narcotics, psychotropics, growth hormones, anabolic steroids, and erythropoietin is illegal and is monitored closely during the Olympic period.

24.14. Summary

Delivering pharmacy services for international games requires significant planning and coordination between the organising committee, local pharmacy services, and national pharmacy organisations. These events present unique professional challenges for pharmacists and pharmacy staff, requiring specialist attention to anti-doping issues and the specific requirements of sports medicine for elite athletes.

Pharmacy services for international games have evolved in recent years in such a way that they are no longer on the periphery, but are now considered a central and integrated part of medical services at these games. As shown at the London 2012 Games, the pharmacy profession is now confidently at the forefront of promoting safe and effective medicine use in sport, and pharmacists have a key role in the education of athletes and other health care professionals in preventing doping in sport.

24.15. Bibliography

Mottram, D., and Stuart, M. (2011). Pharmacy planning gains momentum for the Olympic and Paralympic Games. *Pharmaceutical Journal* 286:77–78.

Stuart, M. C. (2005). Pharmacy for elite athletes at international games. In S. B. Kayne (Ed.), *Sport and exercise medicine for pharmacists* (pp. 269–296). London, UK: Pharmaceutical Press.

Stuart, M. (2012). Delivering pharmacy services for the London 2012 games is no easy task. *Pharmaceutical Journal* 289:61.

Stuart, M., and Mottram, D. (2012). The final preparations of pharmacy services for the London 2012 games. *Pharmaceutical Journal* 289:60.

Stuart, M., and Mottram, D. (2013). The emerging specialty of sports pharmacy. *Aspetar Sports Medicine Journal* 2(1):66–71.

Stuart, M., Mottram, D., Erskine, D., Simbler, S., and Thomas, T. (2013). Development and delivery of pharmacy services for the London 2012 Olympic and Paralympic Games. *European Journal of Hospital Pharmacy* 20(1):42–45.

Stuart, M., Mottram, D., and Thomas, T. (2013). Innovations in Olympic and Paralympic pharmacy services. *British Journal of Sports Medicine* 47(7):404–406.

The extent of doping in sport

Chapter 25

Prevalence of drug misuse in sport

David R. Mottram

25.1. Introduction

Meaningful data on the prevalence of use of performance-enhancing drugs and methods in competitive sport are difficult to obtain. Evidence may be as diverse as statistics on positive dope tests, results of surveys of athletes about either their self-reported use or their perceptions of drug use by others, anecdotal reports, and investigative journalism (Yesalis *et al.* 2001). These sources of evidence are inconsistent (Dimeo and Taylor 2013). Speculation of levels of prevalence of drug use range from less than 1 per cent to more than 90 per cent. A number of studies have been undertaken to evaluate the prevalence of doping within individual countries or sports. However, it has been suggested that such studies generally underestimate the problem due to small sample populations (Lippi *et al.* 2008).

The purpose of this chapter is to evaluate the published evidence and to comment on the validity and accuracy of this evidence. The chapter is divided into a section discussing statistics on prohibited drug use in sport, including statistics from World Anti-Doping Agency (WADA)-accredited laboratories and statistics derived from national and international studies on prevalence, and a section on surveys into drug misuse in sport. Finally, a perspective on the prevalence of drug misuse in sport through medical practitioners and other health care professionals is presented.

25.2. Statistics on the use of prohibited drugs and methods in sport

Statistics from WADA-accredited laboratories

Statistics on doping control are available from WADA, which assumed responsibility for anti-doping in 2003. Prior to this date, responsibility lay with the International Olympic Committee (IOC) Medical Commission. Statistical results from the IOC were reviewed in a previous edition of this book (Mottram 2005).

The statistical data since 2003 are derived from results from the WADA-accredited laboratories, of which there were thirty-two as of 2014 (WADA 2014). Overall, the percentage of positive test results (adverse analytical findings, or AAFs) has remained consistently low, despite a steady increase in the number of tests conducted annually (Table 25.1).

An AAF is defined by WADA, in their World Anti-Doping Code (2009; p126), as follows:

> A report from a laboratory or other WADA-approved entity that, consistent with the International Standard for laboratories and related technical documents, identifies in a

Table 25.1 Adverse analytical findings for all sports by WADA-accredited laboratories, 2003–2012

	A-samples analysed	Number of adverse findings	Percent of adverse findings
2012	267,645	4,723	1.76
2011	243,193	2,885	1.2
2010	258,267	2,790	1.08
2009	277,928	3,091	1.11
2008	274,615	5,061	1.84
2007	223,898	4,402	1.97
2006	198,143	3,887	1.96
2005	183,337	3,909	2.13
2004	169,187	2,909	1.72
2003	151,210	2,447	1.62

sample the presence of a prohibited substance or its metabolites or markers (including elevated quantities of endogenous substances) or evidence of the use of a prohibited method.

These figures include findings from athletes who had received approval to take a drug, having applied successfully for Therapeutic Use Exemption.

Variations exist in the extent of analytical findings both among laboratories and among sports. Generally, there have been few consistent patterns. However, in terms of laboratories, Tokyo consistently recorded a low percentage of adverse findings (0.16–0.61 per cent) between 2003 and 2012, whereas the Paris laboratory (1.97–6.00 per cent) and Ghent laboratory (2.05–4.86 per cent) recorded consistently high findings over the same period. This variation may be accounted for by the extent to which individual laboratories conduct no-notice, out-of-competition testing (OOCT) and the types of sports within the population for which the laboratory conducts tests.

WADA summary statistics for the substances identified, for all sports, in each class of drugs for the years 2003 to 2012, are shown in Table 25.2. It is clear that anabolic agents consistently appear as the class of substance most frequently found in samples analysed.

Stimulants, a large group of drugs with diverse modes of action and clinical uses, have appeared as the second, or occasionally third, most frequently identified class. Stimulants have the potential to impart significant performance-enhancing effects, although this group of drugs includes substances that are used recreationally and drugs that may be taken inadvertently through over-the-counter self-medication.

Cannabinoids, despite their questionable performance-enhancing benefits, appear third on the list of AAFs, probably due to their widespread use as recreational drugs coupled with a long retention time within the body following consumption.

The increased number of AAFs for diuretics and other masking agents may reflect an attempt by athletes to use these substances to counter improvements in anti-doping testing procedures.

The relatively high number of AAFs attributable to beta-2 agonists is, in part, explained by the fact that AAFs include results where athletes have been using the drug legitimately through Therapeutic Use Exemptions, a facility used commonly with beta-2 agonists. A similar rationale may apply to the glucocorticosteroid class of drugs.

Thereafter, in Table 25.2, relatively small numbers of AAFs have been recorded for the other classes of drugs. Details of the specific drugs identified under each class can be viewed on the WADA Anti-Doping Testing Figures Report (https://wada-main-prod.s3.amazonaws.com/resources/files/WADA-2012-Anti-Doping-Testing-Figures-Report-EN.pdf).

Table 25.2 Number of adverse findings for WADA-prohibited substances and methods identified by WADA-accredited laboratories, 2003–2012

	2003	2004	2005	2006	2007	2008	2009	2010	2011	2012
Anabolic agents	872	1,191	1,864	1,966	2,322	3,259	3,297	3,374	3,325	2,279
Stimulants	516	382	509	490	793	472	325	574	718	697
Cannabinoids	378	518	503	553	576	496	399	533	445	406
Diuretics and other masking agents	142	157	246	290	359	436	273	396	368	322
Beta-2 agonists	297	381	609	631	399	350	303	209	225	131
Glucocorticosteroids	286	548	325	282	288	316	265	234	274	365
Peptide hormones, growth factors, and related substances*	79	78	162	42	41	106	100	86	125	181
Hormone antagonists and modulators**	6	8	21	30	18	29	50	75	70	74
Beta blockers	30	25	42	28	27	31	38	30	21	13
Narcotics	26	15	17	16	21	28	24	20	20	26
Enhancement of oxygen transfer	–	2	–	–	3	–	–	–	1	–
Chemical and physical manipulation	2	–	–	4	3	–	5	6	3	1
Alcohol	–	–	–	–	–	–	5	9	5	5
Total	2,716	3,305	4,298	4,332	4,850	5,523	5,084	5,546	5,600	4,500

Note: Some findings correspond to multiple measurements on the same athlete, such as longitudinal studies on testosterone.

* Peptide hormones, growth factors, and related substances were listed as hormones and related substances prior to 2011.

** Hormone antagonists and modulators were listed as Agents with Antioestrogenic Activity prior to 2008.

Statistics derived from Olympic Games

Drug testing during the Olympic Games falls under the remit of the IOC in compliance with international standards for testing. The IOC agrees on the number of tests to perform in collaboration with the international federations (IFs) concerned, the local organising committee of the Games, and the laboratory accredited for the Games.

Statistics on the number of tests carried out and the number of positive cases recorded at Olympic Games between 1968 and 2012 are shown in Tables 25.3 and 25.4.

The figures again show small numbers of positive results compared with the number of samples analysed. However, it should be noted that the IOC asks IFs and national Olympic Committees to intensify their testing and other anti-doping efforts in the build-up to the Games to ensure that only 'clean' athletes make it to the Games.

Statistics derived from national and international studies on prevalence

A limited number of studies have been undertaken into the extent of drug misuse within specific countries or sports. These are listed in Table 25.5.

In the South African study (Van der Merwe *et al.* 1992) samples were taken from athletes in a wide range of sports. The percentage of positive results over the study period was very

Table 25.3 Tests carried out and the number of positive cases recorded at Summer Olympic Games between 1968 and 2012

Year	Place	Number of tests	Number of cases recorded
1968	Mexico City	667	1
1972	Munich	2,079	7
1976	Montreal	2,054	11
1980	Moscow	645	0
1984	Los Angeles	1,507	12
1988	Seoul	1,598	10
1992	Barcelona	1,848	5
1996	Atlanta	1,923	2
2000	Sydney	2,359	11
2004	Athens	3,667	26*
2008	Beijing	4,770	14
2012	London	5,051	9

Source: International Olympic Committee. (2014). The fight against doping and promotion of athletes' health. Available online at http://www.olympic.org/Documents/Reference_documents_Factsheets/Fight_against_doping. pdf (accessed 5 September 2014).

* In Athens, the cases recorded covered not only adverse analytical findings reported by the laboratory but also violations of the anti-doping rules, such as nonarrival within the set deadline for the test, providing a urine sample that did not conform to the established procedures, and refusal to comply with the procedures or to deliver urine.

consistent each year, being relatively high (average 5.5 per cent). The main drugs identified were stimulants (50.4 per cent) and anabolic steroids (41.6 per cent).

In an Italian study, stimulants (55 per cent), anabolic agents (32 per cent), beta blockers (10 per cent), and narcotics (3 per cent) were the main drugs identified (Benzi 1994). Amphetamine was the most frequently identified stimulant, being associated with cyclists. However, the percentage of positive results, overall, in Italy decreased from 0.59 per cent in 1988 to 0.29 per cent in 1992. The author commented on the low number of accredited

Table 25.4 Tests carried out and the number of positive cases recorded at Winter Olympic Games between 1968 and 2012

Year	Place	Number of tests	Number of cases recorded
1968	Grenoble	86	0
1972	Sapporo	211	1
1976	Innsbruck	390	2
1980	Lake Placid	440	0
1984	Sarajevo	424	1
1988	Calgary	492	1
1992	Albertville	522	0
1994	Lillehammer	529	0
1998	Nagano	621	0
2002	Salt Lake City	700	7
2006	Turin	1,200	7
2010	Vancouver	2,149	1

Source: International Olympic Committee. (2014). The fight against doping and promotion of athletes' health. Available online at http://www.olympic.org/Documents/Reference_documents_Factsheets/Fight_against_doping .pdf (accessed 5 September 2014).

Table 25.5 Published statistics on doping control in specific countries

Author	Country	Years data were collected	No. of samples	Percent of positive test results
Rossi and Botrè (2011)	Italy	2000–2009	95,000	1.0–1.8
Bahr et al. (1998)	Norway	1977–1995	12,870	1.2
Ueki et al. (1998)	Japan	1985–1996	~14,000	~1.0
Mottram et al. (1997)	UK	1991–1995	17,193	1.0–1.5
Delbeke (1996)	Belgium	1987–1994	4,374	7.8 in cyclists
Benzi (1994)	Italy	1988–1992	N/A	0.29–0.59
Van der Merwe (1992)	S. Africa	1986–1991	2,066	5.2–5.9 in most years

laboratories worldwide. Few tests are therefore conducted relative to the number of athletes participating in sport. The author concluded that the data generated from the laboratories are only the 'tip of the iceberg.'

In the Belgian study (Delbeke 1996), the percentage of positive results was higher than most other countries, as reported earlier in this chapter under statistics from WADA laboratories. However, this study was confined to cyclists, as cycling was the most popular sport in Belgium and it has a long-standing reputation for being associated with drug misuse. The most frequently used drugs were stimulants, including over-the-counter products and amphetamines. There were also a significant number of positive results for nandrolone. The tests were all conducted unannounced, which may also account for the high level of positive results.

A review of data from the United Kingdom (Mottram *et al.* 1997) showed that anabolic steroids and stimulants are the two main drugs of abuse, with narcotic analgesics also frequently detected. The authors commented on the fact that competitors may have been taking drugs that were undetectable at the time.

Japan has conducted tests both in competition and out-of-competition testing (OOCT) since 1985. In line with international trends, the major abused drugs were stimulants and anabolic steroids. Ephedrine, methylephedrine, and phenylpropanolamine, all available over-the-counter, were the main stimulants, and nandrolone and testosterone the main steroids (Ueki *et al.* 1998). The authors noted the value of testing agencies being independent from sports federations.

Bahr *et al.* (1998) collected data on Norwegian athletes from four accredited laboratories in Germany, Norway, Sweden, and the United Kingdom. The drugs identified were anabolic agents (75 per cent; almost half of which were testosterone), stimulants (17 per cent), narcotic analgesics (8 per cent), diuretics (5 per cent), and 4 per cent manipulation attempts. The majority were unannounced tests. A gradual decrease in the percentage of positive samples was recorded among Norwegian athletes as the frequency of testing in the high-prevalence sports – powerlifting, weightlifting, and track and field athletics – was increased during the period from 1987 to 1995. The authors commented on the beneficial effects of unannounced OOCT.

These national studies generally reflect international trends, with anabolic agents and stimulants being the most frequently identified drugs, although the principal class identified varied from country to country. For example, a study that undertook a 10-year review of AAFs from the WADA-accredited Italian anti-doping laboratory showed that cannabinoids and cocaine were the most frequently detected drugs (Rossi and Botrè 2011). National differences exist where particular sports dominate the scene or where a more extensive regime of OOCT exists.

Of course, infringements involve methods as well as drugs. The International Association of Athletic Federations reported a prevalence of blood doping of 14 per cent for the entire population of samples collected from elite track-and-field athletes between 2001 and 2009 (Sottas *et al.* 2011).

25.3. Athlete surveys into drug misuse in sport

There have been many survey-based studies published on the prevalence of drug misuse. Unfortunately, few have been based on surveys conducted with athletes and even fewer with elite athletes. Surveys are broadly divided into those that ask about self-use of drugs and those that seek information on perceived use by others. Results from the former type of study tend to reflect underreporting (Thevis *et al.* 2008), whilst those on perceived use tend to produce exaggerated claims.

Evidence such as that presented by Franke and Berendonk (1997), relating to the systematic approach to the misuse of drugs in sport by the government of the German Democratic Republic, is rare. The logistical, social, and ethical problems associated with obtaining such data are immense, hence the scarcity of such studies in the literature.

Methods used to question athletes may involve a randomised response technique (RRT), an anonymous indirect interview technique, or a standard questionnaire technique. A study by Striegel *et al.* (2010) favoured RRT rather than a standard questionnaire because the perceived anonymity is higher with RRT. The use of questionnaires as a technique to evaluate doping prevalence has been reviewed by Lentillon-Kaestner and Ohl (2011). This section of the chapter reviews some of the more recently published surveys on drug misuse in athletes (Table 25.6).

University students participating in intercollegiate athletics were the subjects in the Spence and Gauvin (1996) study. Painkillers (17.7 per cent), alcohol (94.1 per cent), anabolic steroids (0.9 per cent), amphetamines (0.7 per cent), marijuana (19.8 per cent), and cocaine (0.8 per cent) were the main drugs from the IOC Prohibited List cited as being used by respondents.

La Torre *et al.* (2001) conducted a study using amateur athletes from a number of sports. Doping was considered to be widespread in high-level sport (27.8 per cent of participants). A total of 16.5 per cent of athletes declared using amino acids and/or creatine, and 28.6 per cent of respondents considered it acceptable to use drugs in order to improve performance.

Table 25.6 Surveys on drug misuse in sport by athletes

Author	Year	Country	Number of subjects
Pitsch and Emrich	2012	Germany	
Lentillon-Kaestner and Ohl	2011	Switzerland	1,810
Streigel *et al.*	2010	Germany	1,847
Tscholl *et al.*	2008	International	2,944
Thevis *et al.*	2008	Germany	964
Pitsch *et al.*	2007	Germany	448
Alaranta *et al.*	2006	Finland	446
Chester *et al.*	2003	UK	112
La Torre *et al.*	2001	Italy	1,056
Spence and Gauvin	1996	Canada	754

The Chester (2003) study looked specifically at over-the-counter stimulants and surveyed regional, national, and international track-and-field athletes. Results showed that 3.4 per cent of respondents declared that they had used OTC stimulants for the specific purpose of performance enhancement.

Alaranta *et al*. (2006) described a self-reported survey of elite athletes in Finland. In this study, 30 per cent of respondents reported that they personally knew an athlete who used banned substances and 15 per cent had been offered banned substances, particularly speed and power athletes. Stimulants were the most frequently offered, followed by anabolic steroids.

Pitsch *et al*. (2007) used a web-based interview of top athletes in Olympic disciplines in Germany to ask about their current use of doping practices as well as their exposure to such practices in the past. In response to the question, 'Have you ever used banned doping substances or methods in order to enhance performance?,' the lower limit of the interval was 25.8 per cent and the upper limit was 48.1 per cent.

Thevis *et al*. (2008) conducted a survey of sports science students but also carried out urine chemical analysis for anabolic steroids, stimulants, and selected drugs covered by doping control regulations. In total, 11.2 per cent of the urine samples contained drugs subject to doping control. Surprisingly, no anabolic steroids were detected. The most frequently detected substance was the major metabolite for tetrahydrocannabinol in cannabis (9.8 per cent), followed by stimulants related to cocaine and amphetamines (1.0 per cent). Cannabis use had not been reported by any participants in the study, highlighting the issue of under-reporting when self-use questionnaire surveys are employed.

Tscholl *et al*. (2008) examined medication use in football players during Fédération Internationale de Football Association (FIFA) World Cups in 2002 and 2006. Each team physician documented all medication and nutritional supplements taken in the 72 hours prior to each match. Results recorded 1.8 substances per player per match, of which 42.9 per cent were medicinal and 57.1 per cent nutritional supplements. The most frequently prescribed medicines were nonsteroidal anti-inflammatory drugs, beta-2 agonists, and corticosteroids. The high intake of these substances led the authors to question whether the medication was taken solely for therapeutic purposes.

Striegel *et al*. (2010) reported that 6.8 per cent of athletes subject to doping controls as members or junior members of German national teams confessed to having practiced doping. Pitsch and Emrich (2012) recorded a prevalence ranging between 10 and 35 per cent in a survey on doping among Germen elite athletes in 2008.

Lentillon-Kaestner and Ohl (2011) questioned the very use of surveys to accurately measure prevalence of doping. In a survey that they conducted in Switzerland, they reported prevalence rates between 1.3 and 39.2 per cent in athletes; however, this depended upon the definition of doping and the types of questions used. Marijuana and drugs for asthma were the most frequently used.

As previously stated, published work on drug use by athletes is scarce. The few studies reported above indicate that results are highly variable. They are based on surveys with widely differing aims and protocols, in some cases seeking information on self-use and in others on predicted use by fellow athletes. Other variables included the type of sport undertaken by respondents and the specificity, or otherwise, of drugs under investigation. Clearly, athlete surveys are an unreliable means of obtaining robust data on worldwide trends in prohibited drug use by athletes.

25.4. A perspective on the prevalence of drug misuse in sport through medical practitioners

A review of elite athletes' attitudes, beliefs, and knowledge about doping in sport indicated that coaches appeared to be the main influence and source of information for athletes, whereas doctors and other specialists did not seem to act as principal advisors (Morente-Sánchez and Zabal 2013). Clearly, this is a situation that should not prevail because general practitioners and sport physicians have particular responsibility in addressing the issue of doping in sport (Lippi *et al*. 2008). This applies particularly in the case of drugs, such as beta-2 agonists and glucocorticosteroids, for which medical practitioners may be required to complete Therapeutic Use Exemption forms for athletes claiming to suffer from asthma or to have inflammatory sports injuries (Orchard *et al*. 2006).

Physicians and pharmacists responsible for athletes' medications need to be aware of the medicines that an athlete is taking because all medicines have adverse effects that may have deleterious effects on athlete performance (Alaranta *et al*. 2008). Unnecessary medication should be avoided in elite athletes.

Dawson (2001), a medical practitioner, identified four general groups of patients that use performance-enhancing drugs: athletes seeking to achieve their sporting goal, gymnasium users, persons in specific high-risk occupations, and recreational drug users.

A study by Gupta and Towler (1997) indicated that 53 per cent of medical practitioners had reported that they had seen at least one patient in the previous year who told them that he or she had used anabolic steroids for nonmedical purposes. A small minority of these doctors were prepared to prescribe anabolic steroids for bodybuilding purposes.

Dean (2000) discussed the professional dilemma faced by medical practitioners with regard to treating athletes who are involved in drug misuse. It is unethical for a doctor to withhold treatment from a patient on the basis of a moral judgement that the patient's activities or lifestyle might have contributed to the condition for which treatment is sought. On the other hand, doctors who prescribe or collude in the provision of drugs or treatment, with the intention of improperly enhancing performance in sport, are equally acting unethically. This was highlighted in the case of six Finnish skiers who tested positive for a masking agent, hydroxy ethyl starch, at the World Nordic Skiing Championships in 2001. It transpired that their head coach and two national team doctors had assisted these athletes in the intravenous administration of this drug (Seiler 2001).

In general, medical practitioners lack knowledge on the issue of drug misuse in sport (Greenway and Greenway 1997; Rosano *et al*. 2005). Consequently, some doctors may be prescribing banned substances to athletes unwittingly. On the other hand, drugs may be prescribed in the full knowledge of the purpose for which they may be used (Laure 1997). Either way, this study by Laure reported that 61 per cent of performance-enhancing drug supplies for amateur athletes were obtained from medical practitioners.

There is certainly scope for improved education for medical practitioners on prohibited substances in sport (Greenway and Greenway 1997; Alaranta *et al*. 2008; Dikic *et al*. 2013).

25.5. General discussion

The number of tests conducted annually by accredited laboratories has steadily increased over the years (Table 25.1). Despite this increase, the percentage of positive results has remained consistently low, below 2 per cent. Thus, only the tip of the iceberg may be perceived by assessing the presence of a prohibited substance or its metabolites or markers in blood or urine samples of an athlete at a given/specific time (Marclay *et al.* 2013). Few people would regard the AAF figures reported by WADA as being an indication of the true prevalence of drug misuse in sport. A survey of public opinion in Australia (Moston *et al.* 2012) showed that the public believed that a quarter of athletes used banned performance-enhancing drugs and that a third of athletes used banned recreational drugs.

Some of the reasons for perceptions on prevalence are as follows:

- Too few tests are conducted relative to the number of athletes competing in sport.
- A large proportion of the drugs do not need to be taken at the time of competing, and the extent of OOCT is inconsistent among sports federations and among national anti-doping organisations.
- Athletes continue to be adept at tailoring their drug use around times when they are least likely to be tested.

Another factor that leads one to believe that statistics are misleading with regard to prevalence is the increasing use of drugs that are naturally occurring in the body. It is extremely difficult to determine what a 'normal' level of such substances is in an 'average' athlete. There must, therefore, be innumerable instances of the use of these drugs that remain undetected. The introduction by WADA of Athlete Biological Passports, which record haematological and steroidal profiles of athletes, goes some way toward addressing this problem (Mareck *et al.* 2008).

What is needed is good quality research on drug use by athletes at all levels of ability, from junior to elite. Unfortunately, ethical constraints and the reluctance of athletes to divulge true and accurate information on the subject makes this an unachievable goal. We are therefore left in the position of mere speculation. This encourages the media to publish unsubstantiated conjecture and rumour. In turn, this fuels misconceptions and fears in the minds of competitors, which itself encourage further drug use in sport.

25.6. Summary

- Meaningful data on the prevalence of doping in sport is difficult to obtain.
- Results derived from statistical data from testing laboratories are very different from those obtained through surveys.
- WADA laboratory statistics suggest that, annually, fewer than 2 per cent of samples analysed produce an adverse analytical finding.
- Independent studies on the prevalence of doping reveal significantly higher levels of drug misuse in sport.
- Many factors lead us to believe that statistics on the prevalence of drug misuse in sport are misleading, including the trend toward the use of prohibited substances and methods that are found naturally in the body.
- The introduction by WADA of Athlete Biological Passports, which record the haematological and steroidal profiles of athletes, goes some way toward addressing this problem.

25.7. References

Alaranta, A., Alaranta, H., and Helenius, I. (2008). Use of prescription drugs in athletes. *Sports Medicine* 38(6):449–463.

Alaranta, A., Alaranta, H., Holmila, J., *et al.* (2006). Self-reported attitudes of elite athletes toward doping: Differences between type of sport. *International Journal of Sports Medicine* 27(10): 842–846.

Bahr, R., and Tjornhom, M. (1998). Prevalence of doping in sports: Doping control in Norway, 1977–1995. *Clinical Journal of Sports Medicine* 8(11):32–37.

Benzi, G. (1994). Pharmacoepidemiology of the drugs used in sports as doping agents. *Pharmacological Research* 29(1):13–26.

Chester, N., Reilly, T., and Mottram, D. R. (2003). Over-the-counter drug use amongst athletes and non-athletes. *Journal of Sports Medicine and Physical Fitness* 43(1):111–118.

Dawson, R. T. (2001). Hormones and sport. Drugs in sport – the role of the physician. *Journal of Endocrinology* 170(1):55–61.

Dean, C. (2000). Performance enhancing drugs: Damned if you do and damned if you don't. *British Journal of Sports Medicine* 34(2):154.

Delbeke, F. T. (1996). Doping in cyclism: Results of unannounced controls in Flanders (1987–1994). *International Journal of Sports Medicine* 17(6):434–438.

Dikic, N., McNamee, M., Günter, H., *et al.* (2013). Sports physicians, ethics and anti-doping governance: Between assistance and negligence. *British Journal of Sports Medicine* 47(11):701–704.

Dimeo, P., and Taylor, J. (2013). Monitoring drug use in sport: The contrast between official statistics and other evidence. *Drugs: Education, Prevention and Policy* 20(1):40–47.

Franke, W. W., and Berendonk, B. (1997). Hormonal doping and androgenization of athletes: A secret program of the German Democratic Republic government. *Clinical Chemistry* 43(7):1262–1279.

Greenway, P., and Greenway, M. (1997). General practitioner knowledge of prohibited substances in sport. *British Journal of Sports Medicine* 31(2):129–131.

Gupta, L., and Towler, B. (1997). General practitioners' views and knowledge about anabolic steroid use: Survey of GPs in a high prevalence area. *Drug and Alcohol Review* 16(4):373–379.

La Torre, G., Limongelli, F., Masala, D., *et al.* (2001). Knowledge, attitudes and behaviour toward doping and food supplementation in a sample of athletes of central-southern Italy. *Medicina Dello Sport* 54(3):229–233.

Laure, P. (1997). Doping in sport: Doctors are providing drugs. *British Journal of Sports Medicine* 31(3):258–259.

Lentillon-Kaestner, V., and Ohl, F. (2011). Can we measure accurately the prevalence of doping? *Scandinavian Journal of Medical Science in Sport* 21(6):e132–e142.

Lippi, G., Franchini, M., and Guidi, G. C. (2008). Doping in competition or doping in sport? *British Medical Bulletin* 86(1):95–107.

Marclay, F., Manglin, P., Margot, P., *et al.* (2013). Perspectives for forensic intelligence in anti-doping: Thinking outside the box. *Forensic Science International* 229(1):133–144.

Mareck, U., Geyer, H., Opfermann, G., *et al.* (2008). Factors influencing the steroid profile in doping control analysis. *Journal of Mass Spectrometry* 43(7):877–891.

Morente-Sánchez, J., and Zabala, M. (2013). Doping in sport: A review of elite athletes' attitudes, beliefs and knowledge. *Sports Medicine* 43(6):395–411.

Moston, S., Skinner, J., and Engelsberg, T. (2012). Perceived incidence of drug use in Australian sport: A survey of public opinion. *Sports in Society* 15(1):64–77.

Mottram, D. R. (2005). Prevalence of drug misuse in sport. In D. R. Mottram (Ed.), *Drugs in sport* (4th ed., pp. 357–380). London, UK: Routledge.

Mottram, D. R, Reilly, T., and Chester, N. (1997). Doping in sport: The extent of the problem. In T. Reilly and M. Orme (Eds), *The clinical pharmacology of sport and exercise* (pp. 3–12). Amsterdam, the Netherlands: Excerpta Medica.

Orchard, J. W., Fricker, P. A., White, S. C., *et al*. (2006). The use and misuse of performance-enhancing substances in sport. *Medical Journal of Australia* 184(3):132–136.

Pitsch, W., and Emrich, E. (2012). The frequency of doping in elite sport: Results of a replication study. *International Review for the Sociology of Sport* 47(5):559–581.

Pitsch, W., Emrich, E., and Klein, M. (2007). Doping in elite sports in Germany: Results of a www survey. *European Journal for Sport and Society* 4(2):89–102.

Rosano, A., Carletti, M., Donini, L. M., *et al*. (2005). Doping and supplements: Awareness and knowledge by the Italian general practitioners. *Medicina Dello Sport* 58(4):265–272.

Rossi, S. S., and Botrè, F. (2011). Prevalence of illicit drug use among the Italian athlete population with special attention on drugs of abuse: A 10-year review. *Journal of Sports Sciences* 29(5):471–476.

Seiler, S. (2001). Doping disaster for Finnish Ski Team: A turning point for drug testing? *Sportscience* 5(1):1–3.

Sottas, P. E., Robinson, N., Fischetto, G., *et al*. (2011). Prevalence of blood doping in samples collected from elite track and field athletes. *Clinical Chemistry* 57(5):762–769.

Spence, J. C., and Gauvin, L. (1996). Drug and alcohol use by Canadian university athletes: A national survey. *Journal Drug Education* 26(3):275–287.

Striegel, H., Ulrich, R., and Simon, P. (2010). Randomised response estimates for doping and illicit drug use in elite athletes. *Drug and Alcohol Dependence* 106(2–3):230–232.

Thevis, M., Sauer, M., Geyer, H., *et al*. (2008). Determination of the prevalence of anabolic steroids, stimulants and selected drugs subject to doping controls among elite sport students using analytical chemistry. *Journal of Sports Sciences* 26(10):1059–1065.

Tscholl, P., Junge, A., and Dvorak, J. (2008). The use of medication and nutritional supplements during FIFA World Cups 2002 and 2006. *British Journal of Sports Medicine* 42(9):725–730.

Ueki, M., Hiruma, T., Ikekita, A., *et al*. (1998). Trends in drug abuse in competitive sports, and the international anti-doping movement. *Journal of Toxicology – Toxin Reviews* 17(1):73–83.

Van der Merwe, P. J., and Kruger, H. S. L. (1992). Drugs in sport – Results of the past 6 years of dope testing in South Africa. *South African Medical Journal* 82(3):151–153.

World Anti-Doping Agency. (2014). Accredited laboratories for doping control analysis. Available online at https://www.wada-ama.org/en/who-we-are/anti-doping-community/accredited-approved-labo-ratories (accessed 9 September 2014).

Yesalis, C. E., Kopstein, A. N., and Bahrke, M. S. (2001). Difficulties in estimating the prevalence of drug use among athletes. In W. Wilson and E. Derse (Eds.), *Doping in elite sport: The politics of drugs in the Olympic movement* (pp. 43–62). Champaign, IL: Human Kinetics.

Chapter 26

Future issues concerning drug use in sport

Neil Chester and David R. Mottram

26.1. Introduction

In this chapter, we will address some of the issues that may influence future attitudes, beliefs, and approaches toward doping and anti-doping in sport.

26.2. Performance-enhancing drugs in sport: Should we permit their use?

The control of doping within sport is a complex process – a key aspect of which is making the decision as to where the line should be drawn between permitted and prohibited performance-enhancing drugs. For some individuals, this has begged the question, 'Should a line be drawn at all?' Is it time to abolish the World Anti-Doping Agency (WADA) Prohibited List?

This section reviews some of the arguments that have been proposed for permitting athletes to use prohibited performance-enhancing drugs in sport. The consequences for making such a radical decision are then presented.

Arguments for permitting athletes to use prohibited performance-enhancing drugs in sport

Proposals in favour of permitting athletes to use prohibited performance-enhancing substances within sport are largely based on three fundamental questions:

1 Are the WADA criteria for the selection of substances for inclusion on the Prohibited List robust?
2 Is there a level playing field within sport?
3 Is the cost of anti-doping becoming prohibitive?

Are the WADA criteria for the selection of substances for inclusion on the Prohibited List robust?

The WADA criteria for selection of substances and methods are as follows:

• They enhance or have the potential to enhance performance.
• They carry a potential risk to health.
• They are against the spirit of sport.

One may ask the question, 'What constitutes performance enhancement?' Athletes have inherent physiological characteristics that are unique to each individual. Athletes therefore undertake extensive fitness and skills regimes to make up for perceived metabolic and physical deficiencies. Most competitive athletes include dietary and ergogenic supplementation to achieve these aims. Why should some supplements be permitted and others prohibited? Can a definitive line be drawn accurately between permitted and prohibited substances?

All drugs have side effects, the severity of which depends to a large extent upon the dose of the drug that is used. Consequently, any drug has the potential to pose a risk to health, whether it is permitted or prohibited.

The ultimate aim for all competitive athletes is to increase their personal performance level until they reach the highest pinnacle of achievement, as encouraged by the International Olympic Committee motto: *Citius, Altius, Fortius* (Faster, Higher, Stronger). Is this not the spirit of sport, and therefore should athletes not pursue this by whatever means are available? Do sports fans really concern themselves as to how their heroes achieve greatness?

Is there a level playing field within sport?

It is evident that there is not a level playing field within sport. Athletes who have access to sponsorship and resources are in the advantageous position of being able to purchase the best equipment, train at altitude, and call upon appropriate expertise from coaches, physiotherapists, sports psychologists, and nutritionists. Why should athletes without recourse to such resources not attempt to redress the balance by using drugs to simulate some of these influences?

Is the cost of anti-doping becoming prohibitive?

The infrastructure required to monitor and operate a comprehensive doping control programme is significant. Could the resources required to support this organisational structure be better utilised in other ways, for the benefit of sport? Some would argue that current programmes are not cost effective. Despite such huge investments, doping control as both a treatment and preventative measure is deemed to have a limited effect on the numbers engaged in doping practice (Hermann and Henneberg 2013).

The consequences of allowing athletes to use prohibited performance-enhancing drugs in sport

The consequences of allowing athletes to use prohibited performance-enhancing drugs may be addressed by asking the following questions:

- Between whom will competition take place?
- What will the impact be on the athlete in the short term and long term?
- Should some limits still be applied?
- How would sports fans and sponsors react?

Between whom will competition take place?

Most athletes are not medical practitioners, pharmacologists, or pharmacists. They are therefore not qualified to make rational decisions as to which drug they should use to achieve the performance that they desire. They may turn to health care professionals for such advice. However, this would lead to ethical dilemmas for professionals who may not wish to encourage the use of drugs for nontherapeutic purposes in healthy individuals, but who have the health and welfare of the athlete as a prime consideration.

The playing field of sport would become even less level between the haves and have-nots as certain athletes may gain access to sophisticated but expensive drug regimes.

The proliferation of a black market in 'designer' drugs, produced by 'backstreet' pharmacologists, would be a source of drugs that would be tempting to many athletes. Sports events may end up as a competition primarily among such pharmacologists, with athletes acting simply as conduits for the marketing of the latest designer drugs.

What will the impact be on the athlete in the short term and long term?

In the short term, regardless of the efficacy of drugs as performance-enhancing agents, athletes would feel compelled to use drugs in order to compete on equal terms with their fellow competitors, whom they would assume were using drugs.

The welfare and safety of fellow competitors may be compromised because some athletes could be competing under the influence of drugs that impair normal patterns of behaviour.

All drugs possess side effects, many of which are serious and in some cases life-threatening when taken at supratherapeutic doses. This will pose a significant threat to athletes, who would be self-medicating and focussed on potential short-term gain from drug use rather than on long-term health and welfare.

Should some limits still be applied?

Suggestions have been made that performance-enhancing drugs should be permitted, but that limits could be applied. Where would one draw the line on these limits? At what age should junior athletes be permitted to use performance-enhancing drugs? Should dose limits apply to certain drugs? Should prohibited methods, such as gene doping, be retained?

There are no simple answers to these questions. If limits, of whatever type, still apply, all the current monitoring and testing procedures would need to be retained, except that the bar would be set at a higher level.

How would sports fans and sponsors react?

Because athletes are often viewed as role models by many people, it could be argued that the use of performance-enhancing drugs by athletes would be widely reflected throughout society as a whole, with serious consequences. However, judging by the reaction to recent revelations with respect to the Lance Armstrong case, it would appear that the majority of sports fans are against the practice of doping in sport. Furthermore, it was interesting to note how rapidly sponsorship from companies was withdrawn following revelations of recent cases of doping by high-profile athletes. How long would professional sport survive without the lifeblood of sponsorship?

Conclusion

Despite our best attempts, we will never completely abolish the use of performance-enhancing drugs in sport. However, the worldwide fight against doping must be sustained and strengthened.

We must continue to support WADA and associated anti-doping organisations. The consequences of relaxing anti-doping regulations would destroy sport as it is currently enjoyed by billions of fans around the world.

26.3. Drug trafficking, criminal activities, and law enforcement connected with drug misuse in sport

In a speech presented at a conference of the National Sports Law Institute of Marquette University Law School in 2012, David Howman (2013), director general of WADA, discussed the issue of corruption in sports. He stated that the attack against the integrity of sport has advanced in the areas of illegal betting, bribery, and corruption, with each of those areas linked or directly associated with doping. Indeed, some have estimated that the criminal underworld now 'controls' at least 25 per cent of world sport in one way or another.

A worldwide research study was performed by Alessandro Donati (2007). This study assembled information and data that may be used as the basis for an estimate of the total volume of traffic of doping substances on a world scale.

WADA has worked very closely with national law enforcement agencies, Interpol (WADA 2006), and other investigators responsible for maintaining integrity in sports. These law enforcement agencies have informed WADA that the same individuals responsible for such trafficking and distribution are responsible for much of the illegal betting and much of the bribery and corruption. As far as trafficking or distribution of prohibited substances (chiefly steroids, human growth hormone, and erythropoietin), the markup available for a simple investment can be anything from ten times to one hundred times.

Clearly, the impact of crime and corruption on sport is a serious threat that needs to be addressed. Howman (2013) warned that WADA is not equipped to deal with the criminal underworld, but that any organisation attempting to attack corruption and bribery in sport will need to have statutory teeth and a willingness on the part of police and prosecutors to act. He did, however, suggest that we may be able to learn from the successful WADA sport/ government model. Perhaps a world sports integrity agency could be established with the same governance as WADA – in other words, an equal sharing of governance between sport and governments. This overarching board could have different arms in terms of the aspects it deals with – namely, doping, betting, bribery, and corruption.

The importance of intelligence gathering to target doping through organisations, which includes law enforcement agencies, was emphasised within the World Anti-Doping Code (2013a), as discussed below.

26.4. The normalisation of drug use in society and the impact on the anti-doping movement

A developing threat to the anti-doping movement is considered to be the normalization of drug use within society. The growing trend toward the use and acceptance of enhancement technologies is likely to have a detrimental effect on anti-doping. As society continues to embrace the 'body beautiful' ideal and continues the quest for the ultimate anti-aging elixir, so too does drug-free sport become an ideal within a subsection of society that is effectively dissociated and eroded.

The normalisation of adolescent recreational drug use is a well-known concept that has been described by several researchers, including Measham *et al.* (1994) and Parker *et al.* (1998).

It refers to the acceptance or justification of what is essentially deviant behaviour by both those who participate in the activity and society at large, to the extent that it enters mainstream culture.

The process in which such behaviour has become normalised may be under discussion; however, it is likely to be in part a consequence of increased imagery relating to drugs and drug use, particularly by major companies to market their products in a positive light (Blackman 2010). The advent of the internet has clearly been a significant landmark in the legitimisation and normalisation of nontherapeutic drug use. For the first time, individuals across a wider sector of society were introduced to and bombarded with images relating to drug use and their availability rocketed. The internet also provided a platform for information and misinformation relating to drug use.

There is a danger that the use of performance- and image-enhancing drugs (PIEDs), which is currently viewed as risky behaviour, will become normalised and therefore accepted behaviour within society. Indeed, subliminal messages from advertising are considered to play a part in normalising drug use. For example, the portrayal of male physiques with heavy musculature and the use of the term *steroids* in a positive light to describe power and muscular bulk all help to change the perception of PIED use within society to one that is more acceptable. Clearly, such a change in perception creates a contradiction in terms of the legislation of PIEDs in sport. The perceived ineffectiveness of doping control is further amplified by the normalisation of PIEDs within society.

There is evidence of a growing acceptance of PIED use as an inevitable part of competitive sport. According to findings from interviews with athletes who had used PIEDs, doping was considered to be an established and essential behaviour in competitive sport, and none viewed their activity as abnormal (Pappa and Kennedy 2013). It is this acceptance of PIED drug use in competitive sport that enables athletes to legitimise their behaviour. Clearly, this ability to rationalise is deemed to have a direct impact on the prevalence of PIED use amongst athletes.

Nevertheless, because the anti-doping rules set out in the World Anti-Doping Code establish a framework for the welfare and safety of athletes and attempt to ensure fair play, such normalisation of doping from an athlete's perspective might be disregarded. However, it might be argued that the normalisation of nontherapeutic drug use within the wider society could have a greater effect on PIED use in sport as a consequence of the impact on the anti-doping movement. Of course, without an effective anti-doping programme, PIED use in sport will inevitably mushroom.

Within the wider society, the following factors are thought to undermine the anti-doping movement:

- Widespread use of recreational, illicit drugs across all classes and ages (although generally centred on the young)
- Increased use of image-enhancing and anti-ageing drugs/products across a wide spectrum of society in response to media-driven images and expectations
- Use of cognitive enhancing drugs amongst students and the workforce alike to maintain or increase achievement
- The increased entertainment value of sport for the general public and the audience attitudes toward doping, such as the ambivalence toward athletes who are caught and their enjoyment of watching high-level performance, however it may be achieved.

As these factors, as well as others, become more accepted or central in daily living, it is likely that the zero-tolerance approach to PIED use in sport will appear ever more alien.

Whilst sport may always be able to justify its position as a 'rule-based' institution, it may become more difficult to justify and indeed legislate against something that is becoming increasingly acceptable elsewhere in society.

26.5. The 2015 World Anti-Doping Code

The Fourth World Conference on Doping in Sport was held in Johannesburg, South Africa, in November 2013. This conference was the culmination of a two-year consultation process on the latest revision of the World Anti-Doping Code, effective 1 January 2015.

Overview of the 2015 draft code

The 2015 World Anti-Doping Code (WADA, 2014) incorporated 2,269 changes to the previous version of the code from 2009. These changes were made following 315 submissions, during the three consultation phases, recommending a total of 3,987 changes to the code.

An overview document (WADA 2013a) of the significant changes between the 2009 code and the 2015 code (version 4) categorises the changes to the code into seven general themes, as described in the following sections.

Theme 1: Longer periods of ineligibility for real cheats and more flexibility in sanctioning

Significant changes have been made to the period of ineligibility for doping offences. Whilst longer periods have been introduced for intentional cheating, more flexibility will apply to sanctions in cases of 'no significant fault.'

For many years, the standard period of ineligibility for those who cheat in sport has been 2 years. There was a strong consensus among stakeholders – and in particular, athletes – toward the view that intentional cheaters should be ineligible for a period of 4 years.

There was also a consensus among stakeholders that more flexibility in sanctioning should be permitted in certain circumstances where the athlete can demonstrate that he or she was not cheating, particularly involving specified substances or a contaminated product.

Theme 2: Consideration of the principles of proportionality and human rights

Legal opinion was sought on the enforceability of various aspects of the code applicable to the principles of proportionality and human rights. The convention for the protection of human rights must acknowledge the balance between the interests of anti-doping organisations and the individual's interests.

Theme 3: Increasing importance of investigations and use of intelligence

Anti-doping rule violations can be proved by any reliable means, which includes both analytical and nonanalytical evidence obtained through appropriate investigations. This has been exemplified in recent high-profile cases, such as the Bay Area Laboratory Cooperative investigations and the US Postal Service/Lance Armstrong investigation.

There was a strong consensus that cooperation of governments and all stakeholders in anti-doping rule violation investigations is important and that the role of investigations should be recognised and highlighted in the code. The importance of intelligence gathering to target doping was emphasised.

Recent cases have demonstrated that it sometimes takes a significant period of time before sophisticated doping schemes may be exposed. Therefore, the statute of limitations has been increased to 10 years from the current 8-year statute.

Theme 4: Amendments to better reach athlete support personnel who are involved in doping

In light of the fact that doping in sport frequently involves athlete support personnel, such as coaches and trainers, the code has been revised to better address this problem. Athlete support personnel will be subject to closer scrutiny with respect to their use or possession, without valid justification, of prohibited substances or methods. For those athlete support personnel who have been involved in doping activities but are currently outside the jurisdiction of anti-doping authorities, the 2015 amendments add a new anti-doping rule violation article entitled 'Prohibited Association.' The Prohibited Association clause has been added to prohibit athletes from associating with athlete support personnel who have previously been involved in doping activities.

Theme 5: Additional emphasis on smart test distribution planning and smart menus for sample analysis

At the present time, some anti-doping organisations do not direct testing laboratories to conduct a full menu analysis on all testing samples collected. Furthermore, not all organisations collect both urine and blood. The 2015 code amendments address this situation by providing a technical document that identifies the prohibited substances or methods that are most likely to be abused in particular sports and sport disciplines. The document may be used in test distribution planning and sample analysis.

Theme 6: Attempts to balance the interests of international federations and national anti-doping organizations

International federations and national anti-doping organisations both play a crucial role in combating doping. It is important that their respective roles are collaborative and coordinated, particularly with respect to major event organisation. The 2015 code has been changed to better clarify and balance these responsibilities. The responsibility for conducting results management and hearings shall be the responsibility of the anti-doping organisation that initiated the sample test or other asserted anti-doping rule violation.

Theme 7: Making the code clearer and shorter

Stakeholders' desire to make the code shorter and less technical, without compromising clarity and comprehension, has been addressed in the 2015 code. Clarification of the code will be enhanced by the creation of an athlete's guide.

Other code changes

Other miscellaneous changes to the code include the following:

- The period to accumulate three missed tests or filing failures that result in an anti-doping rule violation has been reduced from 18 months to 12 months.
- Athletes who 'retire' should give 6 months' notice before returning to competition.
- Anti-doping organisations may impose financial sanctions.
- Educational programs should focus on prevention.

Review of the international standards for testing and investigations, laboratories, protection of privacy and personal information, and therapeutic use exemptions

Few significant changes to the international standards were proposed at the conference, except for the inclusion of intelligence-based investigations as part of the revised standard for testing. In the future, risk assessment of potential anti-doping rules violations should be used to target athletes.

With respect to Therapeutic Use Exemptions (TUEs), international federations must make clear when they consider an athlete to have become an 'international-level athlete' because TUEs issued by national anti-doping organisations may not automatically apply at the international level.

Conference resolution

Following the meeting of the WADA Executive Committee and Foundation Board, the World Anti-Doping Code 2015 was approved and endorsed by the delegates at the conference. The Johannesburg Declaration was then presented to the conference (WADA 2013b). This document concluded with the following declaration:

The Johannesburg World Conference on Doping in Sport reaffirms that the ultimate objective of the fight against doping in sport is the protection of all clean athletes and that all concerned parties should commit all required resources and resolve to achieve that objective by intensifying the fight.

New initiatives

At the conference, WADA also announced some new initiatives to tackle doping in sport, which included the following.

Steroidal module

The Steroidal Module joins the Haematological Module to complement the Athlete Biological Passport, which, overall, aims to identify athletes for further target testing in addition to assisting detection of anti-doping rule violations. The Steroidal Module tests an athlete's urine sample to observe unique steroidal variables such as testosterone, therefore making it a useful technique in spotting athlete abuse of anabolic androgenic steroids.

University project

In collaboration with the International University Sports Federation and Gwangju 2015 Universiade Organizing Committee, WADA has developed an eTextbook and teaching material for first-year university students. The anti-doping eTextbook is part of an initiative to deliver a full 'model curriculum' for university academic staff to educate future practitioners, athletes, coaches, and all leaders of sport on the dangers of doping in sport and their role in combatting the issue.

26.6. Summary

- There are wide-ranging issues that may influence future attitudes, beliefs, and approaches toward doping and anti-doping in sport that need to be addressed.
- Arguments for permitting the use of performance-enhancing drugs in sport are spurious. Although illegal drug use in sport will never be completely abolished, the anti-doping fight must continue.
- The impact of crime and corruption in sport is a serious threat that needs to be tackled. The cooperation of law enforcement agencies with anti-doping organisations should be encouraged and expanded.
- The normalisation of drug use in society may, in the future, make it significantly more difficult to legislate against drug use in sport.
- A number of important changes were introduced to the 2015 World Anti-Doping Code, particularly in the areas of sanctions, a more intelligence-based approach to anti-doping, and a greater emphasis on education relating to drug use in sport.

26.7. References

Blackman, S. (2010). Youth subcultures, normalization and drug prohibition: The politics of contemporary crisis and change? *British Politics* 5(3):337–366.

Donati, A. (2007). World traffic in doping substances. Available online at https://wada-main-prod.s3.amazonaws.com/resources/files/WADA_Donati_Report_On_Trafficking_2007.pdf (accessed 22 August 2014).

Hermann, A., and Henneberg, M. (2013). Anti-doping systems in sports are doomed to fail: A probability and cost analysis. Available online at http://www.adelaide.edu.au/news/binary9861/Doping.pdf (accessed 23 July 2014).

Howman, D. (2013). Supporting the integrity of sport and combatting corruption. *Marquette Sports law Review* 23(2):245–248. Available online at http://scholarship.law.marquette.edu/sportslaw/vol23/iss2/11 (accessed 23 July 2014).

Measham, F., Newcombe, R., and Parker, H. (1994). The normalization of recreational drug use amongst young people in North-West England. *British Journal of Sociology* 45(2):287–312.

Pappa, E., and Kennedy, E. (2013). 'It was my thought...he made it a reality': Normalization and responsibility in athletes' accounts of performance-enhancing drug use. *International Review for the Sociology of Sport* 48(3):277–294.

Parker, H., Measham, F., and Aldridge, J. (1998) *Illegal leisure: The normalization of adolescent drug use*. London, UK: Routledge.

World Anti-Doping Agency. (2006). WADA and Interpol cooperation. Available online at https://www.wada-ama.org/en/what-we-do/investigation-trafficking/trafficking/interpol-cooperation (accessed 22 August 2014).

World Anti-Doping Agency. (2014). World Anti-Doping Code: Draft 2015. Available online at https://wada-main-prod.s3.amazonaws.com/resources/files/wada-2015-world-anti-doping-code.pdf (accessed 9 September 2014).

World Anti-Doping Agency. (2013a). Significant changes between the 2009 Code and the 2015 Code, Version 4.0. Available online at https://elb.wada-ama.org/en/content/significant-changes-between-the-2009-code-and-the-2015-code-0#.VA-RQcstDX4 (accessed 23 July 2014).

World Anti-Doping Agency. (2013b). Johannesburg declaration. Available online at http://wada2013.org/documents/WADA-WCDS-2013-Jburg-Declaration-FINAL.pdf (accessed 9 September 2014).

Appendix: Synopsis of drugs used in sport

David R. Mottram and Neil Chester

A.1. Introduction

The first section of this synopsis presents an overview of the more commonly used classes of drugs and methods on the 2014 World Anti-Doping Agency (WADA) Prohibited List, including

- WADA category
- Use in sport
- Pharmacological action
- Adverse effects.

The second section presents information on drugs that are not prohibited but are commonly used by athletes. The adverse effects of these drugs and the implications for their use in sport are described.

A.2. WADA-prohibited drugs and methods

Anabolic androgenic steroids

WADA category

I. Substances and methods prohibited at all times (in- and out-of-competition). S1. Anabolic Agents 1. Anabolic Androgenic Steroids

Use in sport

Anabolic androgenic steroids (AASs) are used to improve strength by increasing lean body mass, decreasing body fat, prolonging training by enhancing recovery time, and increasing aggressiveness.

Pharmacological action

AASs have two major effects: an androgenic or mascularizing action and an anabolic or tissue-building effect. They may be taken orally or by deep intramuscular injection. Injectable preparations may be water or oil based. In general, oil-based preparations have a longer biological half-life. AASs produce their effect through an action on endogenous androgen receptors. They increase protein synthesis and possibly have an anticatabolic effect by antagonizing the effect of glucocorticoid hormones, such as cortisol, released during intense exercise.

Adverse effects

Acne and water retention are common, reversible side effects. Prolonged use may lead to male-pattern baldness. Cardiovascular side effects associated with AAS use include hypertension and alteration of cholesterol levels. The liver is a target tissue for androgens and it is the principal site for steroid metabolism, especially after oral administration. A number of effects on the liver have been described, including hepatocyte hypertrophy and, at high doses, cholestasis and peliosis hepatis. Androgens also increase the risk of liver tumours. Psychological effects with AASs, such as mania, hypomania, and depression, have been reported.

In women, the extent of AAS use is less well known. The risks of steroid misuse in women are greater than in men, with some side effects being irreversible. Females prefer oral steroids, which are shorter acting than the oil-based injectable steroids, such as testosterone, which are more likely to produce side effects such as acne, unwanted facial hair, cliteromegaly, and a change in the shape of the face, with squaring of the jaw line.

In men, AAS misuse is commonly associated with testicular atrophy and reduced sperm production. Gynaecomastia is a common side effect among male body builders associated with steroid misuse.

Erythropoietin

WADA category

I. Substances and methods prohibited at all times (in- and out-of-competition). S2. Peptide Hormones, Growth Factors and related substances.

Use in sport

The increase in production of erythrocytes by erythropoietin (EPO) improves the oxygen-carrying capacity of the blood. This effect is particularly useful in endurance sports. Misuse normally involves synthetic, recombinant EPO. More recently, the erythropoietin derivative, darbepoietin, and the erythropoietin receptor activator, CERA, have been used, both of which are prohibited by WADA.

Pharmacological action

EPO is a glycoprotein hormone, produced primarily in the kidneys. The stimulus for its production is reduced oxygen delivery to the kidney. Its effect is to increase the number of erythrocytes that are produced from the bone marrow and to increase the rate at which they are released into the circulation.

Adverse effects

EPO can initially produce flu-like symptoms, such as headaches and joint pain, but these usually resolve spontaneously, even with continued use. Up to 35 per cent of patients on EPO develop hypertension and the risk of thrombosis is increased. In sport, the misuse of EPO poses a significant potential risk to health because the raised haematocrit increases blood viscosity, which may be further exacerbated through dehydration.

Growth hormone and insulin-like growth factor I

WADA category

I. Substances and methods prohibited at all times (in- and out-of-competition). S2. Peptide Hormones, Growth Factors and related substances.

Use in sport

Human growth hormone (hGH) is used to increase muscle mass. It allows users to train harder, longer, and more frequently and promotes faster recovery after training.

Pharmacological action

hGH is a polypeptide hormone produced by the pituitary gland to maintain normal growth from birth to adulthood. It has a short (about 20-minute) half-life, during which time it activates hepatic growth hormone receptors, mediating the production of insulin-like growth factor 1 (IGF-1). It is IGF-1 that is responsible for most of the anabolic action of hGH.

Adverse effects

Overuse of hGH in children can lead to gigantism; in adults, it can lead to acromegaly. Features of acromegaly include skeletal deformities, arthritis, and enlargement of organs such as the heart, lungs, liver, intestines, and spleen. Hypertension, diabetes mellitus, peripheral neuropathy, and muscle weakness, despite an increase in size, may develop. Increased protein synthesis also produces thickening and coarsening of the skin. Association between the use of hGH and leukaemia has been reported.

When athletes use IGF-1, adverse effects are the same as for hGH. IGF-1 commonly produces hypoglycaemia, as it promotes the uptake of glucose into cells.

The use of hGH has become more popular among female athletes because there is no risk of developing the androgenic side effects associated with AASs.

Beta-2 agonists

WADA category

I. Substances and methods prohibited at all times (in- and out-of-competition). S3. Beta-2 agonists and S1 Anabolic Agents 2. Other Anabolic Agents

All beta-2 agonists are prohibited, except salbutamol, formoterol, and salmeterol, which are permitted in sport when taken by inhalation in accordance with the manufacturers' recommended therapeutic regimen.

The presence in urine of salbutamol in excess of 1000 ng/ml or formoterol in excess of 40 ng/ml is presumed not to be an intended therapeutic use.

Other drugs used in the treatment of asthma, including corticosteroids (subject to restriction, see below), anticholinergics, methyl xanthines, and cromoglycate, are permitted in sport.

Use in sport

All beta-2 agonists are potent bronchodilators and may therefore improve performance in aerobic exercise. Beta-2 agonists, particularly clenbuterol, possess anabolic activity and are used as an alternative or in addition to anabolic steroids.

Pharmacological action

Bronchodilation is mediated through stimulation of the beta-2 adrenoreceptors in the smooth muscle of the respiratory tract. Beta-2 adrenoreceptors are also found in skeletal muscle, the stimulation of which induces muscle growth. Beta-2 agonists are also capable of reducing subcutaneous and total body fat.

Adverse effects

At the higher doses likely to be experienced by misusers in sport, these drugs lose their selectivity, leading to stimulation of beta-1 adrenoreceptors. This commonly produces fine tremor, usually of the hands, and may produce tachycardia, arrhythmias, nausea, insomnia, and headache.

When clenbuterol is used in doses producing anabolic effects, additional side effects, such as generalized myalgia, asthenia, periorbital pain, dizzy spells, nausea, vomiting, and fever have been reported.

Diuretics

WADA category

I. Substances and methods prohibited at all times (in- and out-of-competition). S5. Diuretics and Other Masking Agents

Use in sport

Diuretics do not have performance-enhancing effects but have been used to increase urine production in an attempt to dilute other doping agents and/or their metabolites. Diuretics are also used to reduce weight in sports where weight classification applies. In this context, they are subject to testing at the time of the weigh-in.

Diuretics are used by body builders to counteract the fluid-retentive effects of androgenic anabolic steroids.

Pharmacological action

Diuretics variably exert their pharmacological effect on the kidney, to produce an increased loss of fluid.

Adverse effects

The primary adverse effect results from induced hypohydration, although concomitant electrolyte disturbances compromise the heart and muscles. These effects are exacerbated where hyperthermia and dehydration accompany fatigue and glycogen depletion.

Blood doping

WADA category

I. Substances and methods prohibited at all times (in- and out-of-competition). M1. Manipulation of blood and blood components.

Use in sport

Blood doping increases the oxygen-carrying capacity of the blood.

Adverse effects

Blood doping may lead to adverse effects associated with hyperviscocity of the blood, as discussed under EPO. Otherwise, autologous blood doping carries no more risk than any other procedure involving invasive techniques. However, risks due to cross-infection and nonmatched blood may occur when nonautologous infusion is carried out.

Amphetamines

WADA category

II. Substances and methods prohibited in-competition. S6. Stimulants a: Nonspecified Stimulants

Use in sport

Amphetamines are used, during competition, to reduce fatigue and to increase reaction time, alertness, competitiveness, and aggression. Amphetamines may be used out-of-competition to intensify training.

Amphetamines and derivatives such as ecstasy are recreational drugs; therefore, competitors may test positive for amphetamines having not intended to use them for performance enhancement.

Pharmacological action

There are four mechanisms of action:

1   Releasing neurotransmitters, such as noradrenaline, dopamine, and serotonin, from their respective nerve terminals
2   Inhibition of neurotransmitter uptake

3   Direct action on neurotransmitter receptors
4   Inhibition of monoamine oxidase activity.

Of these, neurotransmitter release is the most important.

Adverse effects

The adverse effects of amphetamines include restlessness, irritability, tremor, and insomnia with an increase in aggressive behaviour and the potential for addiction. At higher doses, amphetamines may produce sweating, tachycardia, pupillary dilation, increased blood pressure, and heat stroke. Effects on the heart may lead to arrhythmias, of which ventricular arrhythmia is potentially fatal.

Cocaine

WADA category

I. Substances and methods prohibited in-competition. S6. Stimulants a: Nonspecified Stimulants
Cocaine possesses local anaesthetic properties. Other local anaesthetics are permitted in sport.

Use in sport

Studies on the ergogenic effects of cocaine are inconclusive. Cocaine is a recreational drug. Many instances of positive doping results have arisen from residual levels remaining in the body after recreational use rather than an attempt by the athlete to enhance performance. Cocaine is notable for distorting the user's perception of reality; therefore, the athlete may perceive enhanced performance when, in reality, a decrease in endurance and strength due to the drug exists.

Pharmacological action

The pharmacological effects of cocaine on the brain are complex and include inhibition of the uptake of various central neurotransmitters, particularly dopamine.

Adverse effects

The complex pharmacology of cocaine leads to a wide spectrum of adverse effects, including a negative effect on glycogenolysis, paranoid psychosis, seizures, hypertension, and myocardial toxicity, which could lead to ischaemia, arrhythmias, and sudden death, especially following intense exercise. Smoked 'crack' cocaine is more dangerous because the rate of absorption is greater, leading to a more intense effect on the cardiovascular system.

Ephedrine and other sympathomimetics available in over-the-counter (OTC) medicines

This group includes drugs such as ephedrine, methylephedrine, and pseudoephedrine.

WADA category

I. Substances and methods prohibited in-competition. S6. Stimulants b: Specified Stimulants
    WADA regulations define a positive result for these substances if they appear in the urine at concentrations above specified threshold levels.
    Competitors should be aware of the fact that even using the manufacturers' recommended doses may result in exceeding permitted levels.
    Other drugs that are found commonly in OTC medicines, such as antihistamines (e.g. triprolidine, astemizole), analgesics (e.g. paracetamol), imidazole decongestants (e.g. xylometazoline), cough suppressants (e.g. pholcodine), and expectorants (e.g. ipecacuanha), are not prohibited by WADA.

Use in sport

Sympathomimetics produce central stimulant effects.

Pharmacological action

These drugs produce decongestion by decreasing mucus secretion. They are structurally related to amphetamines and therefore produce a similar, though weaker, effect as central stimulants.

Adverse effects

OTC sympathomimetics variably produce side effects such as headache, tachycardia, dizziness, hypertension, irritability, and anxiety.

Narcotics

WADA category

II. Substances and methods prohibited in-competition. S7. Narcotics
    Some less potent narcotics, such as codeine, dihydrocodeine, dextropropoxyphene, and dextromethorphan, are permitted by WADA.

Use in sport

Potent narcotic analgesics are misused in sport for their pain-relieving properties.

Pharmacological action

Alkaloids from the opium poppy and their synthetic analogues interact with the receptors in the brain, which are normally acted upon by the endogenous endorphin transmitters. They have the capacity to moderate pain but also affect emotions. Frequent use may induce tolerance and dependency, the extent of which is variable depending on the narcotic used.

Adverse effects

In high doses, narcotic analgesics can cause stupor and coma, with the possibility of death due to respiratory depression. Where dependency has occurred, withdrawal symptoms include craving, anxiety, sweating, insomnia, nausea and vomiting, muscle aches, and potential cardiovascular collapse.

Cannabinoids

WADA category

II. Substances and methods prohibited in-competition. S8. Cannabinoids

Passive inhalation of cannabinoids has been cited as the reason for a positive test result on a number of occasions. However, the levels of cannabinoids present in the body due to passive inhalation are unlikely to exceed the threshold level used in testing.

Use in sport

Cannabinoid effects are incompatible with most sports; therefore, tests are only conducted in certain sports.

Pharmacological action

The active constituent of marijuana is 1-5-9-tetrahydrocannabinol (THC). When smoked, 60–65 per cent is absorbed; effects are noted within 15 minutes and last for 3 hours or so. It produces a sedating and euphoric feeling of well-being.

Adverse effects

The central depressant effects of THC decrease the motivation for physical effort. Motor coordination, short-term memory, and perception are impaired. In addition to its psychological effects, THC induces tachycardia, bronchodilation, and an increased blood flow to the limbs.

Glucocorticosteroids

WADA category

II. Substances and methods prohibited in-competition, S9. Glucocorticosteroids

Glucocorticosteroids are prohibited when administered orally, rectally, or by intravenous or intramuscular injection. Glucocorticosteroids are permitted, subject to Therapeutic Use Exemption, if the route of administration is limited to inhalation or by intraarticular, periarticular, peritendinous, epidural, or intradermal injection. Topical preparations when used for auricular, buccal, dermatological, gingival, nasal, ophthalmic, and perianal disorders are not prohibited.

Use in sport

Glucocorticosteroids are important in the management of sports injuries due to their potent anti-inflammatory properties.

Pharmacological action

These drugs are related to the adrenocorticosteroid hormone released from the adrenal cortex. They have a widespread effect on the body including glucocorticoid effects on carbohydrate, protein, and fat metabolism and on electrolyte and water balance, as well as their anti-inflammatory effect. As anti-inflammatory agents, they reduce the swelling, tenderness, and heat associated with injury.

Adverse effects

Local damage may be produced at the site of injection due to dosage volume and subcutaneous atrophy, with associated depigmentation. Corticosteroids produce a catabolic effect on skeletal muscle, leading to muscle weakness soon after treatment has begun, even with modest doses.

Alcohol

WADA category

III. Substances prohibited in particular sports. P1. Alcohol
 The sports listed in the 2014 WADA Prohibited List were air sports, archery, automobile, karate, motorcycling, and powerboating.

Use in sport

Alcohol (ethanol) may be used, potentially, as a performance-enhancing drug due to its anti-anxiety effect. In some team sports, where alcohol is part of a social convention, peer pressure may lead to overindulgence, with consequences for the partaker and for fellow competitors.

Pharmacological action

Alcohol affects neural transmission in the central nervous system by altering the permeability of axonal membranes and thereby slowing nerve conduction. Alcohol also decreases glucose utilization in the brain. Overall, alcohol impairs concentration, reduces anxiety, and induces depression and sedation.

Adverse effects

The adverse effects of alcohol have been extensively documented over many centuries.

Beta blockers

WADA category

III. Substances prohibited in particular sports. P2. Beta blockers

Use in sport

Beta blockers have a use in sport where motor skills can be affected by muscle tremor, caused by anxiety. Beta blockers are therefore prohibited in certain sports, such as archery and other shooting events, and in high-risk sports, such as ski jumping and automobile racing.

Pharmacological action

Beta blockers are first-line drugs in the management of angina pectoris, hypertension, some cardiac arrhythmias, hyperthyroidism, and glaucoma and are used occasionally for migraine and essential tremor.

Adverse effects

The adverse effects of beta blockers vary according to the properties of the individual drug. Beta blockers may produce bronchoconstriction, fatigue, cold extremities, sleep disturbances, and nightmares.

Prohibited supplements

Use in sport

Athletes commonly take dietary or nutritional supplements, most of which are not prohibited in sport (see *Nutrition Supplements* in the next section). However, in many countries, the manufacturing of supplements is not appropriately regulated by the government. This means that supplements can contain prohibited substances. For example, the ingredients on the inside of the bottle may not match those listed on the outside label of the package. In some cases, the undeclared substances found in the supplement can include one that is prohibited under anti-doping regulations. Examples include supplements that advertise 'muscle-building' or 'fat-burning' capabilities, which are the most likely to contain a prohibited substances, such as anabolic agents or stimulants, including methylhexaneamine or oxilofrine.

A large number of positive doping results have been attributed to the mislabelling and contamination of supplements. The terms 'herbal' and 'natural' do not necessarily mean that the product is safe or free from prohibited substances. Black market or unlabelled products are a particular concern.

Athletes should be aware of the dangers of potential contamination of supplements and that taking a poorly labelled supplement is not an adequate defence in a doping hearing.

A.3. Drugs used in sport that are not on the WADA Prohibited List

In this section, consideration is given to the use of therapeutic drugs in the management of illnesses that athletes may experience and for which they may self-medicate or seek medical advice from a general practitioner, pharmacist, or other health professional.

Nonsteroidal anti-inflammatory drugs

Use in sport

Nonsteroidal anti-inflammatory drugs (NSAIDs), such as aspirin and indomethacin, are widely used as analgesic and anti-inflammatory drugs for the treatment of sports injuries.

Pharmacological action

The analgesic, anti-inflammatory, and antipyretic activity of NSAIDs is based on their ability to inhibit prostaglandin synthesis.

Adverse effects

The most common adverse effects associated with NSAIDs are gastrointestinal, including nausea, dyspepsia, and ulcers.

Topical administration of NSAIDs may offer an effective and possibly safer alternative route of administration.

Benzodiazepines and other anxiolytics

Use in sport

A number of classes of drugs have been used as anxiolytics, including alcohol, beta blockers, and benzodiazepines. Alcohol and beta blockers have been described above, as they are restricted in certain sports.

Pharmacological action

Benzodiazepines variously reduce the activity of a number of central neurotransmitters, such as acetylcholine, serotonin, and noradrenaline. The antianxiety effect is primarily through release of gamma-aminobutyric acid, which inhibits the release of serotonin.

Adverse effects

Benzodiazepines are relatively free of adverse effects. However, they are liable to produce dependency if used for extended periods. Benzodiazepines may also be used by athletes for insomnia. Under these circumstances, athletes need to be aware of the 'hangover' effect of these drugs.

Caffeine

Use in sport

Caffeine was removed from the Prohibited List by WADA in January 2004. However, WADA continues to monitor for its misuse in sport.

Caffeine may be used primarily for its central stimulant effect, to improve alertness, reaction time, and attention span. In addition, caffeine may increase the mobilization and utilization of fatty acids, leading to a sparing of muscle glycogen.

Pharmacological action

Caffeine inhibits the phosphodiesterase group of enzymes, which activate second messengers such as cyclic AMP. They act as one of the links between receptor activation and cellular responses. Caffeine also directly antagonizes adenosine receptors.

Adverse effects

Mild side effects associated with caffeine include irritability, insomnia, and gastrointestinal disturbances. More severe effects include peptic ulceration, delirious seizures, coma, and superventricular and ventricular arrhythmias.

Cough and cold preparations

Use in sport

The use of medication for these self-limiting conditions is questionable. The only potential use for drugs is for the control of symptoms, such as headache, fever, runny nose, and cough. However, many of the drugs found in OTC cough and cold remedies are sympathomimetics used as decongestants. Some of these, such as ephedrine and pseudoephedrine, are banned by WADA, although there are cut-off concentrations in the urine for these drugs.

Pharmacological action

Apart from the sympathomimetic decongestants discussed previously, cough and cold medicines may contain analgesics (paracetamol, codeine), antihistamines (e.g. triprolidine, astemizole), imidazole decongestants (e.g. xylometazoline), cough suppressants (e.g. pholcodine), and expectorants (e.g. ipecacuanha), all of which are permitted by WADA.

Adverse effects

In general, cough and cold preparations are taken for short periods of time, and therefore side effects are limited. However, nasal decongestants are liable to produce rebound congestion if used for more than 1 week. Sedating antihistamines may have adverse effects on performance in most sports.

Antidiarrhoeals

Use in sport

First-line treatment for diarrhoea is oral rehydration therapy (ORT). Antimotility drugs may be used for short-term symptomatic relief of acute diarrhoea if it is likely to affect performance.

Pharmacological action

ORT enhances the absorption of water and replaces electrolytes. Antimotility drugs (codeine, diphenoxylate, loperamide) are opioids with a direct relaxant effect on the smooth muscle of the gastrointestinal tract.

Adverse effects

Tolerance and dependence may develop with prolonged use of antimotility drugs. Loperamide may produce abdominal cramps, drowsiness, and skin reactions.

Nutritional supplements

Use in sport

Nutritional supplements are used by many athletes to maintain a 'balanced' diet. However, many athletes have used supplements in an attempt to enhance performance through ergogenic aids, without contravening WADA regulations.

The manufacture and sale of nutritional supplements is not as closely regulated as that for drugs. Nutritional supplements may therefore contain banned substances or their precursors, which produce the same metabolites as banned substances in the urine. The use of nutritional supplements may therefore lead to a positive dope test result.

Pharmacological action

Manufacturers may make exaggerated claims regarding the ergogenic properties of their products. There is little, if any, evidence that many nutritional supplements possess ergogenic properties in athletes consuming a balanced diet.

Adverse effects

Some nutritional supplements have the potential for harm. Creatine has been the subject of many studies, but results are equivocal as to whether it produces ergogenic effects. There are few reliable scientific data on possible adverse effects of creatine, but its potential effect on renal dysfunction and electrolyte imbalance, leading to a predisposition to dehydration and heat-related illness, suggests caution in its use.

Index